BLEOMYCIN CHEMOTHERAPY

BLEOMYCIN CHEMOTHERAPY

Edited by

Branimir Ivan Sikic
Department of Medicine
Divisions of Oncology and Clinical Pharmacology
Stanford University School of Medicine
Stanford, California

Marcel Rozencweig
Bristol-Myers Company
Pharmaceutical Research and
Development Division
Syracuse, New York

Stephen K. Carter
Bristol-Myers Company
Pharmaceutical Research and
Development Division
New York, New York

1985

ACADEMIC PRESS, INC.
(Harcourt Brace Jovanovich, Publishers)
Orlando   San Diego   New York   London
Toronto   Montreal   Sydney   Tokyo

ACADEMIC PRESS, INC.
Orlando, Florida 32887

United Kingdom Edition published by
ACADEMIC PRESS INC. (LONDON) LTD.
24–28 Oval Road, London NW1 7DX

LIBRARY OF CONGRESS CATALOGING-IN-PUBLICATION DATA

Main entry under title:

Bleomycin chemotherapy

    Based on a symposium held at the St. Francis Hotel
in San Francisco on Sept. 14 and 15, 1984, sponsored by
the Northern California Cancer Program and Bristol
Laboratories.
    Includes bibliographies.
    1. Bleomycin—Congresses.   2. Cancer—Chemotherapy—
Congresses.   I. Sikic, Branimir Ivan.   II. Rozencweig,
Marcel.   III. Carter, Stephen K., DATE-
IV. Northern California Cancer Program.   V. Bristol
Laboratories.   [DNLM: 1. Bleomycins—therapeutic use—
congresses.   2. Neoplasms—drug therapy—congresses.
QZ 267 B647 1984
RC271.B57B57   1985   616.99'4061   85-11051
ISBN 0-12-643160-4 (alk. paper)
ISBN 0-12-643161-2 (paperback)

PRINTED IN THE UNITED STATES OF AMERICA

85 86 87 88   9 8 7 6 5 4 3 2 1

CONTENTS

v

III. HEAD AND NECK CANCER

IV. THE MALIGNANT LYMPHOMAS

Contents

CONTRIBUTORS

Numbers in parentheses indicate the pages on which the authors' contributions begin.

IDA ACKERMAN, (215), Toronto–Bayview Regional Cancer Centre, Ontario Cancer Treatment and Research Foundation, and Sunnybrook Medical Centre, Toronto,.Ontario, Canada M4N 3M5

DAVID S. ALBERTS, (227), The Cancer Center, College of Medicine, University of Arizona, Tucson, Arizona 85721

SILVIO ARISTIZABAL, (227), The Cancer Center, College of Medicine, University of Arizona, Tucson, Arizona 85721

EMILIO BAJETTA, (127, 181), Division of Medical Oncology, Istituto Nazionale Tumori, 20133 Milan, Italy

SAMUEL C. BALLON, (239), Department of Obstetrics/Gynecology, Section of Gynecologic Oncology, Stanford University School of Medicine, Stanford, California 94305

MARTIN P. BERRY, (215), Toronto–Bayview Regional Cancer Centre, Ontario Cancer Treatment and Research Foundation, and Sunnybrook Medical Centre, Toronto, Ontario, Canada M4N 3M5

MARTIN E. BLACKSTEIN, (215), Mount Sinai Hospital, Toronto, Ontario, Canada

GIANNI BONADONNA, (127, 181), Division of Medical Oncology, Istituto Nazionale Tumori, 20133 Milan, Italy

VALERIA BONFANTE, (127, 181), Division of Medical Oncology, Istituto Nazionale Tumori, 20133 Milan, Italy

ROBERTO BUZZONI, (127, 181), Division of Medical Oncology, Istituto Nazionale Tumori, 20133 Milan, Italy

EDWIN C. CADMAN, (313), Cancer Research Institute, University of California School of Medicine, San Francisco, California 94143

GEORGE P. CANELLOS, (187), Department of Medicine, Harvard Medical School, and Dana–Farber Cancer Institute, Boston, Massachusetts 02115

ROBERT W. CARLSON, (69), Northern California Cancer Program, Palo Alto,

California, and Department of Medicine, Division of Oncology, Stanford University School of Medicine, Stanford, California 94035

STEPHEN K. CARTER, (3), Bristol-Myers Company, Pharmaceutical Research and Development Division, New York, New York 10154

PAMELA A. CATTON, (215), Toronto–Bayview Regional Cancer Centre, Ontario Cancer Treatment and Research Foundation, and Sunnybrook Medical Centre, Toronto, Ontario, Canada M4N 3M5

CHARLES A. COLTMAN, JR., (137), Department of Medicine, Division of Oncology, University of Texas Health Sciences Center, San Antonio, Texas 78284

ROBERT L. COMIS,[1] (277), State University of New York Upstate Medical Center, Syracuse, New York 13210

GEOFFREY M. DAVIES, (215), Toronto–Bayview Regional Cancer Centre, Ontario Cancer Treatment and Research Foundation, and Sunnybrook Medical Centre, Toronto, Ontario, Canada M4N 3M5

EDWARD J. DE PERSIO, (137), Wenatchee Valley Clinic, Wenatchee, Washington 98801

DENNIS O. DIXON, (137), Southwest Oncology Group Biostatistical Center, Houston, Texas 77030

HISAO EKIMOTO, (289), Research Laboratories, Nippon Kayaku Company, Ltd., Tokyo 102, Japan

WILLIAM K. EVANS, (215), Toronto General Hospital, Toronto, Ontario, Canada M5G 1L7

RAYMOND H. FARMEN, (277), State University of New York Upstate Medical Center, Syracuse, New York 13210

C. R. FRANKS, (277), Bristol-Myers International Corporation, Pharmaceutical Research and Development, Brussels, Belgium

KAREN K. FU, (95), Department of Radiation Oncology, University of California, San Francisco, California 94143

AKIO FUJII, (289), Research Laboratories, Nippon Kayaku Company, Ltd., Tokyo 102, Japan

TAKEYO FUKUOKA, (289), Research Laboratories, Nippon Kayaku Company, Ltd., Tokyo 102, Japan

ROBERT C. GAVER, (277), Bristol-Myers Company, Pharmaceutical Research and Development Division, Syracuse, New York 13221

ROBERT B. GOLBEY, (59), Memorial Hospital for Cancer and Allied Diseases, New York, New York 10021

---

[1]Present address: Fox Chase Cancer Center, Philadelphia, Pennsylvania 19111.

PETRE N. GROZEA, (137), University of Oklahoma Health Sciences Center, and Presbyterian Hospital, Oklahoma City, Oklahoma 73104

RICHARD T. HOPPE, (155), Department of Radiology, Division of Radiation Therapy, Stanford University School of Medicine, Stanford, California 94305

SANDRA J. HORNING, (169), Department of Medicine, Division of Oncology, Stanford University School of Medicine, Stanford, California 94305

CHARLOTTE D. JACOBS, (79), Department of Medicine, Division of Oncology, Stanford University School of Medicine, Stanford, California 94305

STEPHEN E. JONES, (137), University of Arizona Health Sciences Center, Tucson, Arizona 85724

MARTIN LEVITT, (215), University of Manitoba Faculty of Medicine, Manitoba Cancer Foundation, Winnipeg, Manitoba, Canada R3E 0V9

BRIAN J. LEWIS, (47), Cancer Research Institute, Department of Medicine, University of California, San Francisco, California 94143

ARTHUR C. LOUIE, (257, 277), Bristol-Myers Company, Pharmaceutical Research and Development Division, Syracuse, New York 13221

AKIRA MATSUDA, (289), Research Laboratories, Nippon Kayaku Company, Ltd., Tokyo 102, Japan

HENSLEY A. B. MILLER, (215), Toronto–Bayview Regional Cancer Centre, Ontario Cancer Treatment and Research Foundation, and Sunnybrook Medical Centre, Toronto, Ontario, Canada M4N 3M5

SEIKI MINAMIDE,[2] (289), Research Laboratories, Nippon Kayaku Company, Ltd., Tokyo 102, Japan

FRANCO M. MUGGIA, (203), Division of Oncology, Rita and Stanley H. Kaplan Cancer Center, New York University School of Medicine, New York, New York 10016

YASUHIKO MURAOKA, (289), Institute of Microbial Chemistry, Tokyo 141, Japan

TOKUJI NAKATANI, (289), Research Laboratories, Nippon Kayaku Company, Ltd., Tokyo 102, Japan

KIYOHIRO NISHIKAWA, (289), Research Laboratories, Nippon Kayaku Company, Ltd., Tokyo 102, Japan

DAVID OSOBA, (215), Toronto–Bayview Regional Cancer Centre, Ontario

---

[2]Present address: Research Laboratories for Applied Toxicology, Nippon Kayaku Company, Ltd., Takasaki, Gunma Prefecture 370-12, Japan.

Cancer Treatment and Research Foundation, and Sunnybrook Medical Centre, University of Toronto, Toronto, Ontario, Canada M4N 3M5

MARCEL ROZENCWEIG, (277), Bristol-Myers Company, Pharmaceutical Research and Development Division, Syracuse, New York 13221

JAMES J. RUSTHOVEN, (215), Toronto–Bayview Regional Cancer Centre, Ontario Cancer Treatment and Research Foundation, and Sunnybrook Medical Centre, University of Toronto, Toronto, Ontario, Canada M4N 3M5

SEI-ICHI SAITO, (289), Institute of Microbial Chemistry, Tokyo 141, Japan

ARMANDO SANTORO, (127, 181), Division of Medical Oncology, Istituto Nazionale Tumori, 20133 Milan, Italy

FRANCES A. SHEPHERD, (215), Toronto General Hospital, Toronto, Ontario, Canada M5G 1L7

BRANIMIR IVAN SIKIC, (37, 69, 239, 247), Department of Medicine, Divisions of Oncology and Clinical Pharmacology, Stanford University School of Medicine, Stanford, California 94305

ARTHUR T. SKARIN, (187), Department of Medicine, Harvard Medical School, and Dana–Farber Cancer Institute, Boston, Massachusetts 02115

MONICA B. SPAULDING, (117), Oncology Section, Buffalo Veterans Administration Medical Center, and State University of New York at Buffalo, Buffalo, New York 14215

EARL A. SURWIT, (227), The Cancer Center, College of Medicine, University of Arizona, Tucson, Arizona 85721

KATSUTOSHI TAKAHASHI, (289), Research Laboratories, Nippon Kayaku Company, Ltd., Tokyo 102, Japan

TOMOHISA TAKITA, (289), Institute of Microbial Chemistry, Tokyo 141, Japan

GLEN A. TAYLOR, (215), Toronto–Bayview Regional Cancer Centre, Ontario Cancer Treatment and Research Foundation, and Sunnybrook Medical Centre, Toronto, Ontario, Canada M4N 3M5

KATHRYN TURNBULL, (215), Toronto–Bayview Regional Cancer Centre, Ontario Cancer Treatment and Research Foundation, and Sunnybrook Medical Centre, Toronto, Ontario, Canada M4N 3M5

HAMAO UMEZAWA, (289), Institute of Microbial Chemistry, Tokyo 141, Japan

PINUCCIA VALAGUSSA, (127, 181), Division of Medical Oncology, Istituto Nazionale Tumori, 20133 Milan, Italy

SIMONETTA VIVIANI, (127, 181), Division of Medical Oncology, Istituto Nazionale Tumori, 20133 Milan, Italy

DANIEL D. VON HOFF, (203), Department of Medicine, Division of Oncology, University of Texas Health Sciences Center, San Antonio, Texas
78284

PETER M. WEBSTER, (215), Toronto–Bayview Regional Cancer Centre, Ontario Cancer Treatment and Research Foundation, and Sunnybrook Medical
Centre, Toronto, Ontario, Canada M4N 3M5

SHELDON WEINER, (227), The Cancer Center, College of Medicine, University of Arizona, Tucson, Arizona 85721

ROBERT E. WITTES, (109, 305), Cancer Therapy Evaluation Program, Division of Cancer Treatment, National Cancer Institute, Bethesda, Maryland
20205

PREFACE

Bleomycin, a group of glycopeptides isolated from *Streptomyces verticillus,* has a unique structure and mechanism of action among anticancer drugs. As such, it continues to fascinate biochemists and pharmacologists. The drug binds to DNA and functions as a minienzyme by forming a complex with iron and oxygen that results in free radical formation and DNA strand breakage.

The focus of this volume is on the clinical uses of bleomycin. More than a decade has passed since the drug was introduced to the clinic. Its remarkable lack of bone marrow toxicity prompted its addition to myelosuppressive regimens and enabled treatment of patients with compromised hematopoietic function. Pulmonary toxicity has emerged as the major limitation of high cumulative bleomycin doses. Studies continue on the optimal scheduling of the drug.

Bleomycin is an integral component of one of the great triumphs of medical oncology of the past decade—the curative treatment of metastatic testicular carcinomas. Similar curative potential has now been demonstrated for bleomycin in combination with cisplatin and vinblastine in germ-cell cancers of the ovary. Bleomycin is included in several important treatment regimens for Hodgkin's disease and non-Hodgkin's lymphomas. The drug also has clinical activity against squamous carcinomas of various sites.

These uses and other aspects, including the development of new bleomycin analogs, are discussed in these chapters, which were first presented in San Francisco on 14 and 15 September 1984, at a symposium jointly sponsored by the Northern California Cancer Program and Bristol Laboratories.

Section I
INTRODUCTION

Chapter 1

BLEOMYCIN: MORE THAN A DECADE LATER

Stephen K. Carter

Bristol-Myers Company
Pharmaceutical Research and Development Division
New York, New York

I. INTRODUCTION

Bleomycin was discovered in Japan by Umezawa (1976) and was brought to the United States in the early 1970s. Initial clinical trials were sponsored jointly by the National Cancer Institute and Bristol-Myers, both simultaneously filing investigational new drug applications with the Food and Drug Administration (FDA). The original Japanese studies, led by Ichikawa (1970a, 1970b, 1976), demonstrated bleomycin activity against a range of squamous-cell tumors and the malignant lymphomas. Subsequent studies in the United States confirmed the drug's activity in squamous-cell carcinomas of the head and neck, the cervix, and the lymphomas (Blum *et al.*, 1973; Carter and Blum, 1976). In addition, important activity in testicular cancer also was discovered (Samuels *et al.*, 1973). As studies in Europe led to similar conclusions, bleomycin rapidly became established worldwide as a major new drug.

Bleomycin also gained importance clinically because of its toxicity spectrum, which was unique among cytotoxic agents. Of greatest interest was its lack of myelosuppressive properties. Thus, bleomycin could be combined with other drugs without reducing doses because of leukopenia or thrombocytopenia. This factor led to the inclusion of bleomycin in an extensive range of combination regimens for a large number of tumor types. The dose-limiting side effects of bleomycin were found to be skin toxicity and pulmonary fibrosis. The occurrence of skin toxicity was observed to be acute, while the lung impact tended to be chronic—although overlap, in terms of time to toxicity, was seen occasionally.

Bleomycin clinical research has moved predominantly along disease-oriented lines. In every disease in which this drug was believed to have any level of meaningful efficacy, the following research thrusts have occurred in various degrees: (1) combination with other active drugs in treating advanced disease; (2) combination with surgery and/or radiotherapy for adjuvant or neoadjuvant therapy; and (3) combination with noncytotoxic therapeutic approaches.

There also has been a drug-oriented approach to the ongoing research. This has involved modifications of administration schedules and routes, in an attempt either to increase efficacy or diminish side effects, and has involved study of the pulmonary toxicity, with the goal of enabling either prediction of its occurrence or amelioration of its impact.

II. TESTICULAR CANCER

For many years, testicular cancer has been treated with combination chemotherapy involving drugs such as actinomycin D, chlorambucil, methotrexate, and mithramycin (Carter, 1983). These combinations yielded approximately 10% complete response rates. Along with cisplatin, bleomycin was one of the key new drugs that led to the development of newer combinations that have made a dramatic impact on cure rates.

Vinblastine had been shown to have important activity as a single agent by Samuels and Howe (1970). They performed a disease-oriented phase II study using vinblastine at the high doses of 0.4 to 0.8 mg/kg/week, and reported 4 complete responses (19%) and 7 partial responses (33%) among 21 evaluable patients, obtaining an overall response rate of 52%. Previous to this study, the published literature related only four cases treated with this drug and two responses.

Bleomycin's single-agent activity in the treatment of testicular cancer first was reported in a cumulative data report of Blum *et al.* (1973) derived from broad phase II studies. In this report, there was a 32% response rate among the 37 patients treated.

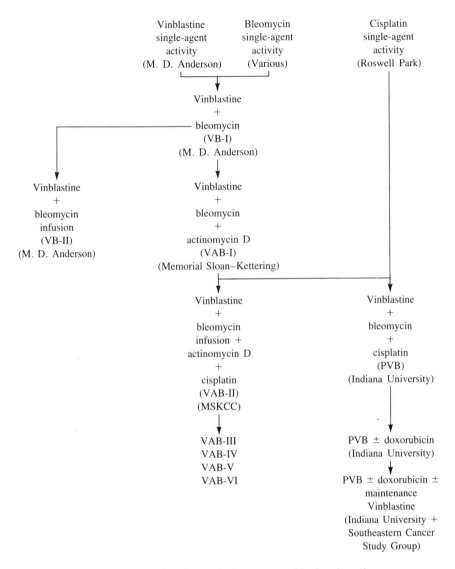

Fig. 1. Historical flow of modern testicular cancer combination chemotherapy.

The first literature report of cisplatin activity came from Higby *et al.* (1974), who related that in 15 evaluable patients the drug achieved 7 complete responses and three partial responses. The 47% complete response rate was the highest ever reported for a single agent, although the experience was small. Cumulative

TABLE I   CRITICAL QUESTIONS IN COMBINATION CHEMOTHERAPY STUDIES OF
TESTICULAR CANCER

Institution and study	Drugs used	Type of study	Critical question(s) posed
I. M. D. Anderson			
1. VB-1	Vinblastine, bleomycin	Phase II	What is the activity of high-dose vinblastine plus bleomycin?
2. VB-2	Same	Phase II	Will changing bleomycin schedule to 120-hr continuous infusion improve the results?
3. VB-3	Same	Phase II	Will changing the sequence of vinblastine usage improve results?
4. VB-3 + sequential cisplatin	Same + cisplatin	Phase II	Will adding cisplatin to VB-3 improve results?
II. Memorial Sloan–Kettering Cancer Center			
1. VAB	Vinblastine, actinomycin, bleomycin	Phase II	What is the activity of VAB?
2. VAB-II	Above + cisplatin	Phase II	Will changing bleomycin schedule to continuous infusion or adding low-dose cisplatin improve results?
3. VAB-III	Induction: VAB-II drugs + cyclophosphamide Maintenance: vinblastine, chlorambucil, actinomycin D, doxorubicin, cisplatin	Phase II	Will changing cisplatin dosage to high dose with hydration, adding cyclophosphamide to induction, and adding a maintenance regimen with chlorambucil and adriamycin improve results?
4. VAB-IV	Same as VAB-III	Phase II	Will giving a second course of bleomycin 16 weeks after start of chemotherapy and a third course with all drugs at 32 weeks improve VAB-III results?
5. VAB-VI	Induction: vinblastine, actinomycin D, bleomycin, cisplatin	Phase II	Will changing the sequence of drug usage in induction and

TABLE I   (*Continued*)

Institution and study	Drugs used	Type of study	Critical question(s) posed
	Maintenance: vinblastine, actinomycin D		simplifying maintenance to two drugs improve VAB-IV results?
III. Indiana University			
1. PVB	Cisplatin, vinblastine, bleomycin	Phase II	What is the efficacy of PVB?
2. Second PVB protocol	PVB ± doxorubicin	Phase III	Will the addition of adriamycin to PVB improve results? Will lowering the vinblastine dose by 25% improve the therapeutic index by lowering toxicity and not lowering efficacy?
3. Third Indiana PVB study + SECSG study	PVB or PVB + doxorubicin ± maintenance vinblastine	Phase III	Will maintenance vinblastine give higher efficacy than no maintenance?

single-agent experience, as derived from six literature reports, totals 70 patients, with a 21% complete response and an overall response rate of 66% (Carter, 1983).

The historical flow of modern combination chemotherapy in testicular cancer (Fig. 1) involves three institutions and is predominantly a series of sequential phase II type, disease-oriented, exploratory studies (Table I). The main thrust was to improve the therapeutic index in the disease by increasing the efficacy, as measured by complete response rate and the duration of disease-free survival. Bleomycin was used in every study shown in Table I. While it was used in different schedules, the relative contributions of these schedule modulations were impossible to determine.

The first randomized phase III study shown in Fig. 1, which represents the second study of the University of Indiana, addressed two drug-oriented questions. The first was related to improving the therapeutic index by increasing efficacy through the addition of doxorubicin to the combination of cisplatin, vinblastine, and bleomycin (PVB). The second addressed improving the therapeutic index by lowering toxicity through reducing the vinblastine dose in PVB. However, neither of these questions focuses on the intrinsic, or relative, activity of the three single-agent components in PVB.

The second randomized study in Fig. 1 is the third-generation study performed at the Indiana University, which focused on the importance of maintenance chemotherapy. In this study, patients achieving complete remission (CR) were randomized either to undergo maintenance with monthly vinblastine or to receive no maintenance after 12 weeks of induction therapy. These patients were joined by those participating in a study of the Southeastern Cancer Study Group (SECSG). Induction was a comparison of PVB versus PVB plus doxorubicin. Results of the study, shown in Table II, demonstrated no advantage to adding doxorubicin and, in addition, demonstrated no advantage to maintenance vinblastine (Einhorn, 1983).

A current study of the SECSG compares PVB with a regimen in which etoposide is substituted for vinblastine (BEP) (Williams *et al.*, 1984). Again, bleomycin is kept as a stable entity of primary induction chemotherapy.

Concurrent to the flow described in Fig. 1, two cooperative groups in the United States were performing randomized phase III studies outlined in Table III. With bleomycin used as a constant, the Southwest Oncology Group (SWOG) compared actinomycin D plus vincristine plus bleomycin (VAB-I) with vinblastine plus bleomycin. The Eastern Cooperative Oncology Group (ECOG) used actinomycin D as a constant and asked whether the addition of bleomycin plus vincristine would improve efficacy.

Once it was established that chemotherapy using combinations of bleomycin, vinblastine, and cisplatin presented a major advance in the primary treatment of metastatic testicular cancer, two additional disease-oriented research thrusts developed: (1) the use of combination chemotherapy as adjuvant treatment for stage II nonseminomatous disease, and (2) the use of second-line chemotherapy on patients who relapsed or failed to respond to PVB- or VAB-type regimens.

TABLE II   INDIANA UNIVERSITY SECSG STUDY IN TESTICULAR CANCER

Parameter	PVB	PVB + doxorubicin	Overall	
Number of patients	87	84	171	
Number of CR	56	57	113	
% CR	64	68	66	
Number of relapses	4	5	9	
% Continuously disease-free	67	70	68	
			Vinblastine maintenance	No maintenance
Number of patients			58	55
Number of relapses			5	4
% Relapses			9	7
% Disease-free			97	95

TABLE III   RANDOMIZED PHASE III TESTICULAR CANCER STUDIES PERFORMED
BY U.S. NATIONAL COOPERATIVE GROUPS (1970s)

Group	Regimens	Critical question(s) asked	Comments
SWOG	1. Vinblastine + bleomycin	Will actinomycin D + vincristine be superior to vinblastine when added to bleomycin	Exact sequence and schedule of bleomycin different in each arm; CR rate higher with VB
	2. Vincristine + bleomycin + actinomycin D		
ECOG	1. Actinomycin D	Will vincristine + bleomycin added to actinomycin D be superior to actinomycin D alone?	Overall, no difference in efficacy
	2. Actinomycin D + vincristine + bleomycin		

A. Adjuvant Treatment for Stage II
Nonseminomatous Disease

Use of these combinations as adjuvant treatment for stage II nonseminomatous disease initially was approached in an exploratory phase II fashion by Indiana University, SWOG, and ECOG. A nonrandomized approach of adjuvant chemotherapy was attempted after retroperitoneal node dissection in patients considered at a high risk for metastatic failure. All patients demonstrated an increased relapse-free survival rate compared with the nonmatched historical controls of past institutional experience.

At Memorial Sloan–Kettering (Vugrin *et al.*, 1979), a modified, less toxic version of VAB-I was administered to 62 patients with stage II disease who had undergone lymphadenectomy and had not received prior radiation. The first report showed that 84% of the patients remained disease-free, and the most potent prognostic variable was the extent of retroperitoneal lymph node involvement. In 29 patients with bulky nodal disease or direct extranodal extension, relapses occurred in 10 (35%) following VAB-I adjuvant treatment, after a median follow-up period of 25+ months. Nine of these 10 relapses occurred within 8 months of lymphadenectomy. In 33 patients with only microscopic nodal involvement, none relapsed during a median follow-up period of 19+ months. The features that constituted good stage II prognosis were ≤5 involved lymph nodes, none larger than 2 cm in diameter, no direct extralymphatic extension, and negative tumor markers after lymphadenectomy.

The VAB-I experience led the investigators to the conclusion that a strategic split was indicated for stage II patients. Those with good prognostic features could continue on the modified VAB-I regimen; those without those features required more aggressive adjuvant chemotherapy. Therefore, 22 stage II patients with poor prognostic signs were given the more aggressive VAB-II regimen after lymphadenectomy. At the time of the report, all 22 patients were disease-free for a median duration of 10+ months.

Testicular cancer raises some crucial questions about adjuvant chemotherapy. Curative chemotherapy is available when patients develop metastatic relapse after initial local and regional control with chemotherapy. In such a situation, the need for adjuvant chemotherapy becomes less urgent. Adjuvant chemotherapy potentially will increase the cure rate when added to the local control modalities of surgery and irradiation. However, it will do so at the cost of unnecessarily treating some patients with drugs. The cure rate of two therapeutic approaches must be compared. The first approach involves optimal treatment with surgery and/or irradiation followed by close observation. At the earliest sign of metastatic relapse, curative intent chemotherapy should be used. In addition, surgical resection of isolated pulmonary metastases could be undertaken as indicated. The second approach would involve initial adjuvant chemotherapy and secondary salvage chemotherapy in patients who relapse. Surgical resection of metastases also could be used when appropriate.

A cost–benefit ratio analysis comparing the two approaches is warranted. The benefit would be seen as the overall cure rate; the cost would be the morbidity and mortality of therapy. It is important to realize that comparing the relapse-free survival of surgery against that obtained with surgery plus adjuvant chemotherapy will not be the crucial endpoint for analysis. Adjuvant chemotherapy may produce a superior initial relapse-free survival rate, but it may not be superior in terms of overall survival. In patients with stage II disease, at least 50% will be cured by their initial surgery; they will be receiving the costs of adjuvant chemotherapy without benefit. These costs involve not only the risks of physical morbidity and treatment mortality, but also a range of psychological, social, and economic costs.

Thus, analysis of adjuvant drug trials in testicular cancer will be complex, involving a range of endpoints and cost–benefit analysis. An initial endpoint will be overall survival versus acute toxicity. The ultimate endpoint will be overall survival versus the acute and chronic toxicities of the treatment. These chronic toxicities will involve such aspects as long-term renal function and auditory function after cisplatin, neurologic function after vinca alkaloids, pulmonary function after bleomycin, and cardiac function after doxorubicin. In addition, the incidence of second malignancies possibly due to treatment must be monitored carefully. It will be tempting, after early analysis of adjuvant trials in testicular cancer, to report positive results based on initial relapse-free survival. However, this should be tempered by the realization that early actuarial analysis can be

TABLE IV   ADJUVANT REGIMENS USED IN THE TESTICULAR CANCER
INTERGROUP STUDY

Drug	Regimen A	Regimen B
Vinblastine	15 mg/kg iv, days 1, 2 every 4 weeks for 8 weeks	4 mg/m², days 1, 29
Bleomycin	30 units (total weekly dose) iv, weekly for 8 consecutive weeks	30 U iv push, then 20 U/m² per 24-hr infusion, 6 days, repeated every 28 days
Platinum	20 mg/m²/day for 5 days once every 4 weeks for two courses	120 mg/m², day 7
Actinomycin D	—	1 mg/m², days 1, 2
Cyclophosphamide	—	600 mg/m², days 1, 2

overly optimistic, and that successful secondary salvage may change the final picture dramatically.

Data currently available indicate that among the 40% of patients who relapse after lymphadenectomy, about 60–80% could be expected to achieve CR with drugs, with 60% of the entire group showing long-term disease-free survival that is indicative of cure. Thus, surgery with delayed chemotherapy at the time of relapse could be expected to salvage 85% of all patients (60% initially, plus 25% at relapse). To show a 10% improvement with surgery plus immediate adjuvant chemotherapy would require 210 patients in a clinical trial. Even if this 10% improvement in cure rate were obtained, it would be necessary to weigh this against the cost of 60% of patients receiving the risks of the drug unnecessarily.

A national study currently is being conducted in the United States, in which many of the major cooperative groups are participating. The study compares adjuvant chemotherapy for stage II patients with resectable lymph nodes with an initial therapeutic approach that eradicates all known disease (surgery), followed by monthly observation of the patient and potentially curative chemotherapy in patients who develop recurrence. Excluded from this study are patients whose markers remain abnormal 4 weeks after lymph node resection and patients whose retroperitoneal nodes are clinically or surgically unresectable. Two chemotherapy regimens are used. One is a modified PVB regimen; the other is a modified VAB-III regimen (Table IV). The regimens overlap in the usage of vinblastine, bleomycin, and cisplatin, but the dosage schedules differ significantly.

B. Second-Line Chemotherapy

The second new research thrust has involved second-line chemotherapy for salvage of patients relapsing after, or failing to respond to, first-line PVB- or

VAB-type regimens. The new drug most commonly added to this equation has been etoposide, or VP-16 (Hainsworth *et al.*, 1984). It has been used in combination with bleomycin, cisplatin, and doxorubicin in various combinations, all of which have been studied, by necessity, in single-arm phase II fashion.

III. HODGKIN'S DISEASE

With the confirmation of bleomycin's activity in Hodgkin's disease through phase II studies conducted in the United States, a wide range of research thrusts followed (Fig. 2). These research strategies were all disease-oriented and assumed the activity of bleomycin. Bleomycin remains a drug that will be used at some point for the great majority of patients with advanced-stage or recurrent disease.

A. Primary Induction Combination Chemotherapy

Two research groups have led the way in using bleomycin as part of primary induction combination chemotherapy for cure (Fig. 3). The Southwest Oncology Group (SWOG) built upon the core of the MOPP (nitrogen mustard, vincristine, procarbazine, and prednisone) combination. In five protocols (Table V), SWOG conducted confirmatory MOPP studies as well as studies adding either bleomycin alone or bleomycin plus doxorubicin (Coltman *et al.*, 1973; Frei and Gehan, 1971; Hersh *et al.*, 1972).

In the most recently reported SWOG study, MOPP plus low-dose bleomycin was compared with the same five drugs plus doxorubicin (MOP–BAP) on two different schedules in patients with advanced Hodgkin's disease (Jones *et al.*, 1982; Jones *et al.*, 1983). A total of 315 patients were randomized and 291 were deemed evaluable in this three-arm study. Overall, the two MOP–BAP schedules resulted in a 77% complete remission rate among 166 patients, as compared with 67% in 125 patients receiving MOPP plus bleomycin (MOPP–Bleo) ($p = .10$). There was no difference between the six- and five-drug approaches in terms of relapse-free and overall survival. The six-drug MOP–BAP regimen did give superior results in patients with more favorable prognoses due to either high initial hemoglobin levels, absence of bone marrow involvement, or absence of "B" symptoms.

Remission induction therapy for responding patients consisted of 10 courses of treatment at 4-week intervals. After completion of 10 courses of therapy, patients who appeared to be in a clinical CR underwent a systematic restaging of their disease. Patients deemed to be in "pathologic CR" after this restaging were left unmaintained. Patients found to have residual microscopic disease, as well as

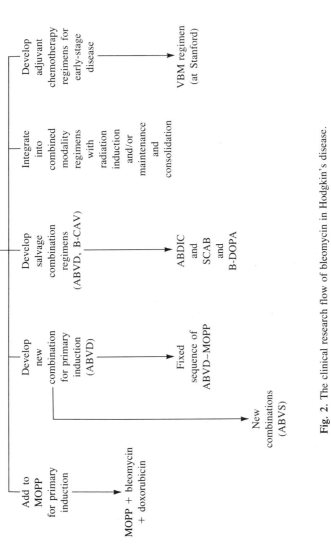

Fig. 2. The clinical research flow of bleomycin in Hodgkin's disease.

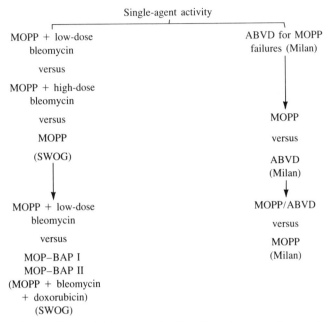

Fig. 3. Historical flow of bleomycin's integration into Hodgkin's disease combination chemotherapy for primary induction.

those in clinical partial remission (PR), were given four additional courses of treatment.

The MOP–BAP 2 regimen was closed to patient entry after only 38 patients received the treatment, since it was considered to be more cumbersome and not likely to be superior to MOP–BAP 1. In the recently published analysis, those 38 patients have been combined with 136 patients receiving MOP–BAP 1 to make a total of 174 treated with MOP–BAP, who are compared with 141 patients receiving MOPP–Bleo. The overall CR rate for all patients treated with MOP–BAP was 77% (76% MOP–BAP 1 or 78% MOP–BAP 2) as compared with 67% for MOPP-Bleo ($p = .05$, one-sided test).

Multivariate analysis demonstrated that the superiority of MOP–BAP over MOPP–Bleo was primarily evident among patients with more favorable prognostic factors, such as higher initial hemoglobin levels, better performance status, no bone-marrow involvement, and asymptomatic disease. In patients with unfavorable pretreatment characteristics, the five- and six-drug regimens gave similar results.

When CR duration was analyzed, both regimens gave comparable results. Only histologic subtype was of prognostic importance, revealing that mixed cellularity disease had a substantially longer duration of CR than did nodular

TABLE V   MOPP PROTOCOLS (SWOG)

Protocol	Induction	Maintenance
SWOG–MOPP 1 and 2 758	MOPP	None MOPP q 2 months
SWOG–MOPP 3 772	MOPP	Actinomycin D, 0.6 mg/m^2/day iv q 2 months × 9 Methotrexate, 12 mg/m^2/day × 5 iv q 2 months × 9 Vinblastine, 10 mg/m^2 iv q wk × 39 (1.5 years)
SWOG–MOPP 4 774	MOPP MOPP + bleomycin 2 mg/m^2, days 1, 8, iv MOPP + bleomycin, 5 U, days 1, 8 of course 1; 10 U/m^2, days 1, 8 of courses 2–6 10 Courses	MOPP q 2 months × 9 + 4000 rad to area of major involvement MOPP q months × 18
SWOG–MOPP 5	MOPP + bleomycin, 2 U/m^2, days 1, 8 MOPP–BAP 1: doxorubicin 30 mg/m^2, day 8, substituted for NH$_2$ in above MOPP–BAP 2: Doxorubicin 15 mg/m^2 added days 1, 8, with NH$_2$ lowered to 3 mg/m^2 days 1, 8	None

sclerosis disease (p = .02). Overall survival for all evaluable patients also was similar in the two treatment programs. Two pretreatment prognostic factors were significantly related to survival: age and performance status.

The Milan Group developed a totally new combination designed to use four drugs not considered to be cross-resistant to the MOPP combination: adriamycin (A), bleomycin (B), vinblastine (V), and dacarbazine or DTIC (D). The resultant ABVD combination was tested in a series of studies (Bonadonna et al., 1975; Bonadonna and Santoro, 1982; Bonadonna et al., 1979; Santoro and Bonadonna, 1979), which began with patients refractory to MOPP, but soon evolved into primary induction strategies. The Milan Group first demonstrated that ABVD can induce a high incidence of CR in MOPP-resistant patients. In 54 consecutive patients defined as resistant to MOPP chemotherapy because of either progressive disease during primary MOPP or relapse within the first 12 months after achievement of complete response, CR was obtained in 59%. Factors that favored achieving CR were the absence of extranodal disease (nodal, 74%, extranodal, 44%; $p = .03$) and the absence of systemic symptoms ("A," 82%; "B," 49%). The ability to achieve CR was independent of whether patients were classified during primary MOPP chemotherapy as failures (52%), partial responders (67%), or complete responders (68%) There also was no statistical evidence that age ($<$ or $\geq$ 40 years), sex, histologic characteristics, or prior irradiation affected the probability of attaining CR with ABVD. The 5-year relapse-free survival was 37%, and the median survival for all patients was 27 months (complete responders, 60 months; partial responders, 12 months; failures, 9 months). When MOPP was given to 16 ABVD-resistant patients, CR was seen in 25% and PR in 12.5%. The median duration of complete remission was 6.5 months and the median survival of complete responders was in excess of 20 months. This initial study indicated that ABVD was an effective salvage regimen when used as initial treatment in MOPP-resistant patients, with a salvage potential of about one-third of complete responders.

The alternating MOPP–ABVD program was started in Milan in 1974. It was designed to maximize the incidence of CR in untreated patients and to minimize relapses. Based on the clinical observation that most patients resistant to MOPP showed progressive disease by the third cycle (DeVita, 1979), MOPP was alternated monthly with ABVD. From 1974 to 1980, 75 patients with initial stage IV Hodgkin's disease (55 cases) or extranodal relapse following primary irradiation (20 cases) were allocated randomly to receive 12 cycles of MOPP or MOPP alternated monthly with ABVD for a total of 12 cycles. If complete response was achieved after 12 cycles of either regimen, no additional treatment was given. If partial response was seen, drug administration was continued at maximum doses until either CR or progressive disease occurred.

The induction of CR was significantly greater after alternating chemotherapy (92%) compared with MOPP alone (71%). Cyclical alternation of chemotherapy appears to prevent all patients from developing progressive lymphoma during the period of drug therapy. The cyclical administration of drug regimens was superior to MOPP alone in all prognostic subgroups. The relapse-free survival at 5 years in the MOPP arm was 37% compared with 70% of those given MOPP plus ABVD, and the median relapse-free survival was 20 months compared with 31 months, respectively. The 5-year survival of patients with no evidence of disease significantly favors the alternating chemotherapy (84%) over MOPP alone (54%). Because of the limited number of patients at risk for 5 years, the difference in total survival was not significant. In both treatment groups, survival curves level off at 2 years after starting treatment. It appears from this study that cyclical delivery of two non–cross-resistant combinations achieved a higher CR rate, longer duration of relapse-free survival, and possibly a higher cure rate in advanced Hodgkin's disease compared with the continuous administration of classical MOPP alone.

A prospective randomized study similar to that carried out in Milan is in progress at the National Cancer Institute (NCI). It employs alternating cycles of MOPP with cycles of a combination of streptozotocin, CCNU (lomustine), doxorubicin, and bleomycin (SCAB). Thus far, only a limited number of patients with stage II, stage III, and stage IV disease have been entered into the trial; therefore, results are premature.

The Eastern Cooperative Oncology Group (ECOG) has combined the SWOG and Milan approaches into a hybrid regimen of six cycles of MOPP and low-dose bleomycin followed by three cycles of ABVD in all responders after the initial six cycles. In a randomized study, ECOG compared this to an approach in which low-dose irradiation is substituted for the three cycles of ABVD (Glick et al., 1984). The results were essentially the same for both approaches, with the exception of a 5-year overall survival (OS) trend favoring the ABVD arm. The OS figure of 92% for those treated with the sequential chemotherapy approach compares quite favorably with all previously reported regimens.

B. Salvage Regimens

The development of salvage regimens for patients failing on MOPP or MOPP-like combinations has focused on the drugs used in ABVD along with the nitrosoureas (CCNU and streptozotocin). A summary of some of these regimens is given in Table VI. Evaluation of these regimens is complicated by the heterogeneity of patients treated and the relatively small patient populations in many literature reports. DeVita defines the criteria of a successful salvage regimen as being a complete remission rate of at least 20% when used in the absence of radiation therapy and maintenance therapy in patients with poor prognosis (as already defined), and a median survival >30 months from the date of relapse for the patients achieving a complete remission.

The regimen to best meet these criteria is ABVD, as seen in the Milan Group's report of a complete remission rate of 59% in MOPP-resistant patients, with a median duration of 17 months and a median survival of 5 years (Bonadonna et al., 1975). Other groups have not been able to reproduce these results. Krikorian et al. (1978) observed that only 5 of 27 patients (22%) who were resistant to MOPP achieved a complete remission with this regimen. Sutcliffe et al. (1979) studied patients failing on MOPP and saw a 7% complete remission rate. In the experience of Case et al. (1977), ABVD gave only a 4% complete response rate in 24 patients.

Other regimens that have given meaningful results as salvage therapy are the ABDIC or SCAB combinations. Both of these combinations produce complete

TABLE VI   SALVAGE REGIMENS IN HODGKIN'S DISEASE
(EXCLUDING MOPP)

Regimens[a]	Investigators	Number of patients	CR[b] (%)
ABVD	Bonadonna et al. (1975)	54	59
ABVD	Krikorian et al. (1978)	27	22
ABVD	Case et al. (1977)	24	29
ABVD	Sutcliffe et al. (1979)	41	7
SCAB	Levi et al. (1977)	17	35
B-CAV	Porzig et al. (1978)	22	50
BVDS	Vinciguerra et al. (1977)	10	30
B-DOPA	Lokich et al. (1976)	15	60
CVB	Goldman and Dawson (1975)	39	25

[a]A, Adriamycin (doxorubicin); B, bleomycin; C, CCNU; D, DTIC; S, streptozotocin; Ve or V, vinblastine.
[b]CR, Complete remission.

remission in about 35% of MOPP-resistant patients, with median survival times
in excess of 28 months.

C. Combined-Modality Strategies with Irradiation

The success of combination chemotherapy in advanced Hodgkin's disease has
led to combined-modality strategies with irradiation. One approach is to employ
the two modalities to improve the cure rate for stage III to stage IV disease. This
involves using irradiation in induction or as a consolidation and/or maintenance
thrust. A second approach is to use chemotherapy as an adjunctive treatment
after induction of complete remission with irradiation. Initially, MOPP was the
chemotherapy used in these two approaches. More recently, bleomycin has been
used in primary drug induction. An example of how drugs and irradiation have
been combined and how bleomycin has entered this picture is shown in Table
VII, which outlines the three combined modality studies of the SWOG (Coltman
et al., 1979; Fuller et al., 1980). These are in addition to the use of "maintenance" irradiation treatment in one maintenance arm of MOPP 4 (see Table VI).

D. Adverse and Toxic Effects

The success of chemotherapy in Hodgkin's disease led to some potentially
adverse consequences among the young people who are cured of this disease.
These consequences were outlined by DeVita (1981) as (1) the long-term effects
of chemotherapy on reproductive capacity, (2) the potential carcinogenic effects

TABLE VII   COMBINED MODALITY HODGKIN'S DISEASE PROTOCOLS (SWOG)

Study[a]	Stages involved	Treatment arms	Results
RAC 1	I, II A, B	Extended field irradiation	Combined response rates similar
		Involved field irradiation + 6 cycles MOPP	Relapse-free survival statistically significantly longer for combined modality
CAR 1	II B, III A, III B	MOPP 3–6 courses followed by total nodal irradiation	Complete response rates: III B 79%, III A 91%, III B 88%
CAR 2	III A, III B	MOPP–Bleo for 10 cycles MOPP–Bleo for 3 cycles followed by total nodal irradiation	No differences in terms of complete response, relapse-free, and overall survivals

[a]RAC, Radiotherapy and chemotherapy; CAR, chemotherapy and radiotherapy

of chemotherapy; and (3) the interaction of the immune system and the immunosuppressive drugs in the drug combinations commonly used.

The late toxic effects of chemotherapy include cardiotoxicity, lung fibrosis, infertility, and second neoplasms. Cardiotoxicity secondary to doxorubicin therapy is a particular concern when the cumulative dose exceeds 550 mg/m^2. Patients with prior radiotherapy to the mediastinum may manifest congestive heart failure after cumulative doses higher than 400 to 450 mg/m^2. Therefore, all regimens containing doxorubicin should be administered with caution. None of the 400 patients treated with ABVD in Milan has exhibited signs and symptoms compatible with cardiomyopathy. In all of these patients, the cumulative doxorubicin dose rarely has exceeded 350 mg/m^2 (Bonadonna and Santoro, 1982). However, long-term follow-up analysis will be required to fully assess the risk of heart damage following the administration of doxorubicin with and without irradiation.

Pulmonary toxicity is a potential side effect after treatment with bleomycin and nitrosoureas. From this point of view, ABVD in men appears to be safe. It is important that the total dose of bleomycin not exceed 200–250 U/m^2 and that its administration be withheld in patients with chronic lung disease or overt pulmonary postirradiation fibrosis.

Male infertility and second neoplasms are of particular concern, especially since many patients with Hodgkin's disease are young and the potential for cure is high. The NCI group (Sherins and DeVita, 1973; Sherins et al. 1978) has noted a high incidence of male infertility following MOPP chemotherapy; this has been attributed to the toxic effect on spermatogenesis by alkylating agents and procarbazine. However, in 25 to 40% of patients treated with MOPP or MOPP-like combinations, spermatogenesis may return approximately 2 years after completion of treatment. The Milan Group (Santoro *et al.,* in press) recently reported that azoospermia occurred in 100% of patients treated with MOPP and in only 15% of patients given ABVD. A similar difference was noticed in the comparative incidence of prolonged amenorrhea. This awaits confirmation from other groups but should be of great importance, since the therapeutic activity of ABVD appears to be equivalent to that of MOPP, at least in the randomized studies carried out thus far in Milan.

Second neoplasms, particularly acute nonlymphocytic leukemia and non-Hodgkin's lymphomas, are now being reported with great frequency among patients subjected to intensive, prolonged chemotherapy with MOPP or MOPP-derived regimens, particularly when combined with irradiation. To date, the updated results with ABVD indicate that this regimen—either when administered alone or when combined with extensive irradiation—appears devoid of carcinogenic activity. However, the follow-up time is still not great enough to make any definite statement.

IV. NON-HODGKIN'S LYMPHOMA

The non-Hodgkin's lymphomas (NHLs) constitute a heterogeneous group of diseases for which chemotherapy may be curative or palliative in intent, depending upon the histologic breakdown. NHL diseases range from those that can be very aggressive and rapidly fatal to some of the most indolent and well-tolerated malignancies of humans. Children with NHL must be considered separately because they present different clinicopathologic problems and require different management programs from adults.

There are numerous histologic classification systems for NHL. A working formulation for clinical usage was reported in a National Cancer Institute–sponsored study (Non-Hodgkin's Lymphoma Pathologic Classification Project, 1982). This international multiinstitutional group performed a clinicopathologic study of 1175 cases of NHL using six different major classifications. Out of this was developed a working formulation of NHL that separates the disease into 10 major types using morphologic criteria only. This formulation is not proposed as a new classification, but rather serves as a means of translation among various systems to facilitate clinical comparisons of case reports and therapeutic trials.

In the United States, the Rappaport classification is deemed most useful for clinicians, and data from all recent trials are based on this system. The Rappaport and other classifications can be used to combine several easily identifiable subgroups into those of good prognosis (favorable) and poor prognosis (unfavorable).

Therapy for favorable NHL is controversial because it is generally accepted that while these tumors are responsive to drugs, they are not curable. This is in contradiction to poor-risk diffuse NHL, which can be cured by therapy that achieves a complete remission. Concerning the good-risk NHL, Rosenberg (1979) has stated, "Early and aggressive treatment programs have failed to result in survival benefits in any study that has been properly controlled."

The low-risk favorable prognosis group of patients with NHL are those with nodular lesions, with NLPD (nodular poorly differentiated lymphocytic lymphoma) being the most common type. Patients with DLWD (diffuse well-differentiated lymphocytic lymphoma) are placed in the good-risk group and may be the most favorable patients of all.

A. Chemotherapy for Good-Risk NHL

The role of chemotherapy in good-risk NHL is dependent on the stage of disease. The great majority of patients with stage III to stage IV disease are probably not curable by any known therapy, including drug treatment, despite very high response rates. Even with documented complete remission, the disease usually recurs at a rate of 10 to 15% annually for a period of 10 years or longer after the end of treatment. Therefore, the role of chemotherapy for these stages is palliative. Some patients require no initial treatment if they are asymptomatic and the size or location of the lymphadenopathy poses no major threat. Some patients will be stable over many months, even years, and treatment can be delayed. For a few, especially the elderly, treatment may never be required.

For the uncommon patient with stage I or stage II disease, the standard treatment is radiation. The potential role of chemotherapy is as an adjunct to increase the cure rate, but as yet, this role has not been established in clinical trials.

Available data indicate that both combination chemotherapy and single-alkylating-agent therapy are capable of achieving pathologically documented complete remissions. With combination chemotherapy, complete remission is achieved more quickly, but this does not appear to have important prognostic significance. With single-agent therapy, a prolonged period of treatment may be required to maximize the complete response rate. Both single-agent and combination regimens show a pattern of late relapse from complete remission in patients with NLPD and DLWD histologies. In spite of this continuous late relapse, the median survival is longer than 5 years, with no obvious differences between combination-induced and single-agent–induced remissions.

Bleomycin's role in good-risk NHL is predominately as a second-line therapy for palliation. No standard regimen exists, and clinical research that specifically addresses this issue has been scant.

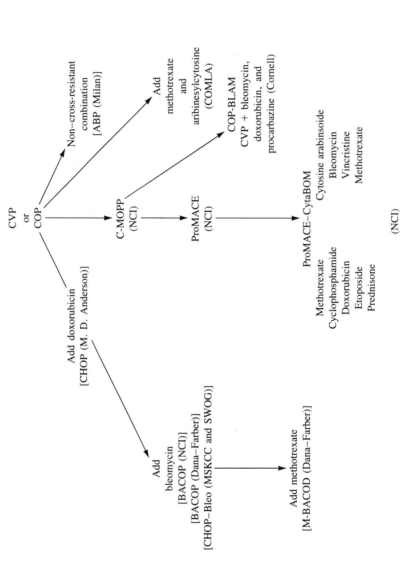

CVP
or
COP

Non—cross-resistant
combination
[ABP (Milan)]

Add
methotrexate
and
aribinesylcytosine
(COMLA)

C-MOPP
(NCI)

COP-BLAM
CVP + bleomycin,
doxorubicin, and
procarbazine (Cornell)

ProMACE
(NCI)

ProMACE–CytaBOM

Methotrexate
Cyclophosphamide
Doxorubicin
Etoposide
Prednisone

Cytosine arabinsoide
Bleomycin
Vincristine
Methotrexate

(NCI)

Add doxorubicin
[CHOP (M. D. Anderson)]

Add
bleomycin
[BACOP (NCI)]
[BACOP (Dana–Farber)]
[CHOP–Bleo (MSKCC and SWOG)]

Add methotrexate
[M-BACOD (Dana–Farber)]

Fig. 4. Bleomycin's integration into combination chemotherapy for poor-risk non-Hodgkin's lymphoma.

B. Chemotherapy for Poor-Risk NHL

In poor-risk disease, the core regimen has been cyclophosphamide, vincristine, and prednisone (CVP or COP). A variety of approaches have been undertaken to improve the therapeutic index of CVP (Fig. 4). Some have included bleomycin and others have not. The main thrust with bleomycin has been to add it to the CHOP (cyclophosphamide, doxorubicin, vincristine, prednisone) regimen to produce either BACOP or CHOP–Bleo.

Two different BACOP schedules have been described. At the NCI, the bleomycin and prednisone were given during the nadir following doxorubicin–cyclophosphamide–vincristine induction. The complete response rate in 25 patients was 48%, with a median survival for the entire group of 14 months. However, none of the 12 patients in CR had relapsed or died at the time of the last report, when the follow-up was as long as 3 years. At the Dana–Farber Cancer Institute (Skarin, 1977), a different schedule of BACOP for 18 patients with NHL resulted in a 50% CR rate, with a median survival of 9 months in the entire group. In this study, maintenance therapy was given to all responders.

SWOG compared CHOP and BCG and CHOP–Bleo with COP–Bleo bleomycin (Jones et al., 1979). In their analysis they combined the two CHOP-based regimens and compared them to the COP–Bleo regimen. In diffuse lymphomas, the CR rate was 58% (65/112) on the CHOP-plus regimens versus 44% (23/52) with COP–Bleo. While the duration of remission and time to remission favored CHOP, the median survival of about 2 years was the same for all three arms.

Regardless of which of the effective combinations is used to treat poor-risk NHL, some generalizations can be made. Patients who do not respond immediately and favorably are unlikely to survive 2 years and will not be cured. Patients who achieve a complete remission and remain disease-free after 2 years appear to be cured of their disease. It is critically important to validate CR through careful restaging, and this is an important component in evaluating literature reports. It also is important to distinguish between CRs that are clinical and those that are pathologic, with restaging. There is no indication that maintenance treatment after pathological CR is of any value.

The NCI Group (Fisher et al., 1983) has been studying a new regimen called proMACE in diffuse aggressive lymphomas. ProMACE comprises prednisone, high-dose methotrexate with leukovorin rescue, doxorubicin, cyclophosphamide, and etoposide (VP-16). Patients receive induction with proMACE, consolidation with MOPP, and late intensification with proMACE. A total of 74 patients have been treated, 17 with stage II disease, 14 with stage III disease, and 43 with stage IV disease. To date, 60 patients have completed therapy and are evaluable for response. Pathologically documented complete responses have been observed in 43 patients (72%). The stage breakdown for CR is 11 in 13 stage II patients (85%), 9 in 10 stage III patients (90%), and 23 in 37 stage IV patients (62%). Relapses have been seen in only 7 of 43 complete responders, with a median study time in excess of 2 years. Actuarial analysis predicts that the 42-month survival will be 62%. Bone marrow toxicity has been significant, with septic deaths occurring in 7 of 74 patients (9%).

The NCI has developed a series of new combinations, which are used in fixed sequential approaches. The primary combination, proMACE, was used initially in sequence with MOPP. A second combination is CytaBOM, which combines cytosine arabinoside, bleomycin, vincristine, and methotrexate. The NCI (Fisher *et al.*, 1984) is comparing proMACE–MOPP versus proMACE–CytaBOM, and preliminary results show the bleomycin-containing regimen to have a higher response rate (89% versus 72%), but also a greater incidence of *Pneumocystis carinii* pneumonia (3 deaths versus 0 deaths).

The M-BACOD regimen (methotrexate, bleomycin, doxorubicin, cyclophosphamide, vincristine, dexamethasone) of the Dana–Farber Cancer Center has been reported to give response rates higher than those previously reported by most groups (Skarin *et al.*, 1983). Among 95 evaluable patients, there were 73 complete remissions (77%), with a 65% 5-year relapse-free survival. The overall 5-year survival was 59%, and 80% in complete responders. Confirmatory and controlled studies are necessary to define the ultimate role of this interesting regimen.

V. HEAD AND NECK CANCERS

Chemotherapy in general, and bleomycin in particular, can be used in a variety of situations to treat squamous-cell cancers of the head and neck. The traditional role is as palliative treatment for advanced or recurrent disease not amenable to therapy with surgery or irradiation. Newer roles are as part of a combined modality strategy. This increasingly involves neoadjuvant or induction chemotherapy, in which drugs are given prior to surgery for patients with operable stage III to stage IV disease. It also involves adjuvant therapy, in which the drugs are given after surgery and become part of the full complexity of the interaction of drugs with radiation. The drug and radiation interaction is complex because the drugs can be used as either sensitizers or as adjunctive cell-killing agents. While these two approaches are conceptually easy to separate, they are difficult to separate in clinical trial data analysis.

In the original Japanese trials, head and neck cancers were reported as responsive to bleomycin. In the early cumulative reviews of U.S. data, response rates were in the range of 15 to 31%, depending upon the stringency of the criteria used. The duration of these responses was short, but the lack of myelosuppression encouraged investigators to pursue combination approaches. Initially, the major drug for combination was methotrexate, but later cisplatin became the critical drug for combination approaches.

A. Combination Chemotherapy for Palliation of
Advanced Disease

One of the most commonly used combinations for palliation of advanced disease has been cisplatin and bleomycin. Unfortunately, while overall response rates are higher than for single agents, complete response rates are low, and the impact on survival is less than dramatic.

An example of a recent trial is that of the Swiss Group for Clinical Cancer Research (SAKK) (Abele *et al.*, 1984). The group compared two bleomycin-containing combinations: bleomycin, methotrexate, and hydroxyurea, and bleomycin, methotrexate, hydroxyurea, and cisplatin. The three-drug regimen achieved 1 complete response and 5 partial responses in 25 patients, yielding a response rate of 24%. The cisplatin-containing regimen resulted in 2 complete responses and 12 partial responses in 23 patients, giving a 61% response rate, which was significantly higher ($p = .01$). The toxicities of nausea and vomiting, stomatitis, and alopecia were more common in the four-drug regimen. No survival or response duration data were available.

Another example is a phase II evaluation by Vogl *et al.* (1984) of another four-drug regimen. This involved cisplatin, bleomycin, sequential 5-fluorouracil (5-FU), and methotrexate, in which the fluorinated pyrimidine was given 1 hr after methotrexate. A total of 49 patients were treated, and 45 were deemed evaluable. The overall response rate was 48%, but the complete response rate was only 4%. The median time to relapse for responders with recurrent or metastatic disease was 24 weeks, and all such patients survived a median of 25 weeks. The toxicity of this regimen was great, and the four-drug results were not considered superior to earlier results with the three-drug approach of cisplatin, bleomycin, and methotrexate.

Lester *et al.* (1984) reported on a similar four-drug approach that also used sequential 5-FU 1 hr after methotrexate, but with somewhat different doses and schedules of the four drugs. They treated 74 patients, of which only 56 were considered to be evaluable. The 18 unevaluable patients had a median survival of 11 months. In the 56 evaluable patients, there were 10 complete responses and 19 partial responses, giving a 52% overall response rate. The median survival for those with partial responses or stable disease was identical—9 months. The median survival of the complete responders was 16 months, while it was only 1 month for those with progressive disease. Toxicity included two deaths from sepsis and one from bleomycin-induced pulmonary fibrosis, but the authors stated that "treatment was generally well-tolerated." The median survival for the entire group was 9 months.

Heyden *et al.* (1984) compared the two-drug regimen of cisplatin plus bleomycin with an investigative combination of vindesine plus methotrexate. A total of 79 patients were treated with one or the other regimen initially, then crossed over at the time of progressive disease. Cisplatin plus bleomycin achieved an overall response rate of 59%, compared with the 26% response rate achieved with the vindesine plus methotrexate regimen ($p = .01$). At crossover, the cisplatin plus bleomycin combination gave a 35% response rate versus no responses with the other combination ($p = .05$). Survival time showed no difference between regimens.

B. Neoadjuvant Treatment

The most commonly used neoadjuvant regimen is cisplatin plus bleomycin. At the time of this writing, six different single-arm series have been reported (Table VIII). The group sizes tend to be small, with 65 being the largest and four of the series involving less than 40 evaluable patients. Three of the series involve one cycle; the other three series involve two cycles. Complete response rates range from 0 to 25%, with no apparent correlation between whether one or two cycles were administered. The overall response rates range from 48 to 88%, with five of six series falling within the 71 to 88% range, indicating reasonable comparability given the great heterogeneity. In none of these six studies are there enough data on long-term survival to judge the actual impact of this type of treatment.

The most interesting combination regimen at this time is cisplatin plus 5-FU, administered by 96- or 120-hr infusion. With continuous infusion of 5-FU, myelosuppression is minimal and, thus, both drugs theoretically could be administered at nearly full therapeutic dose levels. This approach has been pioneered by the group at Wayne State University. In their initial evaluation (Kish *et al.*, 1982) they studied 26 inoperable stage IV disease. Inoperability was based on the surgical evaluation that the primary lesion and/or the regional nodes could not be removed with cancer-free margins. The dose of cisplatin was 100 mg/m² administered by 4-hr infusion (with hydration and mannitol), followed by 1000 mg/m² daily of 5-FU, continuously infused for 4 days. The course was repeated after 3 weeks.

In this initial study, all 26 patients completed two courses. After the second course, 5 complete responses (19.2%) and 18 partial (69.3%) responses were observed, yielding a total response rate of 88.5%. After these two courses, 6 patients underwent radical resection, 6 received radiotherapy followed by resection, and 12 received radiotherapy only. Two patients showed negative histology for tumors at the time of surgical resection after drug therapy, as did one following radiation and surgery after the combination.

The follow-up time was too short and the numbers too small to speak meaningfully about survival. However, the 88.5% response rate was impressive and clearly indicated that this regimen warrants further study in a combined modality setting.

In a follow-up study (Decker *et al.*, 1983), the Wayne State Group adminis-

TABLE VIII CISPLATIN PLUS BLEOMYCIN NEOADJUVANT THERAPY

Reference	Cisplatin dose (mg/m²)	Bleomycin dose (U/m²)	Number of cycles	Local control therapy	Number of evaluable patients	CR[a] no. (%)	PR[b] no. (%)	Overall response (%)
Randolph et al. (1978)	120, day 1	10, days 3–10 infusion	2	Radiotherapy	21	4 (19%)	11 (52%)	71
Hong et al. (1979)	120, day 1	15, days 3–10 infusion	1	Surgery + radiotherapy or radiotherapy alone	39	8 (21%)	22 (56%)	77
Glick et al. (1980)	80–100, day 1; 24-hr infusion	15, days 3–7 infusion	2	Radiotherapy	29	0 (0)	14 (48%)	48
Elias et al. (1979)	100, day 1	15, days 5–9 infusion + methotrexate	1	Surgery + radiotherapy	22	4 (18%)	12 (55%)	73
Spaulding et al. (1982)	80, day 1	Vincristine, 6 hr later; 15, days 3–7 infusion	2	Surgery	50	11 (22%)	33 (66%)	88
Peppard et al. (1980)	100, day 1	15–20, days 2–5 infusion + vincristine	1	Surgery + radiotherapy or radiotherapy alone	65	16 (25%)	36 (55%)	80

[a]CR, Complete remission.
[b]PR, Partial remission.

tered the full dose of 5-FU (1000 mg/m²/day 120-hr infusion) and cisplatin at a dose of 100 mg/m² for three courses every 3 weeks.

Weaver *et al.* (1982) have published the largest experience on neoadjuvant cisplatin plus 5-FU infusion from Wayne State. The patients had stage III and stage IV squamous lesions, with measurable disease and without distant metastases. Patients with a serum creatinine above 1.5 mg/100 m² or a blood urea nitrogen above 20 mg/100 m² were excluded. The cisplatin dose was 100 mg/m² administered with hydration and mannitol diuresis. The 5-FU dose was 1000 mg/m² D × 5 by continuous 24-hr infusion. Three cycles were administered at 3-week intervals.

Of 61 patients entered into the study, 58 completed three cycles. One patient died from aspiration pneumonia after the second course, and 2 patients who were receiving simultaneous radiation for esophageal cancer developed severe leukopenia. Complete responses were observed in 33 patients (54%), and 24 patients (39%) achieved partial response status. Thirteen of the 33 with CR underwent surgery, and 9 showed no histologic evidence of tumor, either in the primary site or in the radical neck specimen. Biopsies of 8 additional patients prior to irradiation also were negative. An additional 15 patients who showed less than total clinical response also underwent resection after drug treatment. Twenty-two received postoperative irradiation and another 23 received irradiation only for local control. According to the authors, the toxicity generally was quite acceptable. Hematologic toxicity was severe in 4 patients and life-threatening in 1.

A total of 13 abstracts on neoadjuvant pilot studies were published at the 1984 meeting of the American Society of Clinical Oncology (Table IX). Only 3 of the 13 included more than 50 patients, and 7 included less than 30 patients. Both of the randomized studies were negative experiences. The NCI Head and Neck Contracts Program three-arm study is the largest. It can be criticized for using only one cycle of cisplatin plus bleomycin, although, as noted earlier, there was no apparent difference between one and two cycles in terms of response induction. The 282 patients are a combination of both induction arms in the three-arm study. However, the 57% 2-year relapse-free survival is reflective only of the arm with neoadjuvant cisplatin. Where approximate 2-year relapse-free survival data are available, the range is from 23 to 61%, with the second highest being from the NCI study, which is not superior to local control therapy only.

At the time of this writing, the greatest excitement in the research community is with the cisplatin plus 5-fluorouracil approach. What is needed are trials that add bleomycin to this two-drug regimen, in the hopes of increasing the efficacy even further.

VI. UTERINE CERVICAL CANCER

In cancer of the cervix, bleomycin's single-agent activity is similar to that found in head and neck cancer, with the durations of response being short. Initial

TABLE IX NEOADJUVANT OR INDUCTION REGIMENS (1984 ASCO)

Reference	Regimen	Number of patients	CR (%)	CR + PR (%)	Local control	Adjuvant chemotherapy	Approximate 2-year relapse-free survival (%)
Perry et al. (1984), Walter Reed Army Medical Center	Sequential 5-FU, methotrexate	18	22	79	Radiotherapy	Yes (cisplatin, vinblastine, bleomycin)	23
Hill et al. (1984), Royal Marsden	Vincristine, 200 bleomycin, 5-FU, methotrexate, hydrocortisone	200	—	66	"Curative"	—	—
Van Rijmenant et al. (1984), Jules Bordet Institut	CABO (cisplatin, methotrexate, bleomycin, vincristine)	27	7	63	Surgery and/or radiotherapy	No	—
Frustaci et al. (1984), Pordenone General Hospital	Cisplatin	34	26	65	Surgery and/or radiotherapy	—	—
Moritmer et al. (1984), University of Washington	Cisplatin	11	18	54	"Definitive local therapy"	No	—
Jacobs et al. (1984a), Radiation Therapy Oncology Group	Cisplatin + 5-FU infusion	23	34	91	Surgery and postoperative radiotherapy	No	—

(continued)

TABLE IX (*Continued*)

Reference	Regimen	Number of patients	CR (%)	CR + PR (%)	Local control	Adjuvant chemotherapy	Approximate 2-year relapse-free survival (%)
Cripps et al. (1984), Ottawa Civic Clinic and Hospital	5-FU, methotrexate, cyclophosphamid, bleomycin; or bleomycin, cisplatin, methotrexate	29	7	50	Surgery and/or radiotherapy	No	—
Jacobs et al. (1984b), NCI Head and Neck Contracts Program	Cisplatin + bleomycin (1 cycle)	282	3	37	Surgery and postoperative radiotherapy	Yes (cisplatin)	57
Holoye et al. (1984), Medical	Bleo–CMF (cyclophosphamide,	43	2	67	Radiotherapy	No	28

College of Wisconsin	methotrexate, 5-FU, bleomycin; 2 cycles)						
Levitan *et al.* (1984), Boston Hospital VA	Cisplatin + bleomycin or bleomycin alone	101	14	51	Surgery and/or radiotherapy	No	—
Spaulding *et al.* (1984), SUNY, Buffalo	Cisplatin, vincristine bleomycin, (2 cycles)	46	24	88	Surgery and/or radiotherapy	No	61
	Cisplatin, vinblastine, 5-FU infusion (2 cycles)	25	4	80	Surgery and/or radiotherapy	No	36
Robinson *et al.* (1984), Israel	Cisplatin, bleomycin, methotrexate (3 cycles)	20	10	55	Radiotherapy	No	—
Laccourrey *et al.* (1984), Paris	Cisplatin, 5-FU, bleomycin (3 cycles)	43	23	84	Surgery	—	—

combination approaches involves mitomycin C with or without vincristine. At Wayne State University and SWOG (Baker *et al.*, 1978), a three-drug combination of mitomycin C, vincristine, and bleomycin (MOB) was tried at several dosage schedules, with disappointing activity at the dosage levels that ultimately were believed to be tolerable.

SWOG treated 130 patients with MOB on three different schedules. The overall response rate was 45%. The schedule of twice-weekly bleomycin and vincristine with a single dose of mitomycin C given every 6 weeks was evaluated in 50 patients. It achieved 8 complete and 14 partial responses for an overall response of 44%. Lymph node, hepatic, and pulmonary metastases responded more frequently than did intraabdominal, pelvic, or skeletal lesions.

Miyamoto *et al.* (1978) reported encouraging results with a sequential combination of 5 U bleomycin daily for 7 days followed by a single injection of 10 mg mitomycin C. They reported a 92% response rate, with responses in 14 of 15 patients and complete responses in 12 patients. Six groups attempted to confirm these positive results but could not (Hugan and Yang, 1981). One such group was the Northern California Oncology Group, which noted only 4 partial responses in 14 evaluable patients for a response rate of 29% (Friedman *et al.*, 1980).

With the discovery of cisplatin activity, this drug became the focus of combination approaches. Several groups added cisplatin to the three drugs in the MOB regimen. Vogl *et al.* (1980) call this "BOMP" and reported responses in 10 of 13 patients, with 3 complete responses. Alberts *et al.* (1981) for SWOG added cisplatin to infusion MOB and observed responses in 6 of 14 patients (43%), with 4 complete responses.

Hakes *et al.* (1981) performed a pilot study of high-dose cisplatin (120 mg/m^2) plus bleomycin and reported responses in 9 of 17 patients, including 9 of 12 patients with extrapelvic disease. No responses were seen in 5 patients with pelvic disease.

The data base for combination chemotherapy in this disease is dominated by small pilot-like or phase II experiences. While some are intriguing, none have enough data from which to draw strong conclusions.

VII. CONCLUSION

After more than a decade of clinical research, many questions about bleomycin remain. The finding of single-agent activity within a disease category starts a cascade of research thrusts—all geared to improving the cure rate or palliation in various disease stages and clinical situations. While the focos of this volume is disease-oriented research with bleomycin, several drug-oriented questions still remain unresolved, including whether continuous infusion is superior to iv bolus or im administration, whether there is a dose–response effect in lymphomas or solid tumors, and whether there are disease- or drug-specific interactions that significantly affect bleomycin pulmonary toxicity in lymphomas or solid tumors. Bleomycin may be more than a decade old, but it is still a vital drug.

REFERENCES

Abele, R., Honegger, H. P., Grossenbacher, R., *et al.* (1984). *Proc. Am. Soc. Clin. Oncol.* **3,** 186.

Alberts, D. S., Martimbeau, P. W., Surwit, E. A., *et al.* (1981). *Cancer Clin. Trials* **4,** 313.

Baker, L. H., Opipari, M. I., Wilson, H., *et al.* (1978). *Obstet. Gynecol.* **52,** 146.

Blum, R. H., Carter, S. K., and Agre, K. (1973). *Cancer* **31,** 903–914.

Bonadonna, G., and Santoro, A. (1982). *Cancer Treat. Rev.* **9,** 21–37.

Bonadonna, G., Zucali, R., Monfardini, S., *et al.* (1975). *Cancer* **36,** 252–259.

Bonadonna, G., Santoro, A., Zucali, R., *et al.* (1979). *Cancer Clin. Trials* **2,** 217–226.

Carter, S. K., and Blum, R. H. (1976). *Prog. Biochem. Pharmacol.* **11,** 158–171.

Carter, S. K. (1983). *Recent Results in Cancer Research* **85,** 70–122.

Case, D. C., Young, C. W., and Lee, B. J. (1977). *Cancer* **39,** 1382–1386.

Coltman, C., Frei, E., and Delaney, F. (1973). *CCR, Cancer Chemother. Rep.* **57,** 109.

Coltman, C., Fuller, L., Fisher, R., and Frei, E. (1979). *In* "Adjuvant Therapy of Cancer II" (S. Jones and S. Salmon, eds.), pp. 129–136. Grune & Stratton, New York.

Cripps, C., Danjoux, E., Nichol, J., *et al.* (1984). *Proc. Am. Soc. Clin. Oncol.* **3,** 181.

Decker, D. A., Drelichman, A., Jacobs, J., *et al.* (1983). *Cancer* **51,** 1353–1355.

DeVita, V. T., Jr. (1979). *Int. J. Radiat. Oncol. Biol. Phys.* **5,** 1855–1867.

DeVita, V. T. (1981). *Cancer* **47,** 1–13.

Einhorn, L. H. (1983). *In* "Urologic Cancer" (D. G. Skinner, ed.), pp. 315–335. Grune & Stratton, New York.

Elias, E. G., Chretien, P. B., Monnard, E., *et al.* (1979). *Cancer* **43,** 1025–1031.

Fisher, R. I., DeVita, V. T., Hubbard, S. M., *et al.* (1983). *Ann. Intern. Med.* **98,** 304–305.

Fisher, R. I., De Vita, V. T., Hubbard, S. M., *et al.* (1984). *Proc. Am. Soc. Clin. Oncol.* **3,** 242.

Frei, E., and Gehan, E. (1971). *Cancer Res.* **31,** 1828.

Friedman, M., Turbow, M. M., and Carter, S. K. (1980). *Proc. Am. Soc. Clin. Oncol.* **21,** 428.

Frustaci, S., Tumolo, S., Veronesi, A., *et al.* (1984). *Proc. Am. Soc. Clin. Oncol.* **3,** 179.

Fuller, L., Gamble, J., Velazquez, W., Rodgers, R., Butler, J., North, L., Martin, R., Gehan, E., and Schullenberger, C. (1980). *Cancer* **45,** 1352.

Glick, J. H., Marcial, V., Richter, M., *et al.* (1980). *Cancer* **46,** 1919–1926.

Glick, J., Tsiatis, S., Prosnitz, L., *et al.* (1984). *Proc. Am. Soc. Clin. Oncol.* **3,** 237.

Goldman, J. M., and Dawson, A. A. (1975). *Lancet* **2,** 1224–1227.

Hainsworth, J. D., Williams, S. D., Einhorn, L. H., *et al.* (1984). *In* "Etoposide (VP-16) Current Status and New Developments" (B. F. Issel, F. M. Muggia, and S. K. Carter, eds.), pp. 233–242. Academic Press, Orlando.

Hakes, T. B., Lynch, G., and Lewis, J. L. (1981). *Proc. Am. Soc. Clin. Oncol.* **22,** 465.

Hersh, E., Frei, E., Coltman, C., and Luce, J. (1972). *Proc. Am. Soc. Clin. Oncol.* **12,** 14.

Heyden, V. H. W., Schroder, M., Scherpe, A., *et al.* (1984). *Proc. Am. Soc. Clin. Oncol.* **3,** 178.

Higby, D. J., Wallace, H. J., Albert, D., and Holland, J. F. (1974). *J. Urol.* **112,** 100–104.

Hill, B. T., Price, L. A., and MacRoe, K. (1984). *Proc. Am. Soc. Clin. Oncol.* **3,** 178.

Holoye, P. Y., Kung, L., Toohill, R., *et al.* (1984). *Proc. Am. Soc. Clin. Oncol.* **3,** 183.

Hong, W. K., Shapshay, S. M., Bhutani, R., *et al.* (1979). *Cancer* **44,** 19–25.

Hugan, M. W., and Yang, R. C. (1981). *In* "Cancer Chemotherapy Annual 3" (H. M. Pinedo, ed.), pp. 333–360. Elsevier, New York.

Ichikawa, T. (1970a). *Proc. 6th Int. Congr. Chemotherapy, Tokyo 1970* Vol. II, 288–290.

Ichikawa, T. (1976). *In* "Gann Monograph on Cancer Research" No. 19, pp. 99–113. University of Tokyo Press, Tokyo.

Ichikawa, T., Nakano, I., and Krokawa, I. (1970). *Proc. 6th Int. Cong. Chemotherapy, Tokyo 1970* Vol. II, 304–308.

Jacobs, J. R., Kinzie, J., Al-Sarraf, M., *et al.* (1984a). *Proc. Am. Soc. Clin. Oncol.* **3**, 180.

Jacobs, C., Wolf, G. T., Makuch, R. W., *et al.* (1984b). *Proc. Am. Soc. Clin. Oncol.* **3**, 182.

Jones, S., *et al.* (1979). *Cancer* **43**, 417.

Jones, S. E., Coltman, C. A., Grozea, P. N., *et al.* (1982). *Cancer Treat. Rep.* **66**, 847–853.

Jones, S. E., Haut, A., Weick, J. K., *et al.* (1983). *Cancer* **51**, 1339–1347.

Kish, J., Drelichman, A., Jacobs, J., *et al.* (1982). *Cancer Treat. Rep.* **66**, 471–474.

Krikorian, J. G., Portlock, C. S., and Rosenberg, S. A. (1978). *Cancer* **41**, 2107–2111.

Laccourrey, H., Brasnau, D., Lacau St. Guily, J., *et al.* (1984). *Proc. Am. Soc. Clin. Oncol.* **3**, 187.

Lester, E. P., Johnson, C. M., Lester, A. K. *et al.* (1984). *Proc. Am. Soc. Clin. Oncol.* **3**, 182.

Levi, J. A., Wiernik, P. H., and Diggs, C. H. (1977). *Med. Pediatr. Oncol.* **3**, 33–40.

Levitan, N., Krueger, S., Bromer, R., *et al.* (1984). *Proc. Am. Soc. Clin. Oncol.* **3**, 183.

Lokich, J. J., Frei, E., Jaffe, N., *et al.* (1976). *Cancer* **38**, 667–671.

Miyamoto, T., Takabe, Y., Watanabe, M., *et al.* (1978). *Cancer* **41**, 403.

Mortimer, J., Cummings, C., Laramore, G., *et al.* (1984). *Proc. Am. Soc. Clin. Oncol.* **3**, 179.

Non-Hodgkin's Lymphoma Pathologic Classification Project (1982). *Cancer* **49**, 2112.

Peppard, S. B., Al-Sarraf, M., Powers, W. E., *et al.* (1980). *Laryngoscope* **90**, 1273–1280.

Perry, D. J., Davis, R. K., Duttenhaver, J. R., *et al.* (1984). *Proc. Am. Soc. Clin. Oncol.* **3**, 178.

Porzig, K. L., Portlock, C. S., Robertson, A., *et al.* (1978). *Cancer* **41**, 1670–1675.

Randolph, V. L., Vallejo, A., Spiro, R. H., *et al.* (1978). *Cancer* **42**, 460–467.

Robinson, E., Zidan, G., Kuten, A., *et al.* (1984). *Proc. Am. Soc. Clin. Oncol.* **3**, 187.

Rosenberg, S. (1979). *N. Engl. J. Med.* **301**, 924.

Samuels, M. L., and Howe, C. D. (1970). *Cancer* **25**, 1009–1017.

Samuels, M. L., Johnson, D. E., and Holoye, P. Y. (1973). *Proc. Am. Assoc. Cancer Res.* **14**, 23.

Santoro, A., and Bonadonna, G. (1979). *Cancer Chemother. Pharmacol.* **2**, 101–105.

Santoro, A., Bonfante, V., Bonadonna, G., *et al.* (1979). *In* "Adjuvant Therapy of Cancer II" (S. Jones and S. Salmon, eds.), Grune & Stratton, New York.

Schein, P. S., DeVita, V. J., Hubbard, S., *et al.* (1976). *Ann. Intern. Med.* **85**, 417–422.

Sherins, R. J., and DeVita, V. T. (1973). *Ann. Intern. Med.* **79**, 216–220.

Sherins, R. J., Olweny, C. L. M., and Ziegler, J. L. (1978). *N. Engl. J. Med.* **299**, 12–16.

Skarin, A., *et al.* (1977). *Blood* **49**, 759.

Skarin, A. T., Canellos, G. P., Rosenthal, D. S., *et al.* (1983). *J. Clin. Oncol.* **1**, 91–98.

Spaulding, M. B., Kahn, A. De Los Santos, R., *et al.* (1982). *Am. J. Surg.* **144**, 432–436.

Spaulding, M. B., De Los Santos, R., Klotch, D., *et al.* (1984). *Proc. Am. Soc. Clin. Oncol.* **3**, 187.

Sutcliffe, S. G., Wrigley, P. F. M., Stansfeld, A. G., *et al.* (1979). *Cancer Chemother. Pharmacol.* **2**, 209–213.

Umezawa, H. (1976). *In* "Fundamental and Clinical Studies of Bleomycin" (S. K. Carter, T. Ichikawa, G. Mathe, and U. Umezawa, eds.), pp. 3–37. University of Tokyo Press, Tokyo.

Van Rijmenant, M. E., Dor, R., Balikdjian, G., *et al.* (1984). *Proc. Am. Soc. Clin. Oncol.* **3**, 179.

Vinciguerra, V., Coleman, M., Jarowski, C. I., *et al.* (1977). *JAMA* **237**, 33–35.

Vogl, S. E., Moukhtar, M., Calanog, N., *et al.* (1980). *Cancer Treat. Rep.* **64**, 1005.

Vogl, S., Komisar, A., Kaplan, B., *et al.* (1984). *Proc. Am. Soc. Clin. Oncol.* **3**, 182.

Vugrin, D., Cvitkovic, E., Whitmore, W. F., and Golbey, R. B. (1979). *Semin. Oncol.* **6**, 94–99.

Weaver, A., Flemming, S., Kish, J., *et al.* (1982). *Am. J. Surg.* **144,** 445–448.
Williams, S. D., Loehrer, P. J., Einhorn, L. H., and Birch, R. (1984). *In* "Etoposide (VP-16) Current Status and New Developments" (B. F. Issell, F. M. Muggia, and S. K. Carter, eds.), pp. 225–232. Academic Press, Orlando.

Bleomycin Chemotherapy
(B. I. Sikic, M. Rozencweig, and S. K. Carter, eds.)

Chapter 2

CLINICAL PHARMACOLOGY OF BLEOMYCIN*

Branimir Ivan Sikic

Department of Medicine
Divisions of Oncology and Clinical Pharmacology
Stanford University School of Medicine
Stanford, California

I. PHARMACEUTICAL PROPERTIES

The bleomycins are cytotoxic glycopeptides produced by a strain of the actinomycete *Streptomyces verticillus*. The mixture of glycopeptides that comprise the clinically used drug bleomycin was isolated, purified, and characterized in Japan by Umezawa *et al.* (1966). The clinical formulation is a mixture consisting predominantly of bleomycins A2 and B2, with each batch of drug standardized for potency using an antimicrobial assay. Dosages of the drug, therefore, are expressed in units, each of which represents 0.6–0.7 mg of bleomycin mixture. The drug is stable in aqueous solution for at least 4 weeks when stored at 4°C, and the powdered drug, which is formulated as the sulfate salt, is stable for at least 1 year at room temperature.

Each of the bleomycin peptides has a molecular weight of ~1500. The bleomycinic acid portion of the molecule contains six nitrogens thought to participate in metal binding, notably chelating iron and copper (Oppenheimer *et al.*, 1979). In addition, the bithiazole moiety is thought to intercalate partially between base pairs of DNA, particularly guanine–cytosine pairs (Povirk *et al.*, 1979). The

*Supported in part by National Institutes of Health grant no. CA-27478 from the Department of Health and Human Services.

peptides differ from each other in their terminal alkylamine, which also partici-
pates in binding to DNA.

II. MECHANISM OF ACTION

The mechanism of action of bleomycin is unique among anticancer drugs and
has been a subject of intense interest to biochemists and molecular biologists.
The drug has the dual properties of binding to DNA and chelating various metal
ions, notably iron and copper. The bleomycin–ferrous complex, in particular,
has been shown to function as minienzyme, catalytically reducing oxygen and
producing various free radicals (Sausville et al., 1976; Caspary et al., 1979).
Grollman and Takeshita (1980) have postulated that DNA breakage occurs by
cleavage of the C_3' to C_4' bond of deoxyribose, and that this cleavage is mediated
by the complex of bleomycin, ferrous iron, and molecular oxygen. Alternatively,
this complex has been shown to produce the superoxide radical and the very toxic
hydroxyl free radical, which could produce similar damage.

The net result is both single- and double-strand breaks in DNA, with resulting
chromosomal deletions and fragmentation. Bleomycin is generally more active
against dividing cells than nondividing cells and demonstrates specificity for the
G_2 and M phases of the cell cycle (Twentyman, 1984).

The chemistry of the DNA breakage is thought to involve abstraction of a
hydrogen atom from deoxyribose at the C_4' position by the free radical species
and subsequent attack by an oxygen molecule to form a peroxide (Grollman and
Takeshita, 1980). The opening of the deoxyribose ring leads to liberation of free
bases, a glycolic acid ester, and a base–propanol, which subsequently can be
degraded to liberate malondialdehyde. Thymine is released preferentially, with
some release of the other three bases as well. There appears to be some prefer-
ence for the GpT sequence of DNA, and cleavage appears to occur specifically at
the 3′ side of guanine.

Very little bleomycin actually enters cells, and the drug appears to localize
eventually to the nuclear envelope (Fujimito, 1974; Fujimoto et al., 1976). The
mode of drug uptake by cells is not well characterized. There does appear to be
preferential breakage of the linker regions of DNA, between nucleosomes (Kuo
and Hsu, 1978). The processes involved in the repair of bleomycin damage also
are not well understood. However, various bacterial and yeast mutants that are
deficient in DNA repair have been shown to be more sensitive to bleomycin
damage. Similarly, human fibroblasts that have an impaired DNA repair mechanism, such as those of ataxia telangiectasia, have been shown to be more sensitive to bleomycin (Taylor et al., 1979). Conversely, it is postulated that an

increased ability to repair DNA damage produced by bleomycin may be a mechanism of resistance to the drug, although there is no direct evidence of this.

It has been proposed that the major mechanism of resistance to bleomycin is an increase in the level of a cytosolic enzyme termed "bleomycin hydrolase" (Umezawa et al., 1966). This aminopeptidase inactivates the drug and is virtually absent in lung and skin, the two normal tissues most susceptible to the drug. Although increased bleomycin hydrolase has been found in some experimental cell lines and tumors resistant to bleomycin, other resistance models do not show such a correlation. Moreoever, there is no correlation between the cytotoxic activity of bleomycin in clonogenic assays of human ovarian carcinomas and the levels of bleomycin hydrolase in those tumors (Lazo et al., 1982).

It has been shown that hypoxia is a mechanism of resistance to bleomycin in cultured cells, and this may be an important resistance mechanism in human solid tumors with a large hypoxic cell fraction (Roizin-Towle and Hall, 1979; Teicher et al., 1981). Since the drug also acts preferentially on cells that are dividing, especially those in the G_2 and M phases of the cell cycle, tumors with a low growth fraction might be expected to be resistant to the drug on a cytokinetic basis.

III. PHARMACOKINETICS

Bleomycin is extremely water soluble, stable in solution, and is not a vesicant agent. Many routes and schedules of administration have been used, including intravenous bolus injection, intramuscular, subcutaneous, intracavitary (for ascites, pleural effusions, and bladder tumors), and continuous intravenous infusion. There is no appreciable plasma protein binding. The pharmacokinetics of the drug has been studied by radioimmunoassay (Broughton et al., 1977; Alberts et al., 1978). The elimination half-life from the serum of patients is approximately 2 hr after intravenous bolus injection, and 3–4 hr after prolonged intravenous infusion. Elimination after prolonged infusion actually may be biphasic, with an initial elimination half-life of ~2 hr, and a longer secondary elimination phase of 8 to 12 hr (Broughton et al., 1977).

Approximately 50–70% of the drug is excreted via the kidneys within the first 24 hr after injection. As might be expected, the drug serum half-life is highly dependent on renal function. The elimination half-life is ~2 hr for patients with creatinine clearance of greater than 40 ml/min. However, in a study of 3 patients with impaired renal function (Crooke et al., 1977), bleomycin half-life rose exponentially with decreasing creatinine clearance (Table I). On the basis of

TABLE I   THE EFFECT OF
RENAL DYSFUNCTION ON THE
SERUM ELIMINATION HALF-
LIFE OF BLEOMYCIN

Creatinine clearance (ml/min)	Bleomycin half-life (hr)
>40	2
35	4
20	6
15	11
10	21

these observations, we recommend that only 50% of the bleomycin dose be given for a creatinine clearance between 20 and 40 ml/min and that only 25% of the dose be given if the creatinine clearance is below 20 ml/min (Table II).

The most significant drug interaction that has been confirmed for bleomycin is with cisplatin, in instances when the latter agent produces renal toxicity. Lethal bleomycin pulmonary toxicity has been reported in the face of severe cisplatin nephrotoxicity, presumably due to the impairment of bleomycin excretion and relative bleomycin overdose (Bennett et al., 1980).

In certain combination regimens for diffuse lymphomas, such as M-BACOD and BACOP, there was an apparent increased incidence of bleomycin pulmonary toxicity at a dose of 15 U/m^2 (Schein et al., 1976). The recommended dose in these regimes, therefore, was reduced to 4 to 5 U/m^2. Studies in mice indicate that vincristine is the agent responsible for increased pulmonary toxicity in those regimes (Louie et al., 1980). Other drugs—notably doxorubicin, cyclophosphamide, methotrexate, and vinblastine—did not appear to increase the risk for pulmonary toxicity with bleomycin in this model. Glucocorticoids do not appear

TABLE II   RECOMMENDED
DOSE MODIFICATION FOR
BLEOMYCIN IN RENAL
DYSFUNCTION

Creatinine clearance (ml/min)	Recommended dose (%)
>40	100
20–40	50
<20	25

to ameliorate bleomycin pulmonary toxicity, and there have been no controlled clinical trials to suggest that glucocorticoids are beneficial.

Increased ambient oxygen concentrations have been shown to increase the risk for bleomycin pulmonary toxicity in model systems. There also have been reports of a delayed interaction of oxygen and bleomycin in patients who have received elevated ambient oxygen concentrations during anesthesia and surgery (Goldiner and Schweizer, 1979). Several cases of adult respiratory distress syndrome have been reported in this situation, and it is recommended that patients who are undergoing general anesthesia after having received bleomycin not receive increased oxygen during ventilation.

IV. CLINICAL USE

Bleomycin is an important drug in the curative PVB and VAB combinations for testicular carcinomas and germ cell cancers of the ovary (Einhorn and Donohue, 1977; Carlson *et al.*, 1983). It also is active in various curative protocols for Hodgkin's disease and non-Hodgkin's lymphomas. Bleomycin is active as a single agent and in combination regimens for squamous carcinomas from various sites, including the skin, head and neck, cervix, and genitalia (Bennett, 1979).

Bleomycin is remarkably devoid of toxicity to the bone marrow. The major dose-limiting toxicity of the drug is pulmonary fibrosis, which is lethal in ~1% of patients who have received the drug and is clinically evident in ~10% of such patients (Comis *et al.*, 1979; Muggia *et al.*, 1983). Other common toxicities include mild fever, which occurs within the first 24 hr of administration in most patients, and a variety of skin changes, which tend to increase in incidence and severity with increasing cumulative dosages of the drug (Cohen *et al.*, 1973). These skin changes are rarely severe enough to discontinue therapy, but include linear hyperpigmentation of the trunk, erythema of the hands and feet, and thickening of the nail beds. Other toxicities reported with single-agent use include mild nausea, mucositis, and alopecia in a minority of cases. Rarely, vascular vasospastic phenomena have been noted after administering bleomycin-containing combinations, especially PVB, but the contribution of bleomycin to such toxicity is not known (Kukla *et al.*, 1982).

A syndrome of acute fulminant collapse, with features of anaphylaxis such as bronchospasm and hypotension, has been observed in up to 1% of patients with lymphomas treated with bleomycin. Only one case of such reaction has been reported in patients with tumors other than lymphomas (Inbar *et al.*, 1984). The mechanism of this reaction is not known, and it has been reported as late as a few hours after the injection of drug. It has been recommended that patients receive a test dose of 1 to 2 units prior to full-dose therapy. Such reactions should be treated as though they were anaphylaxis, with glucocorticoids, antihistamines, epinephrine, and intravenous fluids.

One of the major controversies regarding the clinical use of bleomycin is the issue of schedule dependence. In animal models, it is quite clear that administration of the same dose by continuous infusion is superior to bolus injection (Sikic *et al.*, 1978; Peng *et al.*, 1980). Both increased antitumor efficacy and decreased pulmonary toxicity have been observed with such continuous infusion. The rationale for the prolonged infusion includes the short half-life of the drug and its phase specificity, so that only a small fraction of tumor cells are exposed during a sensitive phase of the cell cycle with bolus injection. Unfortunately, no randomized clinical trials have been performed to address this question (Samuels *et al.*, 1975; Cooper and Hong, 1981). In the past, the major barriers to prolonged infusion therapy have been cost and convenience, with the need for hospitalizing patients. However, recent developments in portable infusion pump technology and physician awareness of the possible advantages of such administration have increased both the feasibility and interest of such controlled trials (Carlson and Sikic, 1983).

REFERENCES

Alberts, D. S., Chen, H.-S. G., Liu, R., Himmelstein, K. J., Mayersohn, M., Perrier, D., Gross, J., Moon, T., Broughton, A., and Salmon, S. E. (1978). *Cancer Chemother. Pharmacol.* **1**, 177–181.

Bennett, J. M. (1979). *Ann. Intern. Med.* **90**, 945–948.

Bennett, W. M., Pastore, L., and Houghton, D. C. (1980). *Cancer Treat. Rep.* **64**, 921–924.

Broughton, A., Strong, J. E., Holoye, P. Y., and Bedrossian, C. W. M. (1977). *Cancer* **40**, 2772–2778.

Carlson, R. W., and Sikic, B. I. (1983). *Ann. Intern. Med.* **99**, 823–833.

Carlson, R. W., Sikic, B. I., *et al.*, (1983). *J. Clin. Oncol.* **1**, 645–651.

Caspary, W. J., Niziak, C., Lanzo, D. A., Friedman, R., and Bachur, N. R. (1979). *Mol. Pharmacol.* **16**, 256–260.

Comis, R. L., Kuppinger, M. S., Ginsberg, S. J., Crooke, S. T., Gilbert, R., Auchincloss, J. H., and Prestayko, A. W. (1979). *Cancer Res.* **39**, 5076–5080.

Cooper, K. R., and Hong, W. K. (1981). *Cancer Treat. Rep.* **65**, 419–425.

Crooke, S. T., Comis, R. L., Einhorn, L. H., Strong, J. E., Broughton, A., and Prestayko, A. W. (1977). *Cancer Treat. Rep.* **61**, 1631–1636.

Einhorn, L. H., and Donohue, J. (1977). *Ann. Intern. Med.* **87**, 293–298.

Fujimoto, J. (1974). *Cancer Res.* **34**, 2969–2974.

Fujimoto, J., Higashi, H., and Kosaki, G. (1976). *Cancer Res.* **36**, 2248–2253.

Goldiner, P. L., and Schweizer, O. (1979). *Semin. Oncol.* **6**, 121–124.

Grollman, A. P., and Takeshita, M. (1980). *In* "Advances in Enzyme Regulation" (G. Weber, ed.), Vol. 18, pp. 67–83. Pergamon Press, Oxford.

Inbar, M. J., Baratz, M., Figer, A., Schpitzer-Reta, E., and Chaitchik, S. (1984). *Cancer Chemother. Pharmacol.* **13**, 17–71.

Krakoff, I. H., Cvitkovic, E., Currie, V., Yeh, S., and LaMonte, C. (1977). *Cancer* **40**, 2027–2037.

Kukla, L. W., McGuire, W. P., Lad, T., and Saltiel, M. (1982). *Cancer Treat. Rep.* **66**, 369–370.

Kuo, M. T., and Hsu, T. C. (1978). *Nature* **271**, 83–84.

˙ Lazo, J. S., Boland, C. J., and Schwartz, P. E. (1982). *Cancer Res.* **42**, 4026–4033.
Louie, A. C., Evans, T. L., and Sikic, B. I. (1980). *Proc. Am. Assoc. Cancer Res.* **21**, 290.
Muggia, F. M., Louie, A. C., and Sikic, B. I. (1983). *Cancer Treat. Rev.* **10**, 221–243.
Oppenheimer, N. J., Rodriquez, L. O., and Hecht, S. M. (1979). *Biochemistry* **18**, 3439–3445.
Peng. Y.-M., Alberts, D. S., Chen, H.-S. G., Mason, H., and Moon, T. E. (1980). *Br. J. Cancer* **41**, 644–647.
Povirk, L. F., Hogan, M., and Dattagupta, N. (1979). *Biochemistry* **18**, 96–101.
Roizin-Towle, L., and Hall, E. J. (1979). *Int. J. Rad. Oncol. Biol. Phys.* **5**, 1491–1494.
Samuels, M. L., Johnson, D. E., and Holoye, P. Y. (1975). *Cancer Chemother. Rep.* **59**, 563–570.
Sausville, E. A., Peisach, J., and Horwitz, S. B. (1976). *Biochem. Biophys. Res. Communic.* **73**, 814–821.
Sikic, B. I., Collins, J. M., Mimnaugh, E. G., and Gram, T. E. (1978). *Cancer Treat. Rep.* **62**, 2011–2017.
Taylor, A. M. R., Rosney, C. M., and Campbell, J. B. (1979). *Cancer Res.* **39**, 1046–1050.
Teicher, B. W., Lazo, J. S., and Sartorelli, A. C. (1981). *Cancer Res.* **41**, 73–81.
Twentyman, P. R. (1984). *Pharmacol. Ther.* **23**, 417–441.
Umezawa, H., Suhara, Y., Takita, T., and Maeda, K. (1966). *J. Antibiot.* **19**, 210–215.

Section II
TESTICULAR AND OVARIAN CANCERS

Bleomycin Chemotherapy
(B. I. Sikic, M. Rozencweig, and S. K. Carter, eds.)

Chapter 3

CHEMOTHERAPY OF TESTICULAR CARCINOMA: AN OVERVIEW

Brian J. Lewis

Cancer Research Institute
Department of Medicine
University of California
San Francisco, California

I. INTRODUCTION

Currently, approximately 65–100% of patients with advanced or residual non-seminomatous testicular cancer (NSTC) enter complete remission after chemotherapy, and the vast majority do not have a recurrence. Twenty-five years ago, there were virtually no long-term survivors among those whose tumor was not cured surgically. Thus, the management of this malignancy has joined the treatment of Hodgkin's disease as a paradigm of how we would like to approach all solid tumors. In both diseases, success has come through two lines of development: the discovery of increasingly effective therapy, and the evolution of a clearer definition of important prognostic features.

II. CHEMOTHERAPY

A. Evolution of Current Treatment

In 1960, Li used combination chemotherapy with methotrexate, chlorambucil, and dactinomycin for advanced-stage NSTC patients. Seven of 23 patients (30%)

entered complete remission, and 3 of these did not relapse subsequently (Li *et al.*, 1960). Until this report, a variety of single agents had produced transient responses but made no real impact upon the natural history of the disease. In 1966, Mackenzie updated the series started by Li (Mackenzie, 1966). Among 90 patients, the complete response rate was 12%, and the overall response rate was 39%. Significantly, roughly half of the patients entering complete remission did not relapse, giving further impetus to the idea that advanced-disease patients were curable. Through the 1960s, other combinations of alkylators, antibiotics, and antimetabolites failed to improve the control rate further (Anderson *et al.*, 1979).

Samuels and colleagues (1975a) introduced the next advance in the early 1970s by combining vinblastine and bleomycin. Preclinical data suggested that the metaphase arrest induced by vinblastine would augment bleomycin, most effective during the G_2 and M phases of the cell cycle. Bolus injection of bleomycin plus vinblastine produced a 33% complete remission rate, which rose to 53% when the bleomycin dosage was given as a 5-day infusion (Samuels *et al.*, 1975b). Toxicity also escalated, as compared with earlier regimens, and included significant myelosuppression, mucositis, hypertension, hyperbilirubinemia, and pulmonary fibrosis.

The current therapeutic era began in 1974, with the demonstration that cisplatin was highly active in previously treated patients (Higby *et al.*, 1974). Because cisplatin was relatively nonmyelotoxic, Einhorn could combine it with vinblastine and bleomycin (PVB), in the hope of adding to the response rate already seen by Samuels, but without summating toxicities (Table I) (Einhorn and Donohue, 1977).

In this initial study of 47 patients, 70% entered a complete remission after four courses of PVB. In addition, 11 partial responders were rendered disease-free by surgical removal of residual tumor after chemotherapy, yielding an overall complete remission of 81%. Of all the patients originally entered into the trial, 51% subsequently were continuously free of recurrence.

Later studies have refined this experience further. A reduction in the dose of vinblastine from an initial level of 0.4 to 0.3 mg/kg per cycle diminished myelotoxicity without compromising antitumor effect (Einhorn and Williams, 1980). The addition of doxorubicin to PVB did not appear to increase the response rate. A randomized trial conducted with the Southeastern Cancer Study Group (Drasga *et al.*, 1982) showed that maintenance treatment with vinblastine did not improve the already substantial relapse-free survival in patients achieving a complete remission with PVB with or without doxorubicin (12% relapse rate with vinblastine maintenance and 7% without vinblastine maintenance).

Concurrent to the development of PVB, workers at Memorial Hospital in New York City initiated a series of sequential studies originally based upon vin-

TABLE I   CURRENT COMBINATION CHEMOTHERAPY FOR GERM-CELL TUMORS OF
THE TESTIS

A. PVB (Drasga *et al.*, 1982) Cisplatin 20 mg/m^2 iv × 5 days q 3 weeks × 4 courses
 Vincristine 0.3 mg/kg iv q 3 weeks × 4 courses
 Bleomycin 30 units iv weekly × 12 doses

B. VAB-VI (Vugrin *et al.*, 1983)
 Day 1:   Cyclophosphamide 600 mg/m^2 iv
            Vinblastine 4 mg/m^2 iv
            Dactinomycin 1 mg/m^2 iv
            Bleomycin 30 U iv push[a]
 Days 1–3: Bleomycin 20 U/m^2/day by 24-hr infusion × 3 days[a]
 Day 4:   Cisplatin 120 mg/m^2 iv
 Given every 3–4 weeks × 3 courses

---

[a]Bleomycin omitted from third course.

blastine, actinomycin D, and bleomycin (VAB-I) (Table I). The addition of various drugs and schedules and an increasing intensity of therapy improved the complete remission rate and disease-free survival from 14 and 12%, respectively, in the VAB-I study, to 64 and 84% in the more recent VAB-VI trial (Vugrin *et al.*, 1983).

B. Integration of Surgery into Primary Treatment

At the end of induction therapy with PVB, residual masses will remain in a small percentage of patients, despite a profound overall reduction in tumor volume. Attempts to debulk the remaining tumor surgically can convert an additional 10–20% of patients into complete responders (Drasga *et al.*, 1982). Histologically, approximately one-third of resected specimens contain fibrous tissue, one-third mature teratoma, and one-third carcinoma. Patients with residual cancer are at high risk for recurrence and require additional chemotherapy. Patients with fibrosis or teratoma appear to have a 90% chance of remaining recurrence-free, and additional treatment is not recommended.

C. Adjuvant Chemotherapy

Ten percent of patients with stage I NSTC and at least 50% of patients with stage II disease will develop recurrent tumor after apparent surgical cure. Given the efficacy of chemotherapy against advanced disease, it would be logical to give postoperative chemotherapy to the higher risk patients (in particular, stage II patients with macroscopic nodal metastases in the retroperitoneum at the time of node dissection). However, the increased ability to survey for recurrence with serum markers and radiology studies, along with the experience that the majority of recurrences arise in the first 12 months after surgery and the remainder within 2 years (Einhorn, 1981), allows intervention when a recurrence is at a low volume in patients followed closely with no postoperative treatment. Among stage III patients, those with minimal-volume tumor have a 95+% complete remission rate and an excellent chance for cure (Einhorn, 1981).

Chemotherapy may be delayed in stage II patients, using it only in those who eventually fail—and do so at an early point in time, when chances for control through chemotherapy are high. At present, a national intergroup study is under-way to resolve the question of when to apply chemotherapy in stage II patients (Jacobs and Muggia, 1980). The study compares close follow-up alone with two cycles of PVB administered postoperatively in patients whose serum markers have returned to normal. Einhorn has reported on 31 stage II patients followed without treatment after surgery. Twelve patients relapsed, and all were cured with chemotherapy (Drasga et al., 1982). Outside the protocol setting, his policy is to employ intensive follow-up during the first 24 months after surgery in stage I and stage II patients and to hold chemotherapy in reserve.

D. Therapy of Poor-Prognosis Patients

Patients with bulky disease have a greater risk of not achieving disease control through standard induction chemotherapy. Complete remission rate among these patients is approximately 50–60% versus 80–90+% among patients with low tumor burdens. In an attempt to upgrade the response rate, workers at the National Cancer Institute compared surgical debulking before chemotherapy with chemotherapy as initial treatment in poor-prognosis patients (Javadpour et al., 1982). There was no advantage to cytoreductive surgery. In a subsequent trial, the NCI group employed very aggressive chemotherapy with high-dose cisplatin (200 mg/m^2), etoposide, vinblastine, and bleomycin (Ozols et al., 1983; Ozols et al., 1984). Partial responders received intensification therapy with higher-dose etoposide (250 mg/m^2 day for 5 days) plus high-dose cisplatin and autologous bone marrow infusion. Of the 20 patients treated, virtually all showed residual masses after chemotherapy and were subjected to attempted resection. At the time of reporting, 84% entered complete remission and 68% remained alive and disease-free. Of 10 comparable patients who received PVB at the standard dose, 60% entered complete remission and only 30% were alive and disease-free. However, differences in overall survival were not statistically significantly different between the two approaches.

For patients receiving chemotherapy who either never enter complete remission or who relapse after a complete response and escape control with first-line regimens, etoposide has shown significant activity, especially in combination with cisplatin. Up to 40% of heavily pretreated patients showed disease control and were probably cured with etoposide plus cisplatin (Williams *et al.*, 1980). This represents a striking shift in the dismal prognosis previously characteristic of these patients.

Ifosfamide, an alkylating agent studied in Europe (Bremer *et al.*, 1982) and more recently reviewed in a U.S. report (Wheeler *et al.*, 1984), has activity in recurrent disease (Anderson *et al.*, 1979). Responses in resistant disease also have been seen with high-dose etoposide (2400 mg/m^2 per course) plus support with autologous bone marrow infusion. In a pilot study (Wolff *et al.*, 1984), 7 of 10 evaluable patients had previously received standard-dose etoposide. Among the 10 patients treated on the high-dose program, there were 2 complete responses and 4 partial responses. Toxicity was significant and the responses were short-lived, but the response among patients refractory to standard-dose etoposide would suggest, along with the NCI experience, a role for high-dose etoposide, at least in the primary treatment of poor-prognosis patients who do not fare optimally with standard chemotherapy.

E. Seminoma

Seminoma, in contrast to NSTC, is extremely radiosensitive. The majority of seminoma patients present with stage I disease. In a review of 1476 patients, 1032 (70%) were stage I and 95% were disease-free after conventional treatment with surgery and radiation therapy. In stage II patients, 78% were disease-free, while the figure fell to 28% for more advanced disease patients. Radiotherapy alone is not adequate postoperative treatment for high-risk stage II patients (those with bulky abdominal nodes or those with disseminated disease) (Caldwell *et al.*, 1980; Ball *et al.*, 1982).

Earlier trials of single agents, usually alkylators, did not have a significant impact upon survival in poor-prognosis patients with seminoma. More recently, the application of PVB (Drasga *et al.*, 1982), BEP (Peckham *et al.*, 1983), and VAB-VI (Stanton *et al.*, 1983) has moved the control rate into the same range as for advanced NSTC. Interestingly, Oliver (1984) and Samuels and Logothetis (1983) have reported promising results with cisplatin alone. For PVB, 37 of 54 patients achieved complete remission (69%), and with somewhat limited follow-up only 3 had relapsed. Prior radiation was associated with severe myelosuppression (Drasga *et al.*, 1982). In this regard, Peckham *et al.* (1983) substituted etoposide for vinblastine (BEP as opposed to PVB) for both NSTC and seminoma to reduce the risk of myelosuppression. All 7 patients with advanced seminoma were disease-free for a median of 15 months after starting chemotherapy. Myelotoxicity appeared diminished only in those patients who did not receive irradiation and dosage schedules of 3 days as opposed to 5 days of etoposide per cycle. The full-dose regimen containing 5 days of etoposide probably offers no advantage over PVB.

Stanton *et al.* (1983) reviewed 21 patients with bulky stage II or stage III disease who received VAB-VI. Seventeen of the 21 patients (81%) were in complete remission with or without additional surgery. At a median follow-up of 14 months, 3 had relapsed. In these trials, the small numbers of patients, relatively short follow-up periods, and lack of direct comparative data between regimens obviate firm conclusions about the optimal drug treatment for advanced seminoma. Clearly, these drug combinations are active and offer the potential of cure. Myelotoxicity in the face of prior radiation therapy remains problematic.

One solution to this particular toxicity may lie in a "retreat" from combination to single-agent treatment. Oliver (1984) used cisplatin alone (50 mg/m^2 every 2–3 weeks for four doses) to induce complete remission in 9 of 10 nonirradiated patients and 1 of 4 previously irradiated patients with metastatic seminoma. Combination chemotherapy controlled three of the four treatment failures. The patients had a median follow-up of 15 months. Samuels and Logothetis (1983) employed more intensive cisplatin at a weekly dose of 100 mg/m^2. Thirty of 32 advanced-stage patients, excluding 5 with elevated alpha fetoprotein (AFP) levels who received combination chemotherapy, were in continuous complete remission, 22 for more than 2 years. Twelve patients had chronic hearing loss, 9 chronic peripheral neuropathy, and 2 of 10 patients with a rise in serum creatinine did not show full correction of the elevation to less than 1.5 mg/dl. It would be interesting to see how the drug combinations compare with cisplatin alone or less toxic platinum analogs.

III. PROGNOSTIC VARIABLES

A. Tumor Bulk and Serum Markers

Analyses of patients who have received PVB therapy indicate that tumor volume is of paramount importance in predicting outcome (Drasga *et al.,* 1982). Other variables, such as serum level of β human chorionic gonadotropin (β-HCG), AFP, and lactic dehydrogenase, are not likely to be independent of or to outweigh the influence of tumor mass, although these variables do correlate with probability of response and survival.

Before the current chemotherapy era, histopathologic subtype was found to be a significant factor. It now would appear that the potency of current drug regimens usually blurs the distinction between histologic groups, although the presence of endodermal sinus tumor elements may correlate with a decreased probability of complete remission (Logothetis *et al.*, 1984). Similarly, extragonadal presentations have carried a worse prognosis than primary tumors in the testis. However, allowing for the bulkiness of extragonadal disease at the time of discovery and considering data showing good control with modern treatment, it seems that bulk disease in itself is the independent prognostic variable, not site of origin. For example, in a series of 31 patients with advanced primary extragonadal germ-cell tumors, 6 of which were seminoma, 21 patients entered complete remission on PVB with or without doxorubicin, and 89% of these were continuously disease-free at a median follow-up of 3 months (Hainsworth *et al.*, 1982).

A recent study suggests that the pattern of decline in β-HCG levels may be as good or better than tumor volume in predicting outcome. Picozzi *et al.* (1984) studied 40 patients and observed that if the ratio of day 22 β-HCG to day 1 β-HCG was greater than 0.005 during the first cycle of chemotherapy, an incomplete response to treatment could be predicted, with a sensitivity of 90% and a predictive value of 94%. The predictive value for tumor volume was, in contrast, only 62%. If this observation is confirmed, it may identify a subset of patients for which induction treatment will have to be intensified mid-course to capture tumors destined to escape control with the original therapy.

B. Disease-Free Survival

It also is apparent that patients who fail after initially successful chemotherapy, or who are followed expectantly after primary surgery, relapse almost entirely in the first 12 months (Drasga *et al.*, 1982). In a small percentage of patients, recurrent disease occurs in the second follow-up year; thereafter, disease recurrence is rare (Terebelo *et al.*, 1983). This has both management and prognostic implications. It indicates, as outlined by Einhorn (1981), that for the first year after surgery or chemotherapy, patients receive monthly examinations, measurement of serum marker levels, and chest X rays. In the second year, the frequency is every 2 months, and thereafter every 6 months. Again, this program will allow for early and, thereby, more effective intervention when there is recurrent tumor. Prognostically, the temporal pattern of recurrence implies that we can speak of cure with a high degree of confidence once a patient has experienced a 2-year disease-free period.

IV. TOXICITY

The drugs currently used in combination chemotherapy for NSTC are cisplatin, vinblastine, and bleomycin. Toxicity is significant and relates to individual properties of each component, as well as to features that arise from the combination.

A. Myelotoxicity

Vinblastine is the major contributor to myelotoxicity. Cisplatin has a much lower level of myelotoxicity. There can be profound granulocyte nadirs on PVB; this occurs less frequently with the reduction in vinblastine dose mentioned earlier. Since patients may require hospitalization and antibiotic therapy during febrile, granulocytopenic episodes, it is mandatory to provide close follow-up and monitoring of peripheral blood counts during treatment.

B. Neurotoxicity

In the doses used in PVB, vinblastine produces a peripheral neuropathy; however, vinblastine as a single agent does not usually produce this toxicity. Cisplatin can cause both central and peripheral neurotoxicity (Loehrer and Einhorn, 1984), and the latter effect has been known to limit therapy when the drug is used alone. Cisplatin also might be, as an additive with vinblastine, a contributor to the overall neurotoxicity of PVB. Most frequently, there is sub-clinical damage to the organ of Corti, but this usually does not require dose modification. Patients receiving PVB have episodes of severe myalgias second-ary to vinblastine.

C. Nephrotoxicity

As with other compounds containing heavy metals, cisplatin causes renal tubular damage. Current regimens of vigorous hydration have minimized the risk of severe renal dysfunction, although it does not appear possible to avoid some degree of measurable decline in the glomerular filtration rate. Hypomagnesemia is a frequent toxicity, secondary to tubular damage and urinary magnesium losses. It is possible that a reduction in the glomerular filtration rate could augment bleomycin pulmonary toxicity (van Barneveld et al., 1984), and it is important to avoid, as much as possible, other nephrotoxic agents, such as the amnioglycosides, during PVB therapy (Loehrer and Einhorn, 1984).

D. Gastrointestinal Toxicity

Cisplatin causes profound nausea and vomiting. There has been considerable study of a variety of antiemetic programs, and substantial gains have been made in the control of cisplatin-induced emesis with metoclopramide, dexamethasone, butyrophenones, and a variety of other agents (Loehrer and Einhorn, 1984).

E. Gonadal Toxicity

Virtually all patients on PVB become azoospermic after treatment, and there is evidence of significant impairment of spermatogenesis prior to chemotherapy. In a prospective analysis of 41 patients (Drasga et al., 1983), only 6.6% were suitable candidates for sperm banking before treatment. The figure was 27% in a Northern California Oncology Group (NCOG) review (Tseng et al., 1984). However, observations to date suggest that 2–3 years after treatment, there may be substantial recovery of spermatogenesis (Drasga et al., 1983; Tseng et al., 1984). The NCOG analysis of 20 PVB-treated patients, as well as a report from Memorial Hospital (Leitner et al., 1984) describing 8 patients in complete remission after VAB-VI therapy, found endocrinologic evidence of compensated testicular failure.

F. Vasotoxicity

One report (Vogelsang et al., 1981) noted a disturbing frequency of Raynaud's phenomenon in 22 of 60 patients who received vinblastine and bleomycin, with or without cisplatin. The symptoms began at a median of 10 months after the start of chemotherapy. A history of cigarette smoking correlated with the syndrome, and in only half of the patients did the symptoms wane with time. Two patients had nonfatal myocardial infarctions at ages 40 and 45. Of note, workers in Houston earlier had reported on severe coronary artery disease in a 20-year-old and a 25-year-old, both of whom had received PVB treatment (Edwards et al., 1979). The mechanisms of induction of vascular toxicity are unclear, but as Vogelsang et al. (1981) have commented, the pathophysiology of Raynaud's phenomenon relates to the rheologic properties of blood, sympathetic control of vascular tone, and intrinsic state of arterial smooth muscle. Since the syndrome has occurred with vinblastine and bleomycin alone, the contribution of cisplatin is unclear. The syndrome has not occurred with cisplatin alone, but it is interesting to speculate whether cisplatin and vinblastine might summate in producing autonomic neurotoxicity. Bleomycin can damage small blood vessels, while vincristine may affect sympathetic tone. All in all, these data raise concern about the magnitude and severity of vascular toxicity that will be seen in the increasing number of long-term survivors after PVB-based treatment.

G. Second Cancers

After unilateral orchiectomy, there is an increased risk for a second primary germ-cell tumor in the remaining testis. The influence of chemotherapy on this tendency and its carcinogenic tendency in other organ sites are unclear. Among 1150 patients followed at Memorial Hospital in New York from 1945 to 1977 (Cockburn *et al.*, 1983), 52 developed second malignancies (4.5%). Given the variation in management and treatment over these years, firm conclusions about causation are impossible. However, the data did suggest a relationship between radiation therapy and the development of sarcoma, and between the chemotherapy of that era and the appearance of leukemia. The carcinogenic potential of PVB is unknown.

H. Pulmonary Toxicity

Pulmonary toxicity is a long-recognized complication of bleomycin therapy. However, with close monitoring and discontinuation of bleomycin at the first symptom or sign of pulmonary dysfunction, pulmonary fibrosis with PVB should be a rare event. It also is important to keep the total cumulative dose of bleomycin as low as possible, certainly below 300 to 400 U. Vinblastine and cisplatin are not associated with pulmonary toxicity, and there is no indication that they are synergistic with bleomycin.

There has been concern that bleomycin-treated patients are at high risk during subsequent surgery for developing respiratory failure, presumably from increased susceptibility to oxygen toxicity at a high inspired oxygen concentration (F_1O_2). A report from the University of Pennsylvania (LaMantia *et al.*, 1984) reviewed 16 testicular cancer patients who had received bleomycin and subsequently underwent surgery between 1976 and 1982. The authors found no increase in respiratory complications and no evidence that an enriched inspired oxygen concentration was hazardous (mean F_1O_2 in their patients was 0.41). Given the postoperative deaths reported in earlier series (Ginsburg and Comis, 1982), the nature and magnitude of an adverse interaction between prior bleomycin treatment and the use of supplemental oxygen remain open to important questions. It would appear prudent to avoid a high F_1O_2 during surgery, but not to deny the patient the benefit of some oxygen enrichment to avoid the risk of hypoxemia (LaMantia *et al.*, 1984).

V. CONCLUSION

The gains in treatment and clinical management of NSTC patients give rise to a concise and rational therapeutic strategy. Pathologic stage I patients with negative serum markers postoperatively require only close observation. The small percentage of patients who relapse can be detected early and cured with chemotherapy. A similar approach appears feasible for surgically treated stage II patients, although current studies will decide the issue of adjuvant versus expectant chemotherapy. Patients requiring chemotherapy are stage II patients whose markers remain elevated after surgery, stage II patients with residual disease, and stage III patients. Those with minimal tumor volume will be cured more than 90% of the time. Those with bulky tumor can be cured with PVB-based chemotherapy, but the probability is lower, and additional steps, such as more intensive chemotherapy, will be required to improve the control rate. Patients who have a partial response after a suitable period of induction treatment require surgical reexploration and debulking of residual masses as well as additional chemotherapy, if cancer is found. Complete responders who relapse may be re-treated successfully with cisplatin and etoposide or with very high-dose chemotherapy regimens. However, more research in the area of new agents, drug combinations, and treatment strategies is needed. With the identification of several potent treatments ranging from single-agent cisplatin to established NSTC regimens such as PVB or VAB-VI, the outlook for patients with advanced or recurrent seminoma appears to be excellent.

The toxicity of current chemotherapy remains considerable. The individual and combined toxicities of PVB should diminish with the introduction of newer analogs, such as platinum derivatives, which are less nephrotoxic. Given the phase II activity of cisplatin and etoposide in combination for relapsed patients, it is logical to ask if etoposide subsequently can be added to primary induction therapy, again with a likely decrease in overall toxicity and increase in efficacy.

REFERENCES

Anderson, T., Waldmann, T. A., Javadpour, N., and Glatstein, E. (1979). *Ann. Intern. Med.* **90,** 373–385.
Ball, D., Barrett, A., and Peckham, M. J. (1982). *Cancer* **50,** 2289–2294.
Bremer, K., Niederle, N., Krischke, W., Higi, M., Scheulen, M. E., Schmidt, C. G., and Seeber, S. (1982). *Cancer Treat. Rev.* **9** (suppl. A), 79–84.
Caldwell, W. L., Kademian, M. T., Frias, Z., and Davis, T. E. (1980). *Cancer* **45,** 1768–1744.
Cockburn, A., Vugrin, D., Macchia, R., Warden, S., and Whitmore, W. (1983). *Proc. Am. Soc. Clin. Oncol.* **2,** 139.
Drasga, R. E., Einhorn, L. H., and Williams, S. D. (1982), *Ca* **32,** 66–77.
Drasga, R. E., Einhorn, L. H., Williams, S. D., Patel, D. N., and Stevens, E. E. (1983). *J. Clin. Oncol.* **1,** 179–189.
Edwards, G. S., Lane, M., and Smith, F. E. (1979). *Cancer Treat. Rep.* **63,** 551–552.
Einhorn, L. H. (1981). *Cancer Res.* **41,** 3275–3280.
Einhorn, L. H., and Donohue, J. (1977). *Ann. Intern. Med.* **87,** 293–298.
Einhorn, L. H., and Williams, S. D. (1980). *Cancer* **46,** 1339–1334.
Ginsberg, S. J., and Comis, R. L. (1982). *Semin. Oncol.* **9,** 34–51.
Hainsworth, J. D., Einhorn, L. H., Williams, S. D., Stewart, M., and Greco, F. A. (1982). *Ann. Intern. Med.* **97,** 7–11.
Higby, D. J., Wallace, H. J., Albert, D. J., and Holland, J. F. (1974). *Cancer* **33,** 1219–1225.

Jacobs, E. M., and Muggia, F. M. (1980). *Cancer* **45,** 1782–1790.

Javadpour, N., Ozols, R., Anderson, T., Barlock, A. B., Wesley, R., and Young, R. C. (1982). *Cancer* **50,** 2004–2010.

LaMantia, K. R., Glick, J. H., and Marshall, B. E. (1984). *Anesthesiology* **60,** 65–67.

Leitner, S., Bosl, G. J., Sealey, Atlas, S., Bajorunas, D., Scheiner, E., and Myers, W. P. L. (1984). *Proc. Am. Soc. Clin. Oncol.* **3,** 159.

Li, M. C., Whitmore, W. F., Golbey, R., and Grabstald, H. (1960). *J. Amer. Med. Assoc.* **174,** 1291–1299.

Loehrer, P. J., and Einhorn, L. H. (1984). *Ann. Intern. Med.* **100,** 704–713.

Logothetis, C. J., Samuels, M. L., Trindale, A., Grant, C., Gomez, L., and Ayala, A. (1984). *Cancer* **53,** 122–128.

Mackenzie, A. R. (1966). *Cancer* **19,** 1369–1376.

Oliver, R. T. D. (1984). *Proc. Am. Soc. Clin. Oncol.* **3,** 162.

Ozols, R. F., Deisseroth, A. B., Javadpour, N., Barlock, A., Messerschmidt, G. L., and Young, R. C. (1983). *Cancer* **51,** 1803–1807.

Ozols, R. F., Ihde, D., Jacob, J., Steis, R., Veach, S. R., Wesley, M., and Young, R. C. (1984). *Proc. Am. Soc. Clin. Oncol.* **3,** 155.

Peckham, M. J., Barrett, A., Liew, K. H., Horwich, A., Robinson, B., Dobbs, H. J., McElwain, T. J., and Hendry, W. F. (1983). *Br. J. Cancer,* **47,** 613–619.

Picozzi, V. J., Freiha, F. S., Hannigan, J. F., and Torti, F. M. (1984). *Ann. Intern. Med.* **100,** 183–186.

Samuels, M. L., and Logothetis, C. J. (1983). *Proc. Am. Soc. Clin. Oncol.* **2,** 137.

Samuels, M. L., Holoye, P. Y., and Johnson, D. E. (1975a). *Cancer* **36,** 318–326.

Samuels, M. L., Johnson, D. E., and Holoye, P. Y. (1975b). *Cancer Chemother. Rep.* **59,** 563–570.

Stanton, G. F., Bosl, G. J., Vugrin, D., Whitmore, W., Myers, W. P. L., and Golbey, R. (1983). *Proc. Am. Soc. Clin. Oncol.* **2,** 141.

Terebelo, H. R., Taylor, H. G., Brown, A., Martin, N., Stutz, F. H., Blom, J., and Geier, L. (1983). *J. Clin. Oncol.* **9,** 566–571.

Tseng, A., Kessler, R., Freiha, F., Broder, S., Rothman, C., and Torti, F. M. (1984). *Proc. Am. Soc. Clin. Oncol.* **3,** 161.

van Barneveld, P. W. C., Sleiffer, D. T., van der Mark, T. W., Mulder, M. N. H., Donker, A. K. M., Meijer, S., Koops, H. S., Sluiter, H. J., and Peset, R. (1984). *Oncology* **41,** 4–7.

Vogelsang, N. J., Bosl, G. J., Johnson, K., and Kennedy, B. J. (1981). *Ann. Intern. Med.* **45,** 288–292.

Vugrin, D., Whitmore, W. F., and Golbey, R. B. (1983). *Cancer* **51,** 211–215.

Wheeler, B., Einhorn, L., Loehrer, P., William, S. (1984). *Proc. Am. Soc. Clin. Oncol.* **3,** 154.

Williams, D. D., Einhorn, L. H., Greco, F. A. Oldham, R., and Fletcher, R. (1980). *Cancer* **46,** 2154–2158.

Wolff, S. N., Johnson, D. H., Hainsworth, J. D., and Greco, F. A. (1984). *J. Clin. Oncol.* **2,** 271–274.

Chapter 4

THE MEMORIAL HOSPITAL EXPERIENCE IN THE MANAGEMENT OF TESTICULAR GERM-CELL TUMORS

Robert B. Golbey

Memorial Hospital for Cancer and Allied Diseases
New York, New York

I. INTRODUCTION

The Memorial Hospital experience involving chemotherapy to treat testicular germ-cell tumors received its impetus from the observation that disseminated trophoblastic choriocarcinoma frequently could be cured by treatment with methotrexate (Li *et al.*, 1958). When the same drug was used to treat testicular tumors that produced elevations in chorionic gonadotropin titers, comparable results were not obtained. However, a subsequent trial of therapy with actinomycin D and chlorambucil in combination did produce major responses, with some complete responses and some cures (Li *et al.*, 1960; Mackenzie, 1966).

Comparable ability to cure was described for treatment with the combination of vinblastine and bleomycin (Samuels *et al.*, 1975). The activity of these combinations led us, in 1972, to incorporate vinblastine and bleomycin at a somewhat reduced dosage into a combination with actinomycin D (VAB I). The three drugs were administered as pulse doses twice in the first week and once weekly thereafter as tolerated. Initially, the program was well tolerated, but pulmonary toxicity was seen with continued administration of bleomycin. An overall response was observed in 32 of 68 patients (47%) and a complete response (CR) was seen in 15 of 68 patients (22%). Six of the 15 patients with a CR relapsed, leaving 9 patients (13%) free of evidence of disease long-term and potentially cured (Wittes *et al.*, 1976).

Sixteen of the patients who failed this regimen were treated with a combination of bleomycin by continuous infusion plus a pulse dose of cisplatin (Higby *et al.*, 1974; Cvitkovic *et al.*, 1974). Of these patients, 68% (11 of 16 patients) achieved partial remissions (PR), with a median duration of 2.5 months. Severe mucositis was seen frequently but was reversible.

II. THE VAB II REGIMEN

VAB II then was designed to replace the original VAB. Administration of vinblastine and actinomycin D on day 1 were followed by a continuous infusion of bleomycin for 1 week and a pulse dose of 1.2 mg/kg of cisplatin on day 8. This induction was followed by a consolidation phase using the first three drugs weekly, with substitution of cisplatin for actinomycin D every third week. The induction program was repeated 4 months after beginning therapy. Following this reinduction, maintenance therapy was begun with chlorambucil daily plus vinblastine and actinomycin D intravenously every 3 weeks, all continuing for 2 to 3 years.

Fifty patients with measurable metastatic disease were treated with VAB II. The CR rate of the entire group was 50% (25 of 50 patients), with a CR rate of 60% (15 of 25 patients) among those not previously treated with drugs. The cure rate was 22%, with 11 remaining alive and free of evidence of disease (Cheng *et al.*, 1978).

While this study was underway, the problem of the dose-limiting nephrotoxicity of cisplatin was confronted. A technique involving prehydration and mannitol-induced diuresis was developed after animal studies (Hayes *et al.*, 1977). Patients who had failed VAB II were treated with high-dose cisplatin (120 mg/m^2). There were 5 PRs and 1 minor remission (MR) among 9 adequately treated patients, all of whom had become resistant to cisplatin at doses of 1.2 mg/ kg. Nephrotoxicity was less severe and was reversible in most cases. Remissions were short-lived but encouraging, since they occurred in previous treatment failures involving the same drug.

III. THE VAB III REGIMEN

VAB III then was designed to include high-dose cisplatin (Reynolds *et al.*, 1981). A pulse dose of cyclophosphamide was added during induction, since when used as a single agent the drug had induced 3 PRs among 5 patients with testicular cancer, and we had noted 4 MRs in 7 patients with testicular cancer who had failed other chemotherapy. The consolidation phase was made less intense by the deletion of bleomycin, the reintroduction of chlorambucil, and by giving the intravenous drugs every 3 weeks instead of weekly. Doxorubicin was added to the consolidation phase because it had been active as a single agent in 14 of 20 patients with testicular cancer. The reinduction at about 5 months was retained, as was the subsequent maintenance program.

VAB III was given to 92 patients with metastatic testicular cancer, with 89 of them adequately treated. The CR rate was 62% (55 of 89 patients). Of these 55 patients, 15 subsequently relapsed, yielding a CR relapse rate of 27%. The potential cure rate was 45%, with 40 of 89 patients still free of evidence of disease. In the previously untreated group of 45 patients, 24 remained alive without evidence of disease, for a potential cure rate of 54%. In the previously treated group of 44 patients, the potential cure rate was 36%, with 16 remaining alive without evidence of disease. This degree of difference in disease-free survival between patients previously treated with chemotherapy and previously untreated is a consistent observation throughout our studies. Only 4 of 89 patients who were adequately treated did not achieve an objective response to the VAB III protocol. Most of the relapses on VAB III occurred in the first 6–8 months of chemotherapy.

IV. VAB IV AND VAB V REGIMENS

VAB IV was designed to deal with relapses from VAB III occurring in the first 6 to 8 months (Vugrin *et al.*, 1981a). The induction was almost identical to VAB III, but a reinduction without bleomycin was introduced at 16 weeks after the initiation of therapy, followed by a full reinduction with bleomycin at 32 weeks. The subsequent maintenance program was the same as with VAB III.

Of 55 patients entered into this treatment program, 29 achieved CR after chemotherapy alone. An additional 11 patients were free of evidence of disease following surgical removal of stable residual tumor after showing some response to chemotherapy. The histologic examination of residual tumor following chemotherapy revealed mature teratoma (5 patients), necrotic tumor (1 patient), and residual tumor (5 patients). The relapse rates, after CRs were achieved through chemotherapy alone (5 of 29 patients, or 17%) and after chemotherapy plus adjuvant surgery (2 of 11 patients, or 18%) are the same. The total CR rate is 73% (40 of 55 patients), with 60% (33 of 55 patients) continuing free from evidence of disease. When the protocols were compared after equal time of follow-up, VAB IV revealed about the same rate of induction of CRs as did VAB III, but had a lower relapse rate. The end results were improved by the use of surgery to remove residual foci of tumor.

In the course of these studies, risk factors were identified that influenced the likelihood of obtaining a complete response and a potential cure. Three adverse factors were noted. One adverse factor was prior chemotherapy and resistance to one or more of the agents in the combination. A second factor relates to histology, in which embryonal carcinoma was observed as more sensitive than teratocarcinoma, which in turn was more sensitive than pure choriocarcinoma. (Choriocarcinoma in a mixed tumor has only a minor impact on prognosis.) The third adverse factor concerns bulk of tumor: the greater the cell burden, the less the expectation of achieving cure. The degree of serum tumor marker elevation parallels the bulk of tumor. VAB V was designed specifically for those patients with adverse risk factors (Vugrin et al., 1983a). It intensified and prolonged the induction treatment phase. This protocol did improve the response rate in these poor-prognosis patients, but not enough to justify the great increase in toxicity that was endured. The major observation that has had an impact on subsequent treatment programs was that it was possible to treat these patients with high-dose cisplatin as frequently as every 3 or 4 weeks without an increase in nephrotoxicity or ototoxicity.

V. THE VAB VI REGIMEN

The VAB VI regimen incorporated the increased frequency of administration of induction cycles (Vugrin et al., 1981b). The drugs and dosages are

Cyclophosphamide, 700 mg/m^2 day 1   Vinblastine, 4 mg/m^2 day 1
Actinomycin D, 1.0 mg/m^2 day 1   Bleomycin, pulse dose 30 U day 1
Cisplatin, 120 mg/m^2 day 4   Bleomycin, 24-hr infusion × 3 days,
                                    20 U/m^2/day

VAB VI originally was administered for three to five cycles at 3- to 4-week intervals, followed by maintenance therapy with vinblastine and actinomycin out to 1 year. Maintenance therapy has proven not to contribute to the end results and has been removed (Vugrin et al., 1983b). The long-term disease-free survival rates in patients treated with and without maintenance are virtually identical and are in excess of 80% (Table I). Treatment now requires 6 months or less in most patients. This compares favorably with the 3 years of treatment used in the earliest of protocols in order to achieve a 10–20% cure rate.

For patients with disseminated pure seminoma, it had long been known that alkylating agents alone could produce an occasional cure when administered after surgery and/or radiation therapy (Blokhin et al., 1958; Whitmore et al.,

TABLE I TESTICULAR GERM-CELL TUMORS: RESULTS OF TREATMENT

Protocol (reference)	Number of patients evaluated	Complete response (%)				% Relapse from CR	No evidence of disease
		Chemotherapy	Chemotherapy and surgery	Total			
VAB (Wittes et al., 1976)	68	22	—	22		40	13
VAB II (Cheng et al., 1978)	50	50	—	50		52	22
VAB III (Reynolds et al., 1981)	74	54	7	61		29	41
VAB IV (Vugrin et al., 1981a)	41	61	20	81		12	68
VAB V[a] (Vugrin et al., 1983a)	30	37	23	60		10	47
VAB VI (Vugrin et al., 1981b)	25	64	28	92		8	84
VAB VI (Vugrin et al., 1983b) (without maintenance)	34	53	38	91		10	82

[a]Poor-risk patients only.

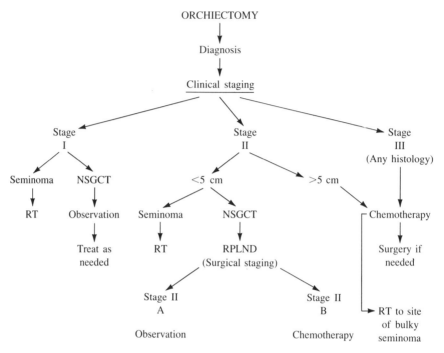

Fig. 1. Conventional therapy for testicular cancer. NSGCT, Nonseminoma germ-cell tumor; RT, radiation therapy; RPLND, retroperitoneal lymph node dissection.

1977; Batata *et al.*, 1982). Cyclophosphamide plus cisplatin was found to achieve better results (Vugrin *et al.*, 1981c), but VAB VI has been shown to be curative for seminomas of extragonadal origin (Jain *et al.*, 1984) and of testicular origin at least as frequently as it is for the other germ-cell tumors (Vugrin and Whitmore, 1984). VAB VI therapy without maintenance is now part of the recommended conventional therapy for some stages of seminoma (Fig. 1).

VI. ADJUVANT SURGERY

Thus far, we have discussed only those changes in chemotherapy that improved the results in patients with advanced disseminated disease (stage III). One other factor that has been basic to the achievement of excellent end results is the increasing awareness of the essential role of adjuvant surgery. After observing that some patients who appeared to have residual tumor after chemotherapy in fact had a transformation of their originally malignant tumor into histologically benign teratoma (Hong *et al.*, 1977), we began to employ surgery in the chest (Bains *et al.*, 1978) and in the retroperitoneum (Whitmore *et al.*, 1981) to provide a diagnosis and to remove the last evidence of neoplasia.

Such adjuvant surgery became a routine part of our protocol after it was demonstrated that a complete response produced by chemotherapy plus surgery was equally as durable as one produced by chemotherapy alone. We were temporarily impeded in the addition of adjuvant surgery to our protocol because several patients died intraoperatively of respiratory failure. This was found to be due to enhanced oxygen toxicity in lungs previously exposed to bleomycin (Goldiner *et al.*, 1978). The problem can be prevented by using a low concentration of oxygen in the anesthetic gas mixture. With this precaution, surgery in these patients is safe and usually well tolerated.

Throughout the years, about one-third of the patients with testicular germ-cell tumors have presented initially in each of three stages (stage I disease shows the tumor confined to the testicle; in stage II disease, the tumor is present in the regional nodes; stage III disease reveals the tumor present beyond the regional nodes).

Historically, 85% of patients with stage I disease have been cured after an orchiectomy, followed by radiation therapy to the retroperitoneal nodes for seminoma or by a retroperitoneal lymph node dissection for other germ-cell tumors. The remaining 15% of patients with stage I disease develop hematogenous metastases and require chemotherapy. Although with very rare exceptions this group can be cured by chemotherapy as simple as actinomycin D alone (Wobler *et al.*, 1983), adjuvant chemotherapy for this group would involve treating 100 patients for every 15 who will benefit from it. This is not a reasonable procedure, since most of the patients who do recur can be cured by appropriate chemotherapy given promptly after the first evidence of recurrence.

In clinical stage I disease, the retroperitoneal lymph node dissection is primarily a staging procedure. Now that the effectiveness of chemotherapy has diminished the importance of precise surgical and pathologic staging and the need for an immediate maximal surgical effort to cure, and as the reliability of our clinical staging procedures has improved, it is possible to avoid the morbidity associated with a node dissection in some patients (Sogani *et al.*, 1984). Node dissection can be deferred if the patient is without evidence of disease after a physical examination; PA and lateral chest X ray; computerized tomography (CAT) of abdomen and pelvis; lymphangiogram in those with a negative CAT scan; serum tumor markers, including α-fetoprotein (AFP), β human chorionic gonadotropin (β-HCG), and lactic dehydrogenase (LDH); routine blood counts; and a screening profile. Twenty percent of these patients will recur with lymphatic or hematogenous metastases and will require surgery and/or chemotherapy later. The importance of close and continuous follow-up for at least 2 to 3 years must be emphasized. Of 59 patients with clinical stage I disease in whom the node dissection was deferred until specific indications arose, 57 patients (96%) are alive and free of disease (47 after orchiectomy alone for a median of 23+ months; 10 after orchiectomy and/or chemotherapy and/or node dissection for a median of 11+ months). One is alive after node dissection and is receiving adjuvant chemotherapy, and one is dead of disease after surgery and chemotherapy.

Patients with stage II disease are heterogeneous in the amount of tumor to be found, ranging from a single microscopic focus to fixed, bulky, unresectable masses. In an early study of adjuvant chemotherapy in stage II patients, we were able to identify good-risk (stage IIA) and poor-risk (stage IIB) groups (Vugrin et al., 1982). According to pathologic staging, the poor-risk group has more than five nodes involved and/or the largest node is larger than 2 cm. In this group, even after an apparently curative node dissection, the likelihood of hematogenous metastases is 50%. With the present simple and effective therapy, initial chemotherapy seems indicated. In stage IIA disease, after a curative node dissection, careful follow-up as in stage I disease is probably the best procedure. In Fig. 1, which summarizes these conclusions, it should be noted that the good-risk/bad-risk division is made on the basis of a clinical estimate of size greater or less than 5 cm. Larger tumors should be treated with chemotherapy before the sites of bulky disease are resected. Smaller tumors should undergo a node dissection, which thereby may avoid the necessity of chemotherapy.

VII. CONCLUSION

Current studies are designed to quantitate the risk factors so that more or less therapy can be prescribed in a selective fashion for each patient (Bosl et al., 1983a,b; Sogani et al., 1983; Vugrin et al., 1984). We are attempting to define the appropriate role for etoposide in the optimal treatment of good- and poor-risk patients (Israel et al., 1984), and we hope to find a platinum analog that will be at least equally as effective as cisplatin but will be easier to administer and tolerate and hopefully can be received on an outpatient basis.

We have come a long way, but there is no reason to think that we have yet achieved the most effective, the safest, the simplest, or the most economic treatment for this disease. That is yet to come. The progress that has been made has depended on the close interaction of surgical, radiation, and medical oncologists, with each contributing maximally as each altered protocol modified their role. The present status of the optimal treatment of germ-cell tumors is a monument to multimodality investigation and therapy and is a model for work on other tumors to follow.

REFERENCES

Bains, M. S., McCormack, P. M., Cvitkovic, E., Golbey, R. B., and Martini, N. (1978). *Cancer* **41**, 850–853.

Batata, M. A., Chu, F., Hilaris, B. S., Papantoniou, P. A., Whitmore, W. F., Jr., and Golbey, R. B. (1982). *Int. J. Radiat. Oncol. Biol. Phys.* **8**, 1287–1293.

Blokhin, N., Larinov, L., and Perevodchikova, A. (1958). *Ann. New York Acad. Science* **68**, 1128–1132.

Bosl, G., Geller, N., Cirrincione, C., Hyck, S., Whitmore, W. F., Jr., Nisselbaum, J., Vugrin, D., and Golbey, R. B. (1983a). *Cancer* **51**, 2121–2125.

Bosl, G., Geller, N. L., Cirrincione, C., Vogelzang, N. J., Kennedy, B. J., Whitmore, W. F., Jr., Vugrin, D., Scher, H., Nisselbaum, J., and Golbey, R. B. (1983b). *Cancer Research* **43**, 3403–3405.

Cheng, E., Cvitkovic, E., Wittes, R. E., and Golbey, R. B. (1978). *Cancer* **42**, 2162–2168.

Cvitkovic, E., Currie, V., Ochoa, M., Pride, G., and Krakoff, I. H. (1974). *Proc. AACR ASCO* **15**, 179.

Goldiner, P. L., Carlon, G. C., Cvitkovic, E., Schweizer, O., and Howland, W. S. (1978). *Br. Med. J.* **1**, 1664–1667.

Hayes, D. M., Cvitkovic, E., Golbey, R. B., Scheiner, E., Helson, L., and Krakoff, I. H. (1977). *Cancer* **39**, 1372–1381.

Higby, D. J., Wallace, H. J. Jr., Albert, D., and Holland, J. F. (1974). *Cancer* **33**, 1219–1225.

Hong, W. K., Wittes, R. E., Hajdu, S. T., Cvitkovic, E., Whitmore, and Golbey, R. B. (1977). *Cancer* **40**, 2987–2992.

Israel, A. M., Bosl, G., and Whitmore, W. F. (1984). *Proc. Am. Soc. Clin. Oncol.* **3**, 159.

Jain, K. K., Bosl, G. J., Bains, M. S., Whitmore, W. F., and Golbey, R. B. (1984). *J. Clin. Oncol.* **2**, 820–827.

Li, M. C., Hertz, R., and Bergenstal, D. M. (1958). *New Engl. J. Med.* **259**, 66–74.

Li, M. C., Whitmore, W. F., Golbey, R. B., and Grabstald, H. (1960). *JAMA* **174**, 1291–1299.

Mackenzie, A. R. (1966). *Cancer* **19**, 1367–1376.

Reynolds, T. F., Vugrin, D., Cvitkovic, E., Cheng, E., Braun, D. W., Hehir, M., Dukeman, M., Whitmore, W., and Golbey, R. B. (1981). *Cancer* **48**, 888–898.

Samuels, M. L., Holoye, P. Y., and Johnson, D. E. (1975). *Cancer* **36**, 318–326.

Sogani, P. C., Whitmore, W. F., Herr, H. W., Bosl, G., Golbey, R. B., Watson, R., DeCosse, J. J. (1983). *Am. J. Med.* **75**, 29–35.

Sogani, P. C., Whitmore, W. F., Herr, H. W., Bosl, G., Golbey, R. B., Watson, R., and DeCosse, J. J. (1984). *J. Clin. Oncol.* **2**, 267–272.

Vugrin, D., and Whitmore, W. F., Jr. (1984). *Cancer* **53**, 2422–2424.

Vugrin, D., Cvitkovic, E., Whitmore, W. F., Jr., Cheng, E., and Golbey, R. B. (1981a). *Cancer* **47**, 833–839.

Vugrin, D., Herr, H. W., Whitmore, W. F., Jr., Sogani, P., and Golbey, R. B. (1981b). *Ann. Intern. Med.* **95**, 59–61.

Vugrin, D., Whitmore, W. F., Jr., and Batata, M. (1981c). *Cancer Clin. Trials* **4**, 423–427.

Vugrin, D., Whitmore, W. F., Herr, H., Sogani, D., and Golbey, R. B. (1982). *J. Urol.* **128**, 715–717.

Vugrin, D., Whitmore, W. F., Jr., and Golbey, R. B. (1983a). *Cancer* **51**, 1072–1075.

Vugrin, D., Willet, F., Whitmore, W. F. Jr., and Golbey, R. B. (1983b). *Cancer* **51,** 211–215.

Vugrin, D., Friedman, A., and Whitmore, W. F., Jr. (1984). *Cancer* **53,** 1440–1445.

Whitmore, W. F., Jr., Smith, D., Yagoda, A., Guthrie, S., and Golbey, R. B. (1977). *Recent Results Cancer Res.* **66,** 244–249.

Whitmore, W. F., Jr., Vugrin, D., Sogani, P. C., Bains, M., Herr, H., and Golbey, R. B. (1981). *Cancer* **47,** 2228–2231.

Wittes, R. E., Yogado, A., Silvay, O., Magill, G., Whitmore, W., Krakoff, I. H., and Golbey, R. B. (1976). *Cancer* **37,** 637–645.

Wobler, T., Eiberger, R., Obdhoff, J., and Schraffordt, K. (1983). *Cancer* **51,** 1076–1079.

Chapter 5

EFFECTIVE TREATMENT OF MALIGNANT OVARIAN GERM-CELL TUMORS WITH CISPLATIN, VINBLASTINE, AND BLEOMYCIN (PVB)

Robert W. Carlson

Northern California Cancer Program
Palo Alto, California
and Department of Medicine
Division of Oncology
Stanford University School of Medicine
Stanford, California

Branimir Ivan Sikic

Department of Medicine
Divisions of Oncology and Clinical
Pharmacology
Stanford University School of Medicine
Stanford, California

I. INTRODUCTION

Although the malignant ovarian germ-cell tumors comprise only 5% of all malignant ovarian neoplasms, they assume an important place in oncology because they occur in patients with a median age of only 19 years and because the majority of patients now can be cured with appropriate therapy. The ovarian germ-cell tumors generally are divided into two categories: (1) the pure dysgerminomas, which are usually curable through surgery, with or without postoperative irradiation, and (2) other histologic types. These latter tumors, which include endodermal sinus tumors, malignant teratomas, embryonal carcinomas, choriocarcinomas, and mixed germ-cell tumors, are usually fatal if treated only by surgery, with or without postoperative irradiation (Asadourian and Taylor, 1969; Krepart et al., 1978; Kurman and Norris, 1976; Norris et al., 1976).

Since the introduction of combination chemotherapy, several drug regimens have been shown to increase the cure rate of patients with ovarian germ-cell

TABLE I   RESULTS OF VAC CHEMOTHERAPY IN THE
TREATMENT OF MALIGNANT OVARIAN GERM-CELL TUMORS
AFTER OPERATIVE CYTOREDUCTION

Series	Number of VAC-treated patients	% Alive without disease
Cangir (1978)		
Stages I–III	16	94
Stage IV	4	0
Slayton (1978)		
Stages I–III	24	54
Gershenson (1983)		
Stages I–III	22	77

tumors significantly if treatment follows operative cytoreduction. The most widely used of the early chemotherapy regimens has been the combination of vincristine, actinomycin D, and cyclophosphamide (VAC), given for 12 to 24 months (Cangir *et al.*, 1978; Slayton *et al.*, 1978). Other effective regimens also have been reported (Gershenson *et al.*, 1983; Bradof *et al.*, 1982; Newlands *et al.*, 1982; Creasman *et al.*, 1979). In uncontrolled studies, postoperative VAC chemotherapy has resulted in an apparent improvement in the survival of patients with ovarian germ-cell tumors, especially in patients with early-stage disease (Table I).

Following demonstration of the pronounced activity of combination cisplatin, vinblastine, and bleomycin (PVB chemotherapy) against testicular germ-cell tumors, reports of the successful treatment of ovarian germ-cell tumors with PVB began to appear (Einhorn and Donohue, 1977; Schlaerth *et al.*, 1980; Julian *et al.*, 1980; Lokey *et al.*, 1981). Since 1978, Stanford University Medical Center has been treating patients with ovarian germ-cell tumors with postoperative PVB chemotherapy (Carlson *et al.*, 1983). This chapter presents an update of our series of patients treated with PVB, as well as a review of the relevant literature.

II. METHODS

All 10 patients with malignant ovarian germ-cell tumors who were treated with PVB chemotherapy at Stanford University since 1978 were identified and their records were examined. Each patient's histopathologic slides were reviewed and each diagnosis was confirmed by the Stanford University Department of

TABLE II   PVB COMBINATION CHEMOTHERAPY
REGIMEN FOR OVARIAN GERM-CELL TUMORS

Drug	Dosage
Cisplatin	100 mg/m^2 by 24-hr infusion, day 1[a]
	or
	20 mg/m^2/day, days 1–5
Vinblastine	0.15–0.18 mg/kg/day, days 1 and 2
Bleomycin	15 U/m^2, days 2, 8, and 15
21-day cycles continued for 4 to 6 cycles	

[a]Method of cisplatin delivery in current series.

Pathology. PVB was administered according to the PVB regimen of the Northern California Oncology Group (Table II). All patients received vigorous hydration before, during, and after each cisplatin infusion. The dose of cisplatin was attenuated in instances of decreased creatinine clearance of severe nausea and vomiting; the dose of vinblastine was decreased in instances of prior episodes of leukopenia with fever, severe arthralgias and myalgias, or severe constipation; and the bleomycin dose was reduced in the presence of pulmonary symptoms, concurrent respiratory tract infection, or sepsis.

All patients were followed by physical examination, chest radiographs, complete blood counts, general chemistries, and serum α-fetoprotein and β human chorionic gonadotropin determinations. Patients underwent pulmonary function testing, audiometry, and second-look laparotomy at their attending physician's discretion.

III. RESULTS

Patient characteristics are recorded in Table III. The median age at diagnosis was 21.5 years (range, 16–33 years). Five stage I patients received PVB chemotherapy for four cycles and 1 stage I patient received it for five cycles. The stage II patient received eight cycles of PVB after failing VAC chemotherapy with ascites and showing an alpha-fetoprotein elevation of greater than 1000 ng/ml. One stage III patient received four cycles of PVB, and two stage III patients received six cycles of PVB.

The acute toxicities experienced by these patients are found in Table IV. All patients developed leukopenia, and 5 patients, while leukopenic, experienced six

TABLE III   PATIENT CHARACTERISTICS

Patient characteristic	Number of patients
Histology	
Endodermal sinus tumor	4
Immature teratoma	
Grade II	1
Grade III	3
Mixed	2
Stage (FIGO)	
I	6
II	1
III	3
Perioperative marker elevation (5 tested)	
α-Fetoprotein	4
β Human chorionic gonadotropin	0
Initial surgical procedure	
Unilateral salpingo-oophorectomy	7
Bilateral salpingo-oophorectomy and hysterectomy	3

episodes of fever that required hospitalization. Two patients required red blood cell transfusions for anemia without evidence of blood loss.

All patients experienced nausea and vomiting secondary to cisplatin, and 5 patients required a total of seven hospitalizations (in addition to routine hospitalization for cisplatin infusion) for control of nausea and vomiting. One patient experienced a transient elevation in the serum creatinine above 1.5 mg/dl, but received subsequent cisplatin without difficulty after a delay in therapy.

Chronic toxicities were not a problem in any of the patients. No patient

TABLE IV   ACUTE TOXICITIES OF PVB

Acute toxicity	Number
Myelosuppression, median (range)	
Lowest leukocyte count	1000/mm^3 (200–1700)
Lowest platelet count	130,000/mm^3 (81–234,000)
Lowest hemoglobin count	9.8 g/dl (8.1–10.3)
Fever and neutropenia	5
Nausea and vomiting	10
Requiring hospitalization	5
Serum creatinine >1.5 mg/dl	1
Hypokalemia (K$^+$ < 3.5 meq/liter)	7
Hypomagnesemia (Mg^{2+} < 1.5 meq/liter)	5
Weight loss ≥10% baseline	4

experienced symptomatic or radiologic bleomycin pulmonary toxicity despite a mean total dose of 165 U/m^2 (range, 112–208 U/m^2). This may reflect, in part, the rapid attenuation of bleomycin dosage when fever with leukopenia or pulmonary symptoms occurred. The patients received a mean of 93% of maximum calculated bleomycin dosage during the first three cycles of treatment. The mean percentages of delivered bleomycin dropped to 64, 50, and 22% during cycles 4, 5, and 6, respectively. Three patients had baseline and follow-up pulmonary function testing, with decreases of 18, 21, and 25% in DL_{CO}, but no patient experienced pulmonary symptoms or limitations of activity that were not present prior to treatment. One patient with severe congenital kyphoscoliosis was given each bleomycin treatment as a 24-hr continuous infusion to decrease bleomycin-associated pulmonary toxicity (Sikic *et al.*, 1978). After receiving a total of 180 U/m^2 of bleomycin, this patient's DL_{CO} decreased from a baseline of 90% of predicted normal to 72% of predicted normal.

All 7 patients who retained an ovary regained normal menstrual function following the PVB regimen. One bore a normal baby 21 months following completion of her therapy, and another is in her third trimester of pregnancy, 45 months following completion of therapy.

Second-look laparotomy was performed on 7 patients. Three of the second-look laparotomies were negative, one revealed necrotic tumor, one a benign ovarian cyst, one mature glial tissue, and one mature teratoma and mature glial tissue. Two patients underwent a third laparotomy, of which one was negative and the other revealed a benign ovarian cyst.

All 10 patients are alive without evidence of disease at last follow-up, with a minimum of 19 months and a median of 28.5 months from initial diagnosis. Nine patients have been followed for 24 or more months since diagnosis.

IV. DISCUSSION

Because the majority of patients with ovarian germ-cell tumors who experience recurrence do so within 1 year of diagnosis, all of the patients in this series probably are cured of their tumors. These excellent treatment results confirm the reports of others documenting the effectiveness of PVB chemotherapy in the ovarian germ-cell tumors (Table V).

Wiltshaw *et al.* (1982) have reported on 8 patients with ovarian endodermal sinus tumors who were treated with PVB chemotherapy. All seven of the patients with stage I, stage II, and stage III disease were alive without evidence of disease at a follow-up of 3 to 33 months. The single patient in this series with stage IV disease died of disease 4 months after diagnosis.

Vriesendorp *et al.* (1984) have reported on 7 patients with ovarian germ-cell tumors treated with PVB. All four of their stage I through stage III patients were

TABLE V   PVB CHEMOTHERAPY FOR THE TREATMENT OF OVARIAN
GERM-CELL TUMORS AFTER SURGICAL OPERATIVE CYTOREDUCTION

Series	Number of patients	Number with prior therapy	% Alive without disease
Schlaerth *et al.* (1980)			
Stages I–III	1	1	100
Julian *et al.* (1980)			
Stages I–III	2	0	100
Lokey *et al.* (1981)			
Stages I–III	2	0	100
Khoo *et al.* (1981)			
Stages I–III	1	1	100
Jacobs *et al.* (1982)			
Stages I–III	4	3	50
Wiltshaw *et al.* (1982)			
Stages I–III	7	0	100
Stage IV	1	0	0
Gershenson *et al.* (1983)			
Stages I–III	2	1	100
Unknown	1	1	0
Vriesendorp *et al.* (1984)			
Stages I–III	4	1	100
Stage IV	3	0	66
Stanford series			
Stages I–III	10	1	100
Total			
Stages I–III	33	8	94
Stage IV	4	0	50

without evidence of disease 21–37 months following diagnosis. Of 3 patients with stage IV disease, 1 died of disease and the others were alive without disease at 17 and 30 months.

Patients treated with PVB chemotherapy experience frequent, moderately severe acute toxicities. The series of Wiltshaw and Vriesendorp document toxicities similar to those reported here. However, the treatment duration is usually short (12–18 weeks), and chronic toxicities should be uncommon when therapy is delivered by experienced oncology teams. In our experience, the cumulative dosage of bleomycin can be limited to prevent significant pulmonary toxicity without apparently losing antitumor efficacy.

Results now achieved with postoperative PVB chemotherapy in patients with stage I ovarian germ-cell tumors suggest that routine second-look laparotomy may no longer be appropriate. However, it would seem prudent to continue performing second-look laparotomy in patients with stage II, stage III, or stage IV ovarian germ-cell tumors, as well as in those with abnormalities revealed by physical, radiographic, or laboratory examination. The necessity of pathologic documentation of treatment failure is underscored by the frequency of benign ovarian cysts, mature teratoma, and negative findings in our patients undergoing laparotomy with suspicion for persistent or recurrent disease.

The retention of ovarian function and fertility following unilateral salpingo-oophorectomy in this young patient population reinforces the appropriateness of consecutive surgical procedures that spare the contralateral ovary in patients without obvious bilateral tumor. In addition, combination chemotherapy may be an appropriate replacement for postoperative abdominopelvic radiotherapy in carefully selected patients with ovarian dysgerminomas (Scott, 1983). Further clinical experience in the use of PVB for dysgerminomas is necessary before definitive recommendations can be made.

The majority of patients with non-dysgerminoma ovarian germ-cell tumors now may be cured if optimal operative cytoreduction is followed by effective combination chemotherapy. In patients reported to be treated with PVB, death from progressive disease has been limited almost exclusively to those with stage IV disease, where optimal operative cytoreduction is unusual. Although we are comparing a small series of patients without randomized controls (Tables I and V), the treatment results with PVB appear at least equal, and probably superior, to those achieved with VAC. Several other chemotherapy regimens also are available, but none appears to be superior to PVB. The acute toxicities of PVB chemotherapy can be moderately severe, but the duration of treatment is short, and significant chronic toxicities are unusual.

ACKNOWLEDGMENTS

We wish to acknowledge and thank Drs. Michael Alexander, Samuel C. Ballon, James Cohen, Robert Levy, William Rogoway, Myron M. Turbow, and Albert Wendt for their professional assistance, and Mrs. Clara Romano for her assistance in preparing the manuscript.

REFERENCES

Asadourian, L. A., and Taylor, H. B. (1969). *Obstet. Gynecol.* 33, 370–379.
Bradof, J. E., Hakes, T. B., Ochoa, M., and Golbey, R. (1982). *Cancer* 50, 1070–1075.
Cangir, A., Smith, J., van Eys, J. (1978). *Cancer* 42, 1234–1238.
Carlson, R. W., Sikic, B. I., Turbow, M. M., and Ballon, S. C. (1983). *J. Clin. Oncol.* 1, 645–651.
Creasman, W. T., Fetter, B. F., Hammond, C. B., and Parker, R. T. (1979). *Obstet. Gynecol.* 53, 226–230.
Einhorn, L. H., and Donohue, J. (1977). *Ann. Intern. Med.* 87, 293–298.
Gershenson, D. M., del Junco, G., Herson, and Rutledge, F. N. (1983). *Obstet. Gynecol.* 61, 194–202.

Jacobs, A. J., Harris, M., Deppe, G., DasGupta, I., and Cohen, C. J. (1982). *Obstet. Gynecol.* **59**, 129–132.

Julian, C. G., Barrett, J. M., Richardson, R. L., and Greco, F. A. (1980). *Obstet. Gynecol.* **56**, 396–401.

Khoo, S. K., Buntine, D. W., Massey, P. F., and Jones, I. S. C. (1981). *Aust. N. Z. J. Obstet. Gynaec.* **21**, 217–225.

Krepart, G., Smith, J. P., Rutledge, F., and Delclos, L. (1978). *Cancer* **41**, 986–990.

Kurman, R. J., and Norris, H. J. (1976). *Cancer* **38**, 2404–2419.

Lokey, J. L., Baker, J. J., Price, N. A., and Winokur, S. H. (1981). *Ann. Intern. Med.* **94**, 56–57.

Newlands, E. S., Begent, R. H. J., Rustin, G. J. S., and Bagshawe, K. D. (1982). *Br. J. Obstet. Gynaecol.* **89**, 555–560.

Norris, H. J., Zirkin, H. J., and Benson, W. L. (1976). *Cancer* **37**, 2359–2372.

Schlaerth, J. B., Morrow, C. P., and DePetrillo, A. D. (1980). *Am. J. Obstet. Gynecol.* **136**, 983–985.

Scott, J. S. (1983). *Br. Med. J.* **286**, 824–825.

Sikic, B. I., Collins, J. M., Mimnaugh, E. G., and Gram, T. E. (1978). *Cancer Treat. Rep.* **62**, 2011–2017.

Slayton, R. E., Hreshchyshyn, M. M., Silverberg, S. G., Shingleton, H. M., Park, R. C., DiSaia, P. J., and Blessing, J. A. (1978). *Cancer* **42**, 390–398.

Vriesendorp, R., Alders, J. G., Sleijfer, D. T., Willemse, P. H. B., Bouma, J., and Mulder, N. H. (1984). *Cancer Treat. Rep.* **68**, 779–781.

Wiltshaw, E., Stuart-Harris, R., Barker, G. H., Gowing, N. F. C., and Raju, S. (1982). *J. R. Soc. Med.* **75**, 888–892.

Section III
HEAD AND NECK CANCER

Bleomycin Chemotherapy
(B. I. Sikic, M. Rozencweig, and S. K. Carter, eds.)

Chapter 6

THE ROLE OF CHEMOTHERAPY IN THE TREATMENT OF HEAD AND NECK CANCER

Charlotte D. Jacobs

Department of Medicine
Division of Oncology
Stanford University School of Medicine
Stanford, California

I. INTRODUCTION

Despite the marked advances of the last decade in the treatment of squamous-cell carcinomas of the head and neck, the morbidity of the disease itself and its therapy is still significant. Following optimal treatment with surgery and/or radiation, at least half of patients with advanced disease will experience recurrence (Snow *et al.*, 1978; Head and Neck Contracts Program, 1984). The ability to salvage and even palliate these patients is poor.

In the past, chemotherapy was used in treating head and neck cancer only as a single agent for selected patients with recurrent disease. With the development of newer agents and combinations, though, a number of potential treatments now are available for patients with recurrent disease. More recently, chemotherapy has been used in primary treatment as part of a combined modality approach, in attempts to improve curability. The oncologist, radiotherapist, and surgeon now must choose among a multitude of combinations of chemotherapeutic agents used in a number of different strategies. It is the task of head and neck cancer investigators to provide guidance in selecting treatment programs that are superior to conventional treatment.

II. SALVAGE TREATMENT

A. Single-Agent Chemotherapy

The single agent used most extensively in the treatment of recurrent head and neck cancer is methotrexate. It has become the standard with which all new agents or combinations are compared. Response rates to conventional-dose methotrexate vary widely, depending upon investigator, patient population, and dose scheduling (Papac *et al.*, 1963; Lane *et al.*, 1968; Leone *et al.*, 1968; Papac *et al.*, 1978; Priestman, 1973). A weekly dose schedule of methotrexate appears to be superior to a monthly schedule (Goldsmith and Carter, 1975). The overall response rate is ~27% (Table I), and most are partial responses of 1 to 2 months duration. Investigators have attempted to improve the efficacy of methotrexate by using higher doses with leucovorin rescue (Levitt *et al.*, 1973). In early studies, this approach appeared to be superior to the use of conventional doses, with response rates averaging 50% (Levitt *et al.*, 1973; Capizzi *et al.*, 1970; Buechler *et al.*, 1979; Frei *et al.*, 1980). However, there were few complete responses, and the response duration was short. Several controlled trials ran-

TABLE I   SINGLE-AGENT CHEMOTHERAPY FOR RECURRENT
HEAD AND NECK CANCER

Agent	Number of patients	Response (%)
Cisplatin[a]	122	30
Methotrexate[b] (conventional dose)	184	27
Methotrexate[c] (moderate dose)	129	50
Bleomycin[d]	360	23

[a]Wittes *et al.* (1977), Jacobs *et al.* (1978), Sako *et al.* (1978), Stephens *et al.* (1973).
[b]Papac *et al.* (1963), Lane *et al.* (1968), Papac *et al.* (1978), Priestman (1973).
[c]Levitt *et al.* (1973), Capizzi *et al.* (1970), Buechler *et al.* (1979), Frei *et al.* (1980).
[d]Turrisi *et al.* (1978).

domizing patients to receive either conventional or moderate-dose methotrexate have concluded that the higher dose is not significantly superior (Kirkwood *et al.*, 1981; Woods *et al.*, 1981; Vogler *et al.*, 1979).

In the early, broad, phase II trials, it became apparent that bleomycin had efficacy in head and neck cancer (Turrisi *et al.*, 1978). Using a number of different doses and methods of delivery, response rates ranged between 6 and 45%, averaging 23%. Most of these were partial responses of 2 to 3 months duration. Because of the drug's relative lack of toxicity and its moderate efficacy, bleomycin has been used frequently in combination chemotherapy for head and neck cancer.

Much of the enthusiasm for the treatment of head and neck cancer emerged with the development of cisplatin. Response rates with this agent averaged 30% (Wittes *et al.*, 1977; Jacobs *et al.*, 1978; Sako *et al.*, 1978; Stephens *et al.*, 1979). The advantages of cisplatin over the other single agents included its rapidity of response and slightly longer response duration of approximately four months.

In a prospective randomized trial, Hong *et al.* (1983) randomized 44 patients with recurrent head and neck cancer to receive either methotrexate (40–60 mg/m^2 iv weekly) or cisplatin (50 mg/m^2, days 1 and 8 every 4 weeks). The overall response rate was 24% for methotrexate and 29% for cisplatin. There was no difference in median duration of response or median survival. The authors concluded that methotrexate and cisplatin were equally effective, although the toxicities differed, with mucositis as the dose-limiting toxicity of methotrexate and vomiting the toxicity of cisplatin.

Several other chemotherapeutic agents have achieved modest response rates for recurrent head and neck cancer, including hydroxyurea (39%), cyclophosphamide (36%), vinblastine (29%), doxorubicin (23%), and 5-fluorouracil (15%) (Carter, 1977). However, most agents have been studied only in a relatively small number of patients.

B. Combination Chemotherapy

A number of chemotherapy combinations have been used to treat recurrent head and neck cancer. Most regimens have been designed for theoretical drug synergy or toxicity considerations. Turrisi *et al.* (1978) reviewed studies of the combination of bleomycin and methotrexate and found the average response rate to be 47% (Table II), with response durations ranging from 1 to 6 months. The authors concluded that the superiority of this combination over single agents had not been established, while toxicity, particularly mucositis, was substantial.

Costanzi *et al.* (1976) studied a kinetically based regimen in which bleomycin was infused over 48 hr to synchronize tumor cells in S phase. It was followed by

TABLE II   COMBINATION CHEMOTHERAPY FOR RECURRENT
HEAD AND NECK CANCER

Combinations[a]	Number of patients	Response (%)
BLM, MTX	81	47
(Turrisi et al., 1978)		
BLM, MTX, or HYD	17	59
(Costanzi et al., 1976)		
BLM, VCR, MTX, H,	85	67
5-FU, DOX		
(Price et al., 1978)		
MTX, 5-FU	23	65
(Pitman et al., 1983)		
CP, BLM, MTX	31	61
(Vogl and Kaplan, 1979)		
CP, 5-FU	30	70
(Kish et al., 1984)		

[a]BLM, Bleomycin; MTX, methotrexate; HYD, hydroxyurea; VCR, vincristine; H, hydrocortisone; 5-FU, 5-fluorouracil; DOX, doxorubicin; CP,
cisplatin.

infusion of S-phase-specific drugs (either methotrexate or hydroxyurea). Both
combinations resulted in a response rate of 59%, but the responses were of brief
duration.

Price et al. (1978) designed a six-drug combination with scheduling such that
cells in each phase of the cell cycle would be killed by one drug, producing
tumor-cell synchrony. Of the 85 evaluable patients, 67% achieved a partial
response without substantial toxicity. Pitman et al. (1983) designed a regimen of
moderate-dose methotrexate with leucovorin rescue, followed in 1 hr by 5-
fluorouracil. The regimen was based on evidence of synergistic tumor kill in
L1210 mice (Cadman et al., 1979). Of 23 patients with recurrent head and neck
cancer, 65% achieved a response, with an 11% complete response rate. The hope
was to develop a regimen that might provide long-lasting palliation for these
patients, but the median response duration for patients with recurrent disease was
only 3.6 months.

Several cisplatin-based combinations are now used to treat the disease. Vogl
and Kaplan (1979) developed a relatively nontoxic outpatient regimen that included the three most effective agents for head and neck cancer: methotrexate (40
mg/m^2, days 1 and 15), bleomycin (10 U, days 1, 8, and 15), and cisplatin (50
mg/m^2, day 4) to be repeated every 3 weeks. Of the initial 37 patients treated,
23% had a complete response, with an overall response rate of 61%. This
regimen was notable for its high complete response rate, a median response
duration of 6 months, and minimal toxicity.

Finally, Kish *et al.* (1984) reported on the use of cisplatin (100 mg/m^2) with a 96-hr infusion of 5-fluorouracil (1000 mg/m^2/day), a combination that has marked efficacy as an induction regimen. Of 30 patients treated, 27% achieved a complete response and 43% a partial response for an overall response rate of 70%. The average duration of response was 11.3 months for complete responders and 6.5 months for partial responders. Major toxicities included vomiting and leukopenia in 50% of patients.

C. Combination Chemotherapy versus Single Agents

Although combination chemotherapy appears to be superior to single agents, it is important to establish this in randomized trials because of the increased expense and toxicity of combination chemotherapy.

Two randomized trials have compared regimens containing cisplatin and methotrexate with single-agent cisplatin (Table III). Davis and Kessler (1979) compared a combination of cisplatin (3 U/kg), methotrexate (15 mg/m^2, days 1 and 5), and bleomycin (15 mg/m^2, twice weekly) with cisplatin. The overall response rate was very poor in both arms, and myelosuppression was significant. Jacobs *et al.* (1983) randomized 80 patients with recurrent head and neck cancer to receive cisplatin (80 mg/m^2 every 3 weeks) or cisplatin plus weekly methotrex-

TABLE III   COMBINATION CHEMOTHERAPY VERSUS SINGLE AGENTS FOR RECURRENT HEAD AND NECK CANCER

Combinations[a]	Number of patients	Response (%)
CP, BLM, MTX		11
versus	57	
CP		13
(Davis and Kessler, 1979)		
CP, MTX		33
versus	80	
CP		18
(Jacobs *et al.*, 1983)		
CP, BLM, VCR		41
versus	51	
MTX		33
(Drelichman *et al.*, 1983)		
CP, BLM, MTX		46
versus	122	
MTX		26
(Kaplan *et al.*, 1981)		

[a]CP, Cisplatin; BLM, bleomycin; MTX, methotrexate; VCR, vincristine.

ate $(250 \text{ mg}/\text{m}^2)$ with leucovorin rescue. The overall response to cisplatin alone was 18%, with 10% complete responses, and the overall response rate to the combination was 33%, with 18% complete responses. There was no significant difference in the response rate, time to progression, or survival, but there was significantly more myelosuppression and mucositis in the combination arm. Finally, Drelichman *et al.* (1983) conducted a randomized trial to compare cisplatin, vincristine, and bleomycin with methotrexate administered weekly. Again, there was no significant difference in overall response rate, complete response rate, or survival.

The only study in which combination chemotherapy has been shown to be superior to a single agent is the study of Kaplan *et al.* (1981). In this study for the Eastern Cooperative Oncology Group, 122 patients were randomized to undergo the outpatient regimen of cisplatin, bleomycin, and methotrexate as previously described (Vogl and Kaplan, 1979); the results were compared against a weekly regimen of methotrexate. The overall response rate in the combination group (46%) was significantly better than that of single-agent methotrexate (26%). Unfortunately, there was no significant difference in survival.

Thus, for recurrent head and neck cancer the most effective agents are cisplatin, bleomycin, and methotrexate, with cisplatin and methotrexate producing equivalent response rates. Although many combinations appear to be superior to single agents, only one randomized trial has shown significant improvement in response rate.

Future approaches to recurrent head and neck cancer could include improvement in the therapeutic index of current drugs by innovative methods of delivery or use of concurrent chemosensitizers and chemoprotectors, new combinations of agents, new drug development, and biologic modifiers.

III. PRIMARY TREATMENT

For the majority of patients with early stages of head and neck cancer, the disease is curable through surgery and/or radiation therapy. However, for patients with locally advanced disease or nodal involvement, the 5-year survival is unacceptably low, despite optimal treatment with surgery and radiation (Snow *et al.*, 1978; Head and Neck Contracts Program, 1984). Chemotherapy has been added in a combined modality approach in attempts to improve curability.

To improve survival for advanced head and neck cancer, the various reasons for shortened survival in these patients must be addressed, including local recurrence, distant metastases, second primaries, and other medical problems. Despite optimal treatment, local recurrent or persistent disease will appear in 20 to 40% of patients. Up to 20% of patients will develop distant metastases, and some sites, such as the nasopharynx and pyriform sinus, have an even higher incidence of distant metastases. Second primaries may be synchronous or metachronous. A summary of four large series indicates that the incidence of second primaries is ~16% (Decroix and Ghossein, 1981; Fu *et al.*, 1977; Gilbert *et al.*, 1975; Nakissa *et al.*, 1978). Of these second primaries, 8% occurred in the head and neck, 2% in the esophagus, 2% in the lung, and 4% in other sites, including nonsquamous histologies. Schottenfeld *et al.* (1974) have shown that the chance of developing a second primary is higher in patients who continue smoking. Finally, this patient population has a high incidence of other medical problems, many of which contribute to their decreased survival. In one series of 733 patients with head and neck cancer (Schottenfeld *et al.*, 1974), the underlying cause of death in up to 30% of cases was other medical problems, predominately atherosclerotic and thromboembolic disease.

There are three theoretic ways in which chemotherapy could be used in a combined modality approach. These include induction chemotherapy prior to surgery or radiation, concurrent chemotherapy with radiotherapy, and adjuvant or maintenance chemotherapy following surgery and/or radiation.

A. Induction Chemotherapy

Induction chemotherapy may be used prior to surgery and/or radiation to reduce tumor size and facilitate standard therapy. Tumor models have shown that the greater the tumor mass, the lower the chance of cure (Griswold, 1975), and this may be due in part to shedding of tumor cells beyond the surgical margins or radiation field. There are several potential advantages to using chemotherapy prior to other therapies. First, the blood supply to the tumor at this point is undisturbed, thus facilitating drug delivery. Second, patients may have a superior performance status, which has been associated with a better response to chemotherapy. Third, when chemotherapy is used prior to other therapy, the response rate can be assessed more accurately. Finally, induction chemotherapy could eradicate micrometastases that occur prior to tumor removal.

However, there are some potential disadvantages to induction chemotherapy. Standard therapy must be delayed—often up to several months—and if the chemotherapy is only partially effective or is ineffective, there is potential for tumor spread. Also, chemotherapy might blur the definition of tumor margins, making it difficult for the surgeon to determine surgical planes. The surgeon may be tempted to perform a lesser surgical procedure in the patient who has had an excellent chemotherapy response, and there may be even more of a temptation for the patient not to undergo morbid treatment if the tumor has decreased in size. Chemotherapy could result in increased postoperative complications, and some of the acute and long-term toxicities are yet to be defined.

Methotrexate was one of the first agents to be used in an induction regimen (Tarpley *et al.*, 1975) (Table IV). A dose of 240 mg/m² of methotrexate was

TABLE IV   INDUCTION CHEMOTHERAPY FOR HEAD AND NECK CANCER

Agents	Number of patients	Response[a]	
		CR	CR + PR
Methotrexate (240 mg/m^2) + leucovorin days 1, 5 (Tarpley *et al.*, 1975)	30	—	20
Cisplatin (3 U/kg) days 1, 22 + bleomycin (0.25 mg/kg) days 3–10 (Randolph *et al.*, 1978)	21	19	71
Cisplatin (100 U/m^2) day 1 + bleomycin (15 mg/m^2) days 3–7 (Head and Neck Contracts Program, 1984)	282	3	37
Cisplatin (100 mg/m^2) day 1 + 5-fluorouracil (1 g/m^2) days 1–15 (Decker *et al.*, 1983)	35	63	94

[a]CR, Complete response; PR, partial response.

given on days 1 and 5, followed by leucovorin. Surgery was performed on days 12–15. Response, defined as tumor shrinkage, occurred in 77% of patients at the primary or nodes; 20% had response at the primary and nodes. When compared with historical controls, this group did not have a significantly improved survival. However, the authors did establish the feasibility of this approach with a low incidence of postoperative complications.

One of the most common induction regimens in clinical trials has been cisplatin followed by a 5- to 7-day infusion of bleomycin (Randolph *et al.*, 1978; Hong *et al.*, 1979). Response rates of 70%, with up to 20% complete responses, have been reported, and many of these patients showed no residual disease at surgery. Histopathologic specimens often demonstrated cellular differentiation and keratin formation (Shapshay *et al.*, 1978). In a larger clinical trial using slightly lower doses of cisplatin and bleomycin, the Head and Neck Contracts Program (1984) reported an overall response rate of 37% and a complete response rate of 3% in 282 patients with advanced, resectable head and neck cancer.

An alternate induction regimen that has been reported is cisplatin (100 mg/m^2) followed by a 5-day infusion of 5-fluorouracil (1 g/m^2/day by constant infusion) (Decker *et al.*, 1983). The authors noted that as the number of induction cycles was increased from one to three, the response rate continued to improve to an overall response rate of 94%, with a 63% complete response rate.

These, in addition to many other induction chemotherapy regimens, demonstrate that induction chemotherapy is highly effective in head and neck cancer and has acceptable toxicity. However, many of these trials are pilot studies from which conclusions about subsequent curability cannot be drawn. Before the superiority of a combined-modality approach can be established, randomized clinical trials with large patient numbers must be performed to account for the various important prognostic factors. Such a study has been undertaken by the Head and Neck Contracts Program (1984), in which patients with advanced squamous-cell head and neck cancer were randomized to receive either standard therapy with surgery and postoperative radiotherapy; induction chemotherapy with cisplatin and bleomycin followed by standard therapy; or induction chemotherapy, standard therapy, and maintenance chemotherapy with cisplatin for 6 months. Results of this trial are forthcoming.

B. Concurrent Radiotherapy and Chemotherapy

Several chemotherapeutic agents have been shown to act as radiation sensitizers *in vitro,* and early clinical trials also suggested synergy between radiation and concurrent chemotherapy (Goffinet and Bagshaw, 1974). However, to date, only a few randomized trials have shown superiority of concurrent chemotherapy and radiation over radiotherapy alone (Table V).

Methotrexate can produce an S-phase block of the cell cycle, resulting in accumulation of cells in the radiosensitive G_1 phase (Berry, 1965). Three large randomized trials using methotrexate immediately prior to radiation therapy have shown no improvement in overall response rate or survival compared to a control group (Knowlton *et al.,* 1975; Lustig *et al.,* 1976; Fazekas *et al.,* 1980). In one large study by the Radiation Therapy Oncology Group (Fazekas *et al.,* 1980), 712 patients were randomized to undergo radiotherapy alone or radiotherapy plus pretreatment methotrexate (25 mg every third day for five doses). There was no significant difference in survival between the two groups, although more patients in the combined therapy group failed to complete radiation therapy.

Theoretically, hydroxyurea can cause increased sensitivity to radiotherapy by killing cells in S phase and synchronizing cells into the more radiosensitive G_1 phase (Elkind and Kano, 1971). To date, though, three randomized trials have shown no advantage to using hydroxyurea over radiotherapy alone (Richards and Chambers, 1969; Stefani *et al.,* 1971; Hussey and Abrams, 1975). Stefani *et al.* (1971) randomized 126 patients with advanced head and neck cancer to radiotherapy alone or radiotherapy plus hydroxyurea at 80 mg/kg biweekly throughout the radiation course. Although the complete response rate was similar in both groups, the survival was inferior in the combination group. In addition, 8% of those receiving radiation alone developed distant metastases, compared with 23% of patients in the combined treatment arm. Enhanced normal tissue toxicity was observed with concurrent hydroxyurea.

One of the first agents shown in a randomized trial to have efficacy when used in combination with radiotherapy was 5-FU (Ansfield *et al.,* 1970). The study

TABLE V RADIOTHERAPY AND CONCURRENT CHEMOTHERAPY FOR HEAD AND NECK CANCER

Agent	Number of patients	% Complete response		% Survival	
		Radiotherapy	Radiotherapy & chemotherapy	Radiotherapy	Radiotherapy & chemotherapy
Methotrexate (Fazekas et al., 1980)	712	—	—	5–21	12–27
Hydroxyurea (Stefani et al., 1971)	126	47	42	51	29
5-Fluorouracil (Ansfield et al., 1970)	134	—	—	15	36
Bleomycin (Cachin et al., 1977)	186	68	67	50	50
Bleomycin (Shanta and Krishnamurthi, 1977)	145	21	77	20	50

randomized 134 patients with advanced head and neck cancer to receive radiotherapy alone or radiotherapy plus 5-FU (10 mg/kg/day $\times$ 3 days, then 5 mg/kg/day $\times$ 1 day, then 5 mg/kg/day three times weekly). The 5-year survival was superior in the combination treatment arm at 36%, as compared with the 15% survival rate for the radiotherapy alone arm. However, the improvement in survival was limited to patients with primary lesions in the tonsil or tongue.

In early pilot studies, bleomycin was noted to be an effective radiosensitizer (Goffinet and Bagshaw, 1974). Cachin *et al.* (1977) reported for the European Organization for Research on the Treatment of Cancer on 186 patients with advanced oropharyngeal carcinoma who were randomized to receive radiotherapy alone or radiotherapy plus bleomycin (15 mg twice weekly for 5 weeks). There was no difference in response rate or survival, and the combination treatment was not well tolerated, with significant mucositis observed.

In contrast, Shanta and Krishnamurthi (1977) reported favorable results for combined modality treatment of 136 patients with oral-cavity cancers, predominantly buccal mucosa, who were randomized to receive radiotherapy alone or radiotherapy plus bleomycin (10–15 mg three times weekly for 6 weeks). The complete response rate in the combined modality group was significantly superior to the radiotherapy group (77 versus 21%). Survival also was significantly improved. The Northern California Oncology Group recently completed a randomized trial of concurrent bleomycin and radiotherapy, followed by maintenance bleomycin and methotrexate (Fu *et al.*, 1983).

Cisplatin has demonstrated activity as a radiosensitizer *in vivo* and *in vitro* (Zak and Drobnik, 1971; Wodinsky *et al.*, 1974). Several mechanisms have been postulated for this interaction, including hypoxic cell sensitization, inhibition of radiation-induced sublethal repair, conversion of lesions to chromosomal aberrations, cell-cycle perturbations, toxic ligand release, and reaction with nonprotein SH groups (Douple and Richmond, 1979; Muggia and Glatstein, 1979). Haselow *et al.* (1982), in a study of the Eastern Cooperative Oncology Group, treated 23 patients with advanced head and neck cancer with cisplatin (10–30 mg/m^2) weekly during radiotherapy. They found the optimal dose to be 20 mg/m^2 weekly, and, because of encouraging results, a randomized trial is underway.

A number of drugs could be used as radiosensitizers, but the ideal sensitizer is one that can increase tumor response without increasing toxicity for normal tissue from radiation. In the future, hypoxic cell sensitizers may be more efficacious than conventional chemotherapy.

C. Adjuvant or Maintenance Chemotherapy

Data from animal models have demonstrated that chemotherapy is most effective when the tumor-cell burden is small and cells have their highest growth fraction (Griswold, 1975). Adjuvant or maintenance chemotherapy could be used in the treatment of head and neck cancer to decrease distant metastases, which represent the only site of recurrence in 20% of patients (Head and Neck Contracts Program, 1984). Several large combined-modality trials of induction chemotherapy or chemotherapy concurrent with radiotherapy have included a maintenance chemotherapy arm. However, investigators have noted difficulties that preclude completion of maintenance chemotherapy, including patient compliance, disease progression, death from other causes, and toxicity limitations.

Thus, numerous studies have been performed using chemotherapy in the combined modality approach, but it is difficult to make specific recommendations. Many investigations are pilot studies with small numbers of patients and short follow-up periods. Often there is a lack of comparability between the various studies reported, particularly regarding conventional therapy. Finally, there are a number of prognostic factors that are known to influence response to therapy, and most reported series include a mixture of these factors.

IV. PROGNOSTIC FACTORS

Several patient characteristics can influence response rates and survivals in head and neck cancer, and these are important stratification variables for randomized trials. Squamous-cell cancer of the head and neck is a heterogeneous disease, and outcome following surgery, radiation, and chemotherapy is known to vary with primary site (Cachin *et al.*, 1977; Snow *et al.*, 1978). Response rates to initial treatment and survival also vary with primary tumor status, nodal status, and disease stage. Baker *et al.* (1981) reported for the Head and Neck Contracts Program that the most useful factor in predicting tumor response was tumor staging. Karnofsky performance status also has been shown to influence response to chemotherapy and survival (Amer *et al.*, 1979). Differing results among pilot studies and conflicting conclusions from randomized clinical trials may be attributed to patient populations displaying various prognostic factors.

V. CONCLUSIONS

For new combined-modality programs that include chemotherapy to be accepted as standard therapy, the programs should be shown to be superior to conventional treatment. Induction chemotherapy can be highly effective and without significant toxicity, but no study to date has shown a significant improvement in outcome with this approach. Although chemotherapy can increase the efficacy of concurrent radiotherapy, only bleomycin and 5-fluorouracil have produced a significant improvement in outcome and only for selected sites. Adjuvant or maintenance chemotherapy has not been shown to improve survival, and it is difficult to deliver in this patient population.

New approaches are needed to improve curability of advanced head and neck cancer through combined-modality treatment. First, primary therapy could be optimized with improved surgical techniques and radiotherapy techniques, such as the use of radiation sensitizers, interstitial implants, and hyperthermia. Detection of residual disease with monoclonal antibodies may help select patients who might benefit from adjuvant therapy. Better chemotherapy programs currently are being developed for induction chemotherapy. The role of biologic modifiers in the combined modality treatment is yet to be defined. Clinical trials may need to involve a more homogeneous patient population or large enough numbers of patients to evaluate various sites and stages. Although all patient groups may not benefit from a new therapy, patients with a particular site, primary tumor status, or nodal status may benefit. Finally, the death rate from second primaries must be reduced.

REFERENCES

Amer, M. H., Al-Sarraf, M., and Vaitkevicius, V. K. (1979). *Cancer* **43**, 2202–2206.

Ansfield, F. J., Ramirez, G., Davis, H. L., Korbitz, B. C., Vermund, H., and Gollin, F. F. (1970). *Cancer* **25**, 78–82.

Baker, S. R., Makuch, R. W., and Wolf, G. T. (1981). *Arch. Otolaryngol.* **107**, 683–689.

Berry, R. J. (1965). *Nature* **208**, 1108–1110.

Buechler, M., Mukherji, B., Chasin, W., and Nathanson, L. (1979). *Cancer* **43**, 1095–1100.

Cachin, Y., Jortay, A., Sancho, H., Eschwege, F., Madelain, M., Desaulty, A., and Gerard, P. (1977). *Eur. J. Cancer* **13**, 1389–1395.

Cadman, E., Heimer, R., and Davis, L. (1979). *Science* **205**, 1135–1137.

Capizzi, R. L., DeConti, R. C., Marsh, J. C., and Bertino, J. R. (1970). *Cancer Res.* **30**, 1782–1788.

Carter, S. K. (1977). *Semin. Oncol.* **4**, 413–424.

Costanzi, J. J., Loukas, D., Gagliano, R. G., Griffiths, C., and Barranco, S. (1976). *Cancer* **38**, 1503–1506.

Davis, S., and Kessler, W. (1979). *Cancer Chemother. Pharmacol.* **3**, 57–59.

Decker, D. A., Drelichman, A., Jacobs, J., Hoschner, J., Kinzie, J., Loh, J. J. K., Weaver, A., and Al-Sarraf, M. (1983). *Cancer* **51**, 1353–1355.

Decroix, Y., and Ghossein, N. (1981). *Cancer* **47**, 503–508.

Douple, E. B., and Richmond, R. C. (1979). *Int. J. Radiat. Oncol. Biol. Phys.* **5**, 1335–1339.

Drelichman, A., Cummings, G., and Al-Sarraf, M. (1983). *Cancer* **52**, 399–403.

Elkind, M. M., and Kano, E. (1971). *Int. J. Radiat. Biol.* **19**, 547–560.

Fazekas, J. T., Sommer, C., and Kramer, S. (1980). *Int. J. Radiat. Oncol. Biol. Phys.* **6**, 533–540.

Frei, E., III., Blum, R. H., Pitman, S. W., Kirkwood, J. M., Henderson, I. C., Skarin, A. T., Mayer, R. J., Bast, R. C., Garnick, M. B., Parker, L. M., and Canellos, G. P. (1980). *Am. J. Med.* **68**, 370–376.

Fu, K. K., Eisenberg, L., Dedo, H. H., and Phillips, T. L. (1977). *Cancer* **40**, 2874–2881.

Fu, K. K., Phillips, T. L., Silverberg, I. J., Friedman, M. A., Kohler, M., and Carter, S. K. (1983). *Proc. Am. Soc. Clin. Oncol.* **2**, 159.

Gilbert, E. H., Goffinet, D. R., and Bagshaw, M. A. (1975). *Cancer* **34**, 1517–1524.

Goffinet, D. R., and Bagshaw, M. A. (1974). *Cancer Treat. Rev.* **1**, 15–26.

Goldsmith, M. A., and Carter, S. K. (1975). *Cancer Treat. Rev.* **2**, 137–158.

Griswold, D. P., Jr. (1975). *Cancer Chemother. Rep.* **5**, 187–204.

Haselow, R. E., Adams, G. S., Oken, M. M., Goudsmit, A., Leiner, H. J., and March, J. C. (1982). *Proc. Am. Soc. Clin. Oncol.* **1**, 201.

Head and Neck Contracts Program, *et al.* (1984). *Proc. Am. Soc. Clin. Oncol.* **3**, 182.

Hong, W. K., Shapshay, S. M., Bhutari, R., Craft, M. L., Ucmakli, A., Yamaguchi, K. T., Vaughn, C. W., and Strong, S. (1979). *Cancer* **44**, 19–25.

Hong, W. K., Schaefer, S., Issell, B., Cummings, C., Luedke, P., Bromer, R., Fofonoff, S., D'Aoust, J., Shapshay, S., Welch, J., Levin, E., Vincent, M., Vaughan, C., and Strong, S. (1983). *Cancer* **52**, 206–210.

Hussey, D. H., and Abrams, J. P. (1975). *Prog. Clin. Cancer* **6**, 79–86.

Jacobs, C., Bertino, J. R., Goffinet, D. R., Fee, W. E., Goode, R. L. (1978). *Cancer* **42**, 2135–2140.

Jacobs, C., Meyers, F., Hendrickson, C., Kohler, M., and Carter, S. (1983). *Cancer* **52**, 1563–1569.

Kaplan, B. H., Schoenfeld, D., and Vogl, S. E. (1981). *Proc. Am. Assoc. Cancer Res.* **22**, 532.

Kirkwood, J. M., Canellos, G. P., Ervin, T. J., Pitman, S. W., Weichselbaum, R., and Miller, D. (1981). *Cancer* **47**, 2414–2421.

Kish, J. A., Weaver, A., Jacobs, J., Cummings, G., and Al-Sarraf, M. (1984). *Cancer* **53**, 1819–1824.

Knowlton, A. H., Percarpio, B., Bobrow, S., and Fischer, J. J. (1975). *Radiology* **116**, 709–712.

Lane, M., Moore, J. E. III, Levin, H., and Smith, F. E. (1968). *JAMA* **204**, 561–564.

Leone, L. A., Albala, M. M., and Rege, V. B. (1968). *Cancer* **21**, 828–837.

Levitt, M., Mosher, M. B., DeConti, R. C., Farber, L. R., Skeel, R. T., Marsh, J. C., Mitchell, M. S., Papac, R. J., Thomas, E. D., and Bertino, J. R. (1973). *Cancer Res.* **33**, 1729–1734.

Lustig, R. A., Demare, P. A., and Kramer, S. (1976). *Cancer* **37**, 2703–2708.

Muggia, F. M., and Glatstein, E. (1979). *Int. J. Radiol. Oncol. Biol. Phys.* **5**, 1407–1409.

Nakissa, N., Hornback, N. B., Shidnia, H., and Sayoc, E. (1978). *Cancer* **42**, 2914–2919.

Papac, R. J., Jacobs, E. M., Foye, L. V., and Donohue, D. M. (1963). *Cancer Chemother. Rep.* **32**, 47–54.

Papac, R., Minor, D. R., Rudnick, S., Solomon, L. R., and Capizzi, R. L. (1978). *Cancer Res.* **38**, 3150–3153.

Pitman, S. W., Kowal, C. D., and Bertino, J. R. (1983). *Seminars in Oncology* **10** (suppl. 2), 15–19.

Price, L. A., Hill, B. T., Calvert, A. H., Dalley, M., Levene, A., Busby, E. R., Schachter, M., and Shaw, H. J. (1978). *Oncology* **35**, 26–28.

Priestman, T. J. (1973). *Br. J. Cancer* **27**, 400–405.

Randolph, V. L., Vallejo, A., Spiro, R. H., Shah, J., Strong, E. W., Huvos, A. G., and Wittes, R. E. (1978). *Cancer* **41**, 460–467.

Richards, G. J. Jr., and Chambers, R. G. (1969). *Am. J. Roentgenol.* **105**, 555–565.

Sako, K., Razack, M. S., Kalnins, I. (1978). *Am. J. Surg.* **136**, 529–533.

Schottenfeld, D., Gantt, R. C., and Wynder, E. L. (1974). *Preventive Medicine* **3**, 277–293.

Shanta, V., and Krishnamurthi, S. (1977). *Clin. Radiol.* **28**, 427–429.

Shapshay, S. M., Hong, W. K., Incze, J. S., Yamaguchi, K., Bhutani, R., Vaughn, C. W., and Strong, M. S. (1978). *Am. J. Surg.* **136**, 534–538.

Snow, J. B., Kramer, S., Marcial, V. A., Gelber, R. D., Davis, L. W., and Lowry, L. D. (1978). *Ann. Otol. Rhinol. Laryngol.* **87**, 686.

Stefani, S., Eells, R. W., and Abbate, J. (1971). *Radiology* **101**, 391–396.

Stephens, R., Coltman, C., Rossof, A., Samson, M., Panettiere, F., Al-Sarraf, M., Alberts, D., and Bonnet, J. (1979). *Cancer Treat. Rep.* **63**, 1609–1610.

Tarpley, J. L., Chretien, P. B., Alexander, J. C., Joye, R. C., Block, J. B., and Ketcham, A. S. (1975). *Am. J. Surg.* **130**, 481–486.

Turrisi, A. T. III, Rozencweig, M., Von Hoff, D. D., and Muggia, F. M. (1978). *In* "Bleomycin[:] Current Status and New Developments" (S. K. Carter, S. T. Crooke, and H. Umezawa, eds.), pp. 151–163. Academic Press, New York.

Vogl, S. E., and Kaplan, B. H. (1979). *Cancer* **44,** 26–31.

Vogler, W. R., Jacobs, J., Moffitt, S., Velez-Garcia, E., Goldsmith, A., Johnson, L., and Mackay, S. (1979). *Cancer Clin. Trials* **2,** 227–236.

Wittes, R. E., Cvitkovic, E., Shah, J., Gerold, F. P., and Strong, E. W. (1977). *Cancer Treat. Rep.* **61,** 359–366.

Wodinsky, I., Swinjarski, J., Kensler, C. J., and Venditti, J. M. (1974). *Cancer Chemother. Rep.* **4,** 73–97.

Woods, R. L., Fox, R. M., and Tattersall, M. H. N. (1981). *Br. Med. J.* **282,** 600–602.

Zak, M., and Drobnik, J. (1971). *Strahlentherapie* **142,** 112–115.

Bleomycin Chemotherapy
(B. I. Sikic, M. Rozencweig, and S. K. Carter, eds.)

Chapter 7

HEAD AND NECK CANCER: BLEOMYCIN PLUS RADIOTHERAPY*

Karen K. Fu

Department of Radiation Oncology
University of California
San Francisco, California

I. INTRODUCTION

Bleomycin is an antitumor antibiotic that is similar to radiation in some of its mechanisms of action. It causes single- and double-strand DNA breaks, inhibits DNA synthesis, and is most effective against cells in M and G_2 phases of the cell cycle (Crooke and Bradner, 1976).

In clinical studies, bleomycin has demonstrated effectiveness against a variety of human tumors, especially squamous-cell carcinoma (Blum *et al.*, 1973; Crooke and Bradner, 1976). In the treatment of advanced squamous-cell carcinoma of the head and neck, bleomycin alone has an overall response rate of 31% (Blum *et al.*, 1973). It has been one of the chemotherapeutic agents most frequently combined with radiotherapy for head and neck cancer, either as a single agent or in combination with other chemotherapeutic agents.

In *in vitro* studies, bleomycin has been shown to decrease the width of the shoulder, as well as the mean lethal dose D_0, of the radiation dose response

---

*Supported, in part, by National Institutes of Health grant CA 21744-06.

curves of mammalian cells (Matsuzawa *et al.*, 1972, Terasima *et al.*, 1975). However, Bleehen *et al.* (1974) observed only an additive effect when bleomycin was combined with radiation on the EMT6 tumor cells *in vitro*. In *in vivo* studies, Jorgensen (1972) observed a synergistic effect with simultaneous radiation and a bleomycin injection, but an additive effect with intermittent bleomycin and radiotherapy on a murine epidermoid carcinoma. Finally, Sakamoto and Sakka (1974) observed only an additive effect on another mouse squamous-cell carcinoma treated *in vivo* with radiation before or after administering bleomycin. Bleomycin has been shown to increase the degree of differentiation in human and experimental squamous-cell carcinomas (Michaels *et al.*, 1973).

II. RANDOMIZED STUDIES

There have been at least 14 studies combining bleomycin and radiotherapy in the treatment of advanced head and neck cancer. However, only five of these were randomized, including one in which bleomycin was combined with preoperative radiotherapy (Table I).

The largest randomized study was conducted by the European Organization for Research on Treatment of Cancer (EORTC), involving carcinoma of the oropharynx (Cachin *et al.*, 1977). There was no significant difference between the control and combined treatment groups in either the tumor regression rate evaluated 6 weeks after completion of radiotherapy or in survival. The prescribed bleomycin dose was 15 U im or iv 2 hr before radiotherapy twice weekly to a total dose of 150 U. However, only 68% of the patients received the prescribed total dose. The incidence of severe mucositis and epidermitis was significantly greater in the combined treatment group, necessitating delay of radiotherapy in 22% of the patients and interruption of treatment in 5%. Severe mucositis also led to the reduction of the radiation dose from the prescribed 7000 rad in 7 to 8½ weeks to 6288 ± 168 rad in 52 ± 2 days.

In the randomized study reported by Kapstad (1978), bleomycin was administered during preoperative radiotherapy. Although clinical evaluation at 2 weeks after irradiation showed a more favorable response rate for the group receiving bleomycin, pathologic examination showed no significant difference in the incidence of negative surgical specimens. Four of 15 patients (27%) in the combined treatment group had negative specimens, compared with 2 of 14 patients (14%) in the radiation alone group. Data on survival are not available.

The randomized study showing the most significant difference in tumor response and survival between the combined treatment and radiation alone groups was reported by Shanta and Krishnamurthi (1980) from India. Favorable re-

TABLE I RANDOMIZED CLINICAL TRIALS OF COMBINED BLEOMYCIN (BLEO) AND RADIOTHERAPY (XRT) FOR ADVANCED HEAD AND NECK CANCER

Reference	Primary site	Number of patients	XRT dose schedule	BLEO dose schedule	Response rate [a] (%)				Survival	
					CR		PR			
					XRT	XRT + BLEO	XRT	XRT + BLEO	XRT	XRT + BLEO
Cachin et al. (1977)	Oropharynx	220 (186 evaluable) XRT: 87 XRT + BLEO: 99	XRT alone: 6403 ± 204 rad/47 ± 2 days XRT + BLEO: 6288 ± 168 rad/52 ± 2 days	15 U im or iv 2 hr before XRT biweekly × 5 weeks to a total dose of 150 U	Primary site 67.9	67	13.1	17.0	Median survival (months) 15	15
					Nodes 49	62	26	14	2-Year actuarial survival (%) 45	42
					Evaluated 6 weeks after XRT					
Kapstad (1978a)	Various sites	32 (29 evaluable) XRT: 14 XRT + BLEO: 15	3000 rad/5 weeks at 150 rad × 5/week during wk 1, 2, 4, and 5; no XRT during week 3 Surgery performed 2 weeks after XRT	15 U im 1 hr before XRT 3×/wk to a total dose of 180 U	7	27	21	33	NA[b]	
					Evaluated 2 weeks after XRT					
Shanta and Krishnamurthi (1980)	Oral cavity, primarily buccal mucosa	157 XRT: 73 XRT + BLEO: 84	XRT alone: 6500 rad/6.5–7 weeks; 5 treatments/week XRT + BLEO: 5500–6000 rad/6.5–7 week; 3 treatments/week	10–15 U ia or iv 2×/week or 3×/week on nonirradiation days to a total dose of 150 to 250 U or 30 U im 2×/week × 2 weeks before XRT and 30 U im × 1 during XRT to a total dose of 150 U	19.2	78.6			5-Year disease-free survival (%) 23.5	65.5
					Evaluated 8 weeks after XRT					

(continued)

TABLE I (*Continued*)

Reference	Primary site	Number of patients	XRT dose schedule	BLEO dose schedule	Response rate [a] (%) CR XRT	CR XRT + BLEO	PR XRT	PR XRT + BLEO	Survival XRT	Survival XRT + BLEO
Morita (1980)	Tongue	45 XRT: 23 XRT + BLEO: 22	XRT alone: 400 rad/4 wk + 4000–6000 rad/5–7 days with radium implant XRT + BLEO: 2000–2400 rad/2 weeks + 4000–6000 rad/5–7 days with radium implant	5 U/day im just before XRT 5×/week to a total dose of 50–60 U	2-Year local control rate (%) 65	73			NA	
Fu et al. (1984)	Various sites	93 XRT: 50 XRT + BLEO: 43	7000 rad at 180 rad/day 5 days/week	5 U iv 2×/week during XRT 15 U/week + MTX 25 mg/m²/week × 16 weeks after completion of XRT	42 Evaluated at 4 wk after XRT 2-Year local-regional control rate (%) 21 ($p=.001$)	54 69	20	30	2-year actuarial survival 36 ($p=.32$)	48

[a]CR, Complete response; PR, partial response.
[b]NA, Not available.

sponse, defined as total healing within the irradiated volume at 8 weeks after completion of radiotherapy, was 78.6% in the combination group and 19.2% in the radiation-only group. The 5-year recurrence-free rate was 71.8 and 17% and the 5-year actuarial disease-free survival was 65.5 and 23.5% for the combination and radiation-only groups, respectively. The difference was statistically significant among patients who received intraarterial or intravenous bleomycin, but not among patients who received intramuscular bleomycin. There also was a significant difference in survival rates with respect to site and tumor stage: the survival was greater when disease was in the buccal mucosa than when it was in the gingiva, and greater in T3 disease as compared with T4 disease. It should be noted, however, that the total bleomycin dose varied for the different routes of administration, and the radiation dose fractionation also differed between study groups.

In the study reported by Morita (1980), patients with carcinoma of the tongue were randomized to receive external-beam radiation therapy with or without bleomycin, followed by interstitial radium implant. Although the total dose of external-beam irradiation was greater for the control group than for the combined-treatment group (4000 rad per 4 weeks versus 2000–2400 rad per 2 weeks), a substantial tumor regression rate of greater than 50%, as evaluated at 2 weeks after external-beam irradiation, was achieved in both the control and combined treatment groups (61 versus 64%). Therefore, the dose effect factor (DEF = isoeffect radiation dose without drug/isoeffect radiation dose with drug) for 50% tumor regression was 1.3/1.5. Two-year local control rates also were not significantly different between the two groups (65 versus 73%). Both groups received the same dose of radium needle implant following the external-beam irradiation. The incidence of osteonecrosis was 20% in the control group but 0% in the group receiving bleomycin. Thus, it would appear that the therapeutic ratio is greater in the combined treatment group.

The Northern California Oncology Group (NCOG) trial differed from most of the other studies, in that the bleomycin dose during irradiation was 5 U iv twice weekly instead of the 10 to 15 U iv or im two to three times weekly used in most other studies (Fu et al., 1984). In contrast to most studies, which showed marked enhancement of radiation mucositis in combined treatment groups, necessitating interruption of radiation and decrease of total radiation dose, there was no significant difference in radiation dose or number of treatment days between the radiation alone and combined treatment groups in this study. Results thus far show a significantly greater 2-year local–regional control rate in the combined-treatment group than the control group (69 versus 21%, $p = .001$). However, the difference in survival was not statistically significant.

Although patients randomized to the combined treatment group should have received maintenance chemotherapy with bleomycin 15 U iv and methotrexate

25 mg/m iv weekly for 16 weeks after irradiation, less than one-third of the patients actually received greater than 50% of the prescribed maintenance chemotherapy dose. Thus, the observed difference in the local–regional tumor response was probably due primarily to the bleomycin administered during irradiation.

III. NONRANDOMIZED STUDIES

Results of nine nonrandomized studies combining bleomycin and radiotherapy in squamous-cell carinoma of the head and neck are summarized in Table II. The patient populations in these studies were quite heterogeneous: most series included patients with advanced disease from various primary sites in the head and neck, although some series (Berdal, 1976; Kapstad et al., 1978) also included patients with T1 N0 or T2 N0 carcinoma of the larynx. Most patients had received no previous treatment, although some patients with recurrent disease were included (Berdal, 1976; Tanaka et al., 1976; Kapstad et al., 1978; Seagren et al., 1979).

In addition, the bleomycin dose schedule varied significantly. Although in most series it was administered at 10 to 15 U iv or im two or three times weekly, not all patients received the prescribed total bleomycin dose because severe mucositis developed during radiotherapy.

The radiation dose schedule also was quite variable. The total radiation dose in some studies was significantly lower than that commonly used without the drug. This was due, at least in part, to the severe mucositis that developed during the combined treatment.

Complete response rates ranged from 38 to 58%. Long-term local–regional control rates were not available. Survival statistics also varied significantly, although the median survival usually was less than 2 years. However, Tanaka et al. (1976) reported a 2-year survival rate of 76.9% among patients who had undergone additional surgery, radiotherapy, or other chemotherapy. Because of the nonrandom nature of these studies, as well as patient heterogeneity and variations in bleomycin and radiation dose schedule, it is not possible to draw any firm conclusions from these studies.

IV. NORMAL TISSUE EFFECTS OF COMBINED TREATMENT

Mild to moderate enhancement of radiation mucositis and skin reaction by bleomycin has been commonly reported when combined radiation and chemo-

TABLE II NONRANDOMIZED CLINICAL TRIALS OF COMBINED BLEOMYCIN (BLEO) AND RADIOTHERAPY (XRT) FOR ADVANCED HEAD AND NECK CANCER

Reference	Primary site	Number of patients	XRT dose schedule	BLEO dose schedule	Response rate[a] (%) CR	PR	Survival (%)
Matsumura et al. (1973)	Paranasal sinuses	22	300 rad/3 week preop rad/4 weeks postop → surgery → 4000	15–30 U im or iv 2×/week or 3×/week to a total dose of 75 to 300 U; 4 patients received BLEO	2-Year local control 40		2-Year survival 40
Berdal (1976)	Various sites	>300; 210 patients observed 1–3.5 years	350 rad/day Mon.–Sat., rest 1 wk, 350 rad/day Mon.–Sat.; total dose 4200 rad to skin, 2500 rad to tumor	15 U/day im 1 hr before XRT Mon.–Sat. first week, then 15 U/day im on Mon., Wed., Fri. for 2 weeks, total dose 180 U (Nov. 1971–May 1973) BLEO dose subsequently lowered to 45 to 80 U given before and during the early part of XRT at 15 to 30 U 2×/week until Dec. 1973; changed to total dose of 0.7/U/kg/week in 3 weekly injections	54	32	Surviving 1–3.5 years Larynx: 83 Hypopharynx: 43 Oral cavity: 43 Tongue: 62
De La Garza et al. (1976)	Various sites	20	4000–6000 rad	15 U iv 2×/week, total dose 150–300 U	CR + PR 70		5 alive NED 9–16 months; 5 alive with disease 6–16 months; 10 died at 1 to 11 months

(*continued*)

TABLE II (*Continued*)

Reference	Primary site	Number of patients	XRT dose schedule	BLEO dose schedule	Response rate[a] (%) CR	PR	Survival (%)
Tanaka et al. (1976)	Oral cavity	39	2500 rad/2 week–3000 rad/3 weeks + further treatment with surgery (15 patients), XRT (17 patients), chemotherapy (4 patients)	7.5 U im 3×/week (4 patients) 10 U iv 2×/week (2 patients) 15 U iv 2×/week (33 patients)	38 Histologically proven		2-Year survival rate 76.9
Kapstad et al. (1978)	Various sites	30 (17 initial and 13 recurrent disease)	Initial disease: 4000–5000 rad at 150 rad × 5/wk during wk 1, 2, 4, 5, 6, and 7 Recurrent disease: 0–4000 rad	15 U im 1 hr before XRT 3×/week to total dose of 60 to 300 U in initial disease and 30 to 225 U in recurrent disease	Initial 41 0 Recurrent	29 15	NA[b]
Rygard and Hansen (1979)	Primarily larynx and oral cavity	33 (simultaneous BLEO and XRT) 68 (sequential BLEO and XRT)	1630 ± 85 to 1720 ± 75 CRE, reu at 160 to 200 rad/day, 5 days/week 1700 ± 96 to 1799 ± 140 CRE, reu at 160–200 rad/day, 5 days/wk	1970–1972: 10–15 U im ½–1 hr before XRT 2–3×/week 1972 on: 0.7 U/kg/week im Mean total dose: 103–156 U	45		Median survival 15 months
				10–15 U im 3×/week before and during the first week of XRT Mean total dose: 115–	44		16–47 months, depending on response to BLEO

Reference	Site	No. of patients	Radiotherapy dose	Bleomycin dose	Response (%)	Survival
Seagren et al. (1979)	Various sites	19	5040 rad + surgery (2 patients), 1–192 implant (7 patients), further XRT (6 patients)	15 U im 2×/week to a total dose of 165 to 180 U	58 / 37 (After 5000 rad)	1-Year crude survival 68 Disease-free survival 57
Shah et al. (1981)	Oral cavity	59 XRT: 36 XRT + BLEO: 23	4000–6000 rad at 200 rad/day 6 days/week	15 U iv ½ hr before XRT 3×/week	XRT alone 50 / 8.3 XRT + BLEO 47.8 / 17.4	Median survival Responders / Nonresponders XRT 6 months / 6 months XRT + BLEO 7 months / 5 months 12 days / 22 days
Silverberg et al. (1981)	Various sites	42	Prescribed dose: 6500 rad at 180 rad/day 5 days/week; Actual dose: 4997–7546 rad; Median: 6649 rad in complete responders, 4620–7360 rad (median 6480 rad) in partial responders	15 U iv 2×/week (19 patients); 5 U iv 2×/week (18 patients); 2 U iv 3×/week (2 patients); 15 U iv weekly (1 patient); 10 U iv 2×/week (1 patient); Total dose: 20–255 U (mean 93 U) in complete responders, 36–180 U (mean 91 U) in partial responders	52 / 43	Median survival 392 days (85–1076 + days in complete responders, 212 days (59–581 days) in partial responders

aCR, Complete response; PR, partial response.
bNA, Not available.

TABLE III   NORMAL TISSUE EFFECTS OF COMBINED BLEOMYCIN AND
RADIOTHERAPY IN THE HEAD AND NECK

| Reference | Normal tissue effect | | Degree of enhancement[c] |
	Type (grade)[a,b]	Incidence (%)	
Randomized studies	Mucositis	47.4	2+
Cachin et al. (1977)	Mucositis + epidermitis	22.2	2+
	Profound weakness	19.1	2+
	Weight loss	18.1	2+
Kapstad (1978a)	Mucositis	53	0
	Skin reaction	20	0
Shanta and Krishnamurthi (1980)	Mucositis	—	2 → 3+
Morita (1980)	Mucositis	—	2+ DEF = 1.5
Fu et al. (1984)	Mucositis (2)	21	0
	Mucositis (3)	63	2+
	Mucositis (4)	16	2+
	Epidermitis (1)	23	1+
	Epidermitis (2)	28	1+
	Epidermitis (3)	35	1+
	Moderate fibrosis	7	0
	Severe fibrosis	5	1+
	Soft-tissue necrosis	5	1+
	Trismus	2	±
Nonrandomized studies			
Matsumura et al. (1973)	Mucositis	—	1+
Berdal (1976)	Mucositis	—	1+
De la Garza et al. (1976)	Mucositis	—	2+
Tanaka et al. (1976)	Mucositis (2)	25–29	1+
	Mucositis (3)	53–75, depending on BLEO dose	2+
Kapstad et al. (1978b)	Mucositis + epidermitis	20	±
	Necrosis	7	2+
Rygard and Hansen (1979)	Mucositis	62	2+
	Mucositis	—	1+
Seagren et al. (1979)	Mucostis (1)	5	0
	Mucositis (2)	26	±
	Mucositis (3)	63	2+
	Epidermitis (1)	11	0
	Epidermitis (2)	63	±
	Epidermitis (3)	21	2+
	Soft-tissue necrosis	21	2+

TABLE III (*Continued*)

| Reference | Normal tissue effect | | Degree of enhancement[c] |
	Type (grade)[a,b]	Incidence (%)	
Shah *et al.* (1981)	Mucositis	83	2+
	Mucositis (3–4)	22	2+
	Epidermitis	17	0
Silverberg *et al.* (1981)	Mucositis (3–4)	33–53, depending on BLEO dose	1 → 2+

[a]Mucositis: grade 1, erythema; grade 2, patchy; grade 3, confluent; grade 4, confluent, necrosis, requiring hospitalization.

[b]Epidermitis: grade 1, erythema; grade 2, dry desquamation; grade 3, moist desquamation; grade 4, necrosis.

[c]Degree of enhancement: 0, no enhancement; ±, equivocal enhancement; 1+, mild enhancement; 2+, moderate enhancement; 3+, severe enhancement.

therapy are administered for head and neck cancer (Table III). In some patients severe mucositis necessitated interruption of treatment, reduction of total radiation dose, and prolongation of overall treatment days.

The degree of enhancement depended on the total bleomycin dose, as well as on the timing of bleomycin administration in relation to radiotherapy. In general, the degree of mucositis increased with increasing bleomycin doses and with concurrent drug and radiation administration. In the study reported by Shanta and Krishnamurthi (1980), more severe mucositis was seen in patients who received bleomycin intraarterially or intravenously than intramuscularly; the total bleomycin dose was 150–250 U in the former group and 150 U in the latter. Rygard and Hanson (1979) noted a decrease of mucositis when most of the bleomycin dose was administered before beginning radiotherapy.

A grading system to describe acute and late normal tissue effects was used in only a few series (Seagren *et al.*, 1979; Silverberg *et al.*, 1981; NCOG, unpublished data). The incidence of grade 3 or confluent mucositis was in the range of 22 to 63%, and the incidence of grade 3 skin reaction or moist desquamation was in the range of 21 to 35%.

Quantitative estimation of the modification of radiation mucositis was available from the report by Morita (1980). The DEF was 1.5 for a 50% incidence of confluent mucositis.

Late normal tissue effects, including increased soft-tissue fibrosis and soft-tissue necrosis, were described in a few series (Kapstad *et al.*, 1978b; Seagren *et al.*, 1979; Fu *et al.*, 1979, 1984). The incidence of soft-tissue necrosis was in the range of 7 to 21% and was the major cause of death in 1 of the patients reported by Seagren *et al.* (1979).

V. DISCUSSION

It is apparent that bleomycin appears to enhance both tumor and normal tissue effects of radiation therapy in the head and neck. Available experimental and clinical data suggest that the enhancement most likely results from an additive effect rather than a supraadditive drug and radiation interaction.

One of the major limitations of combining bleomycin and radiotherapy to treat head and neck cancer is the markedly enhanced radiation mucositis that occurs during concurrent drug and radiotherapy administration. This often has led to a decrease in total bleomycin and/or radiotherapy doses administered as well as interruption of radiation. Review of the normal tissue effects of combined chemotherapy and radiotherapy for head and neck cancer suggests that enhanced normal tissue effects most often are seen with concurrent chemotherapy and radiotherapy; they are less likely to occur when the two modalities are administered sequentially (Fu, 1979). Therefore, to minimize normal tissue toxicity, it may be preferable to administer bleomycin and radiotherapy in a sequential or alternating manner, provided that the enhanced tumor response does not require concurrent administration. This also may allow delivery of a higher dose of bleomycin and radiation or the addition of other chemotherapeutic agents.

Although most studies suggest an improvement in local–regional control with combined bleomycin and radiation, only one randomized study showed a statistically significant improvement in survival (Shanta and Krishnamurthi, 1980). Some of the recent studies using bleomycin in combination with other chemotherapeutic agents as induction therapy prior to surgery and/or radiotherapy have shown encouraging local–regional response rates (Randolph *et al.*, 1978; Peppard *et al.*, 1980; O'Connor *et al.*, 1982; Pennacchio *et al.*, 1982; Ervin *et al.*, 1983; Spaulding *et al.*, 1984; Weaver *et al.*, 1980). Whether these bleomycin-containing combination chemotherapy regimens would lead to improved survival needs further investigation through randomized clinical trials.

REFERENCES

Berdal, P. (1976). *Gann* **19,** 133–149.
Berdal, P., Ekroll, T., Iversen, O. H., and Weyde, R. (1973). *Acta Otolaryngol.* **75,** 318–320.
Bleehen, N. M., Gillies, N. E., and Twentyman, P. R. (1974). *Br. J. Radiol.* **47,** 346–351.
Blum, R. H., Carter, S. K., and Agre, K. (1973). *Cancer* **31,** 903–914.
Cachin, Y., Jortay, A., Sancho, H., Eschwege, F., Madelain, M., Desaulty, A., and Gerard, P. (1977). *Europ. J. Cancer* **13,** 1389–1395.
Crooke, S. T., and Bradner, W. T. (1976). *J. Med.* **7,** 333–428.
De la Garza, J. G., Olivares, F. G., Armendariz, C., and Flores, F. A. M. (1976). *J. Int. Med. Res.* **4,** 158–164.
Ervin, T. J., Weichselbaum, R. R., Miller, D., Posner, M. R., Fabian, R. L., Tuttle, S. A., and Frei, E. III. (1983). *Proc. Am. Soc. Clin. Oncol.* **2,** 164.

Eschwege, F., Richard, J. M., and Sancho-Garnier, H. (1978). *J. Radiologie* **59**, 43–44.

Fu, K. K. (1979). *Front. Radiat. Ther. Onc.* **13**, 113–132.

Fu, K. K. (1984). Unpublished Preliminary Results of Northern California Oncology Group Trial.

Jørgenson, S. J. (1972). *Europ. J. Cancer* **8**, 531–534.

Kapstad, B. (1978). *Int. J. Radiat. Oncol. Biol. Phys.* **4**, 91–94.

Kapstad, B., Bang, G., Rennaes, S., and Dahler, A. (1978). *Int. J. Radiat. Oncol. Biol. Phys.* **4**, 85–89.

Matsumura, Y., Soda, T., and Motomura, K. (1973). *EENT Month.* **52**, 25–34.

Matsuzawa, T., Onoaqwa, M., Morita, K., and Kakehi, M. (1972). *Strahlentherapie* **144**, 614–617, 1972.

Michaels, L., Grey, P. A., and Rowson, K. E. K. (1973). *J. Pathol.* **109**, 315–321.

Morita, K. (1980). *Strahlengherapie* **156**, 228–233.

O'Connor, D., Clifford, P., Edwards, W. G., Dalley, V. M., Durden-Smith, J., Hollis, B. A., and Calman, F. M. (1982). *Int. J. Radiat. Oncol. Biol. Phys.* **8**, 1525–1531.

Pennacchio, J. L., Hong, W. K., Shapshay, S., Gillis, T., Vaughan, C., Bhutani, R., Ucmakli, A., Katz, A. E., Bromer, R., Willet, B., and Strong, S. M. (1982). *Cancer* **50**, 2795–2801.

Peppard, S. B., Al-Sarraf, M., Powers, W. E., Loh, J. K., and Weaver, A. W. (1980). *Laryngoscope* **90**, 1273–1280.

Randolph, V. L., Vallejo, A., Spiro, R. H., Shah, J., Strong, E. W., Huvos, A. G., and Wittes, R. E. (1978). *Cancer* **41**, 460–467.

Rygard, J., and Hansen, H. S. (1979). *Acta. Otolaryngol. Suppl.* **360**, 161–166.

Sakamoto, K., and Sakka, M. (1974). *Br. J. Cancer* **30**, 463–468.

Seagren, S. L., Byfield, J. E., Nahum, A. M., and Bone, R. C. (1979). *Int. J. Radiat. Oncol. Biol. Phys.* **5**, 1531–1535.

Shah, P. M., Shukla, S. N., Patel, K. M., Patel, N. L., Baboo, H. A., and Patel, D. D. (1981). *Cancer* **48**, 1106–1109.

Shanta, V., and Krishnamurthi, S. (1980). *Clin. Radiol.* **31**, 617–620.

Silverberg, I. J., Phillips, T. L., Fu, K. K., and Chan, P. Y. M. (1981). *Cancer Treat. Rep.* **65**, 697–698.

Spaulding, M. B., De Los Santos, R., Klotch, B., Khan, A., Sundquist, N., and Lore, J. (1984). *Proc. Am. Soc. Clin. Oncol.* **3**, 187.

Tanaka, Y., Wada, T., Fuchihata, H., Makino, T., Inoue, T., and Shigematsu, Y. (1976). *Int. J. Radiat. Oncol. Biol. Phys.* **1**, 1189–1193.

Terasima, T., Takabe, Y., and Yasukawa, M. 1975). *GANN* **66**, 701–703.

Weaver, A., Loh, J. J. K., and Vandenberg, H. (1982). *Am. J. Surg.* **140**, 549–552.

Bleomycin Chemotherapy
(B. I. Sikic, M. Rozencweig, and S. K. Carter, eds.)

Chapter 8

THE ROLE OF INDUCTION CHEMOTHERAPY IN COMBINED-MODALITY TREATMENT PROGRAMS

Robert E. Wittes

Cancer Therapy Evaluation Program
Division of Cancer Treatment
National Cancer Institute
Bethesda, Maryland

I. INTRODUCTION

Chemotherapy is incorporated into combined-modality treatment programs to improve survival. Although other worthy endpoints—disease-free survival, patterns of relapse, quality of life—may be measured in the course of such trials, the major impetus for combined-modality trials has been the prospect that the addition of chemotherapy to local treatment may cure a substantial number of patients who otherwise would not be cured. Clearly, this objective may be very difficult to achieve, particularly for diseases such as head and neck cancer. This patient population is predominantly elderly men with a high prevalence of major medical illnesses other than the index cancer. Therefore, such a high rate of competing causes of death may well obscure any beneficial effect of the chemotherapy. These observations notwithstanding, if chemotherapy does not decrease all-cause mortality following the diagnosis of cancer, it will have failed to achieve its ultimate goal.

In principle, chemotherapy may be given either after completion of local therapy, before the start of local therapy, or simultaneously with local treatment (radiotherapy). Obviously, combinations of these strategies are possible and produce more complex treatment programs. Since the mid-1970s, chemotherapy has been used in earnest as initial treatment (or so-called induction or neoadjuvant chemotherapy) in a variety of tumor types.

II. EFFECT ON TREATMENT AND SURVIVAL

A. Potential Benefits

Induction chemotherapy has several potential benefits. First, it provides immediate treatment for occult distant metastases that are responsible for treatment failure. Therefore, it may be expected that the more effectively one can kill distant microfoci of disease, the more likely it is that there will be a beneficial effect on survival. Second, induction chemotherapy may improve control of local and regional disease by decreasing bulk prior to local therapy. Since the efficacy of local therapy for previously untreated patients is determined, in part, by extent of disease, reducing the stage of the cancer prior to local therapy may improve results. Chemotherapy may improve the cosmetic and functional results of cancer treatment by permitting a decrease in the radical extent of certain operations. In addition, as has already been shown in the treatment of extremity bone sarcomas, the time required to deliver several cycles of chemotherapy may be used to good advantage in the construction of a limb prosthesis, which, in turn, permits more conservative surgery. Finally, response or nonresponse to initial chemotherapy in an individual patient may predict the value of the same chemotherapy when given postoperatively to that patient as maintenance.

B. Potential Disadvantages

Induction chemotherapy also has certain potential disadvantages. Theoretically, at least, it may promote the selection of drug-resistant cells, simply because patients are being exposed to chemotherapy when there is maximum body burden of tumor. Second, if there should be tumor progression during induction chemotherapy, previously resectable locoregional disease may become unresectable; even less dramatic disease progression possibly may prejudice chance of cure. Although this possibility was a very real concern during the early years of such trials, experience suggests that the problem is rare in practice, at least with those regimens that have been tested. Finally, the experience of the group at Wayne State University suggests that a high complete response rate to chemotherapy may be accompanied by a substantial rate of refusal of subsequent surgery, despite vigorous advocacy on the part of the responsible physicians (Weaver *et al.*, 1982). Although it may well be that extremely active chemotherapy may obviate the need for standard local modes of therapy, one certainly cannot assume that this is the case without evidence from controlled trials.

III. TESTICULAR CANCER

The value of induction chemotherapy has been explored in several tumor types. Patients with testicular cancer whose retroperitoneal disease is bulky and presumed difficult or impossible to resect have been treated in this manner at several centers. Most investigators have employed surgery after several cycles of chemotherapy; the intent of the operation is to remove all remaining bulk disease both to assess completeness of response and to remove residual malignant elements (Vugrin *et al.*, 1981). The clinical results of such regimens are discussed in detail elsewhere in this volume.

IV. OSTEOSARCOMA

Perhaps osteosarcoma provides the most promising example of the potential of regimens incorporating induction chemotherapy. Over the past decade, several institutions have engaged in trials of induction chemotherapy, either systemically or intraarterially, in combination with surgery and postoperative systemic chemotherapy. Advances in prosthesis technology have permitted the fabrication of a prosthesis during the induction chemotherapy courses (Marcove and Rosen, 1980), an approach that promotes limb conservation where anatomically feasible.

At the Memorial Sloan–Kettering Cancer Center (MSKCC), Rosen and colleagues have utilized preoperative high-dose methotrexate at weekly intervals; chemotherapy following resection or amputation consists of combinations of bleomycin, cyclophosphamide, and dactinomycin, alternated with high-dose methotrexate and doxorubicin. Once the endoprosthesis is in place, patients are treated with one of two regimens, depending on response to the initial courses of methotrexate. Patients whose tumors show striking pathologic evidence of necrosis receive a sequence of drugs including high-dose methotrexate. Those showing less impressive degrees of necrosis are treated without methotrexate. As previously reported (Rosen *et al.*, 1982), disease-free survival resulting from this complex treatment policy is in excess of 80%. To date, there has been no difference in disease-free survival among those patients showing impressive necrosis with methotrexate and patients not showing such necrosis.

Attempts to confirm these encouraging results are in progress within the Children's Cancer Study Group (CCSG) (Study CCG 782). By the very nature of the design of both the MSKCC trial and the follow-up CCSG study, however, it will be impossible to sort out the relative contributions of preoperative versus postoperative therapy, much less the contribution of individual agents or combinations to the end results.

V. HEAD AND NECK CANCER

Trials of induction chemotherapy in stage III and stage IV squamous-cell head and neck cancer have been in progress for several years, mostly as pilot studies in single institutions. High response rates (60–100%) may be achieved with various combinations containing methotrexate and/or cisplatin (Eisenberger *et al.*, in press). Most responses have been partial rather than complete. The preliminary reports of most of these trials have not documented any obvious interference with subsequent local therapy. However, reliable assessments of interactions among modalities are admittedly difficult to document, particularly in uncontrolled studies. Some surgeons have observed that surgery may be technically easier after induction chemotherapy than after preoperative radiotherapy; presumably, drugs have less effect on surrounding normal tissue. On the other hand, if the original extent of disease has not been meticulously documented prior to chemotherapy, the surgeon may lack reliable anatomic guideposts for judging a suitable extent of resection.

VI. DISCUSSION

Needless to say, strong statements about the effect of induction chemotherapy on survival are impossible from small uncontrolled pilot studies. Several years ago, in response to the promising activity of induction chemotherapy, the National Cancer Institute (NCI) organized a multicenter trial to test the efficacy of this approach. Patients with operable stage III and stage IV epidermoid carcinoma from six sites in the oral cavity, the larynx, and the piriform fossa were randomized to one of three treatment policies: (1) surgery followed by postoperative radiotherapy; (2) induction chemotherapy with cisplatin plus bleomycin, followed by local therapy as in (1); and (3) induction chemotherapy followed by local therapy as in (2), followed by six treatments at monthly intervals with continuous-infusion cisplatin. Analysis of the results has shown no effect of induction chemotherapy on disease-free interval or survival (Wolf *et al.*, 1984).

In addition, the trial demonstrated that cisplatin as maintenance therapy was not feasible as originally planned; for a variety of reasons, only a small percentage of the total number of patients randomized to receive maintenance chemotherapy actually received six cycles of it.

This trial may be criticized on several grounds. By current standards, the choice of agents may not be optimal, either in terms of dose of the constituent agents (lower than in the pilot studies) or of number of cycles administered (one). Second, as already stated, the maintenance chemotherapy chosen for testing turned out to be undeliverable in all but a few patients. Nevertheless, this study is a landmark in cancer clinical trials. It demonstrated clearly that multiinstitutional multimodality trials of primary therapy may be done with rigorous quality control in head and neck cancer patients. Moreover, it showed that there is a high level of interest in such questions among head and neck cancer clinicians in the United States. In the past, the clinical cooperative groups have not distinguished themselves in head and neck cancer trials. Only the Radiation Therapy Oncology Group has successfully initiated and concluded trials of this type. More recently, the Eastern Cooperative Oncology Group and the Northern California Oncology Group have demonstrated their capability of adequate performance in clinical trials of primary head and neck cancer therapy. Because there seems to be wider capability and interest among investigators now than in the past, the NCI has strongly encouraged such trials continue on an intergroup basis.

Several centers also have been exploring the potential role of induction chemotherapy in patients with locally advanced (stage III and stage IV) breast cancer. Generally, combination chemotherapy given for a few cycles is followed by surgical resection, which, in turn, is followed by postoperative chemotherapy. These studies have all been small and have lacked simultaneous controls (Table I). There is a suggestion that this approach may result in an increased resectability rate. However, since there are no uniformly accepted criteria for what constitutes resectability in breast cancer, such data are very difficult to interpret without simultaneous controls. In addition, the design of these studies does not permit any statement about the effect of initial chemotherapy upon disease-free interval or survival.

VII. SUMMARY

In summary, definitive conclusions concerning the value of induction chemotherapy are not possible, despite years of clinical trials. In osteosarcoma, where positive effects of systemic treatment on survival appear plausible in certain trials, the specific effect of induction chemotherapy cannot be isolated. It seems clear, however, that the use of induction chemotherapy has permitted the evolution of a far more acceptable cosmetic and functional surgical procedure than has existed in the past. Certainly, this is a worthy therapeutic objective in itself. In

TABLE I   CHEMOTHERAPY BEFORE LOCAL THERAPY IN BREAST CANCER OF
STAGE III AND STAGE IV

Institution	Design[a]	Number of patients	Control group	Reference
University of Maryland	CT → S → CT	27	None	Aisner et al. (1982)
Washington University	CT → RT → CT	22	Historical	Bedwinck et al. (1983)
Instituto Nazionale Tumori	CT → RT → CT versus CT → S → CT	67 65	Randomized	De Lena et al. (1981)
Mt. Sinai	CT → S → CT	17	None	Perloff and Lesnick (1982)
M. D. Anderson	CT → IT → Local CT	52	Historical	Hortobagyi et al. (1983)
Hôpital Tenon et Bichot	CT → S → CT	15	None	Zylberberg et al. (1982)

[a]CT, Chemotherapy; S, surgery; RT, radiotherapy.

head and neck cancer, occasional trials have alleged a substantial impact on disease-free interval and survival, but the vast majority of trials have been inconclusive. If it should turn out that induction chemotherapy improves local control rates, studies to assess the feasibility of reducing the scope of surgery would seem logical. In fact, pilot studies to assess this question are currently in progress. In addition, the Veterans Administration has recently activated a controlled trial to assess whether patients with advanced laryngeal cancer who respond to induction chemotherapy can be treated with radiotherapy but without laryngectomy.

ACKNOWLEDGMENT

The author thanks Mr. William Soper and Ms. Candia Hench for technical and secretarial assistance.

REFERENCES

Aisner, J., Morris, D., Elias, E. G., and Wiernik, P. H. (1982). Arch. Surg. 117, 882–887.
Bedwinck, J. M., Ratkin, G. A., Philpott, G. W., Wallack, M., and Perez, C. A. (1983). Am. J. Clin. Oncol. 6, 158–165.

Children's Cancer Study Group. Study CCG 782.

DeLena, M., Varini, M., Zucali, R., Rovini, D., Viganotti, G., Valagussa, P., Veronesi, U., and Bonadonna, G. (1981). *Cancer Clin. Trials* **4**, 229–236.

Eisenberger, M., Posada, J., Soper, W., and Wittes, R. E. (in press). *In* "Investigative Approaches in the Staging and Management of Head and Neck Cancer" (R. E. Wittes, ed.), Wiley, Chichester, England.

Hortobagyi, G. N., Spanos, W., Montague, E. D., *et al.* (1983). *Int. J. Radiat. Oncol. Biol. Phys.* **9**, 643.

Marcove, R. C., and Rosen, G. (1980). *Cancer* **45**, 3040–3044.

Perloff, M., and Lesnick, G. J. (1982). *Arch. Surg.* **117**, 879.

Rosen, G., Caparros, B., Huvos, A. G., *et al.* (1982). *Cancer* **49**, 1221–1230.

Vugrin, D., Whitmore, W. F. Jr., Sogani, P. C., *et al.* (1981). *Cancer* **47**, 2228–2231.

Weaver, A., Flemming, S., Kish, J., *et al.* (1982). *Am. J. Surg.* **144**, 445–448.

Wolf, G. T., Jacobs, C., Makuch, R. W., and Vikram, B. (1984). *Proc. Int. Conf. Head Neck Cancer.*, p. 43.

Zylberberg, B., Salat-Baroux, J., Ravina, J. H., *et al.* (1982). *Cancer* **49**, 1537–1543.

Chapter 9

INDUCTION CHEMOTHERAPY IN THE TREATMENT OF HEAD AND NECK CANCER: SUNY BUFFALO AND VAMC EXPERIENCE

Monica B. Spaulding

Oncology Section
Buffalo Veterans Administration Medical Center
and State University of New York at Buffalo
Buffalo, New York

I. INTRODUCTION

Head and neck cancer is a devastating illness for the majority of patients with the disease. Current standard treatment requires extensive surgery and large-field radiation therapy, and for those who present with advanced tumors treatment is not a guarantee of cure. In fact, with percentages varying slightly according to the anatomic site of the primary lesion, less than half of those with stage III and stage IV disease may be cured by current surgery and radiation therapy (*Management Guidelines for Head and Neck Surgery,* 1979). Also, in spite of aggressive treatment of the local tumor and its regional nodes, recurrence within the local–regional site is the major site of treatment failure (Snow, 1981).

In 1978, in an attempt to improve the results of such locally directed therapy, our institution began a pilot study of induction or neoadjuvant therapy for patients with advanced head and neck cancer. Patients with advanced, resectable disease and a less than 30% estimated chance of cure with standard therapy alone were considered eligible for the study. The chemotherapeutic regimen was a non-myelosuppressive combination of cisplatin, bleomycin, and vincristine, which we believed would give a high response rate without adding unacceptable toxicity to the usual treatment. In addition, the absence of myelosuppression meant that patients could undergo surgery immediately on completion of chemotherapy. If there was no tumor response, or tumor growth occurred during chemotherapy, surgery could be undertaken immediately. To obtain a response rate high enough to offer benefit but not unduly delay definitive therapy, patients were to receive two courses of the chemotherapy, thereby adding 4 weeks to their usual treatment schedule.

II. METHODS

The study included 93 patients with advanced, biopsy-proven squamous-cell carcinoma arising from sites in the head and neck area. Each patient had a creatinine clearance of >60 cm^3/min, adequate bone marrow function (determined by a WBC of >3500/mm^3 and a platelet count of $>150,000$/mm^3), and adequate pulmonary function, with an FEV$_1$ of ≥ 1.5, if pulmonary function tests could be obtained. Many patients could not perform these tests because of tumors causing upper airway obstruction. In such cases, we relied on a history of no prior significant dyspnea with normal activities. Before therapy, all patients underwent direct and indirect laryngoscopy. Lesions were photographed and their outlines tattooed on the mucosa when possible. Appropriate plain and contrast X-ray films were obtained.

All patients were presented at a multidisciplinary conference attended by the medical staff of Head and Neck Surgery, Medical Oncology, and the other disciplines involved in the patient's care. Indirect laryngoscopy was repeated at this conference to obtain agreement from those attending that the patient was appropriate for study. A complete description of the surgery to be performed was written at this time.

Chemotherapy consisted of two courses of the regimen (Fig. 1). After overnight hydration and during a mannitol-induced diuresis, cisplatin was administered at a dose of 80 mg/m^2. On day 3, vincristine was given by bolus injection, followed 6 hr later by a continuous infusion of bleomycin at a dose of 15 U/m^2/day for 4 days. Patients then were discharged for 2 weeks and readmitted for a second course on day 21. A repeat creatinine clearance was obtained before the second dose of cisplatin was administered, and the dose was modified appropriately if creatinine clearance was impaired. Response to chemotherapy was determined after completion of the second course. Surgery was performed $\sim$30 days after initiating chemotherapy. Postoperative radiotherapy was given to patients who had positive margins and disease in multiple lymph nodes at multiple levels, and to those with disease eroding through the capsule of the lymph node into the soft tissues of the neck.

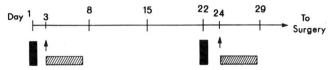

Fig. 1. Two-regimen courses of induction chemotherapy for head and neck cancer. ■, Platinum, 80 mg/m^2; ↑, vincristine, 1 mg/m^2; ▨, bleomycin, 15 U/m^2/day.

Following the completion of definitive therapy, patients were followed at monthly intervals for the first year, every 2 months for the second year, every 3 months for the third year, every 4 months for the fourth year, and every 6 months thereafter.

III. RESULTS

Of the 93 patients admitted into this study, two had two T4 primaries each. There were 29 patients with stage III disease, 63 with stage IV disease, and one with a stage II hypopharyngeal primary (Table I).

The overall response to chemotherapy was 89%, with 19 patients showing complete responses and 10 patients showing less than 50% tumor shrinkage. Clinically complete responses rarely were confirmed pathologically, generally due to microfoci of residual tumor found deep to normal-appearing mucosa. Of the 87 patients who underwent surgery, 6 received postoperative radiotherapy because of disease at the margins of resection (4 patients) or disease breaking

TABLE I DISEASE SITES
AND STAGES

Tumor sites[a]	Number of patients
Oral cavity	21
Oropharynx	22
Hypopharynx	27
Larynx	22
Paranasal sinus	3
Stage	
II	1
III	29
IV	63

[a]Two patients each had two T4 primary tumors.

through the lymph node capsule to invade soft tissue (2 patients). Of the 6 patients who were treated with full-course radiotherapy alone, 2 underwent this regimen because of failure to obtain medical clearance, while 4 refused the required operative procedure. The surgical procedure performed was that which was indicated prior to administration of chemotherapy.

Toxicity was minimal. Nausea and vomiting were controlled by the administration of antiemetics and dexamethasone. All patients developed total alopecia. There were no episodes of pulmonary insufficiency. A decrease in creatinine clearance prior to the second course of chemotherapy was observed in six patients, four of whom showed a clearance of 40 to 60 cm³/min and received a 50% reduction in the second dose of cisplatin. Two patients showed a creatinine clearance of less than 40 cm³/min and did not receive a second course of cisplatin. The renal insufficiency was reversible in all, and no patient required dialysis.

At the time of this writing, disease recurrence had appeared in only 17 of the 93 patients (18%), with 14 of these patients dying of disease. Twenty-three patients died of other causes, 55 remained alive and disease free, and one alive with disease. Follow-up on many of these patients is short; however, a >36-month follow-up has been attained for 46 patients who were treated between 1978 and May 1981. Of these 46 patients, only 12 (26%) showed disease recurrence. Two developed marginal recurrence only and underwent a second resection, remaining disease free at longer than a 40-month follow-up since their marginal recurrence. The other 10 died of recurrent disease, all showing local–regional recurrence at death. Although autopsies were not performed on all patients, 3 had gross evidence of distant disease, as well. Recurrence was evident within the first 18 months of follow-up in all but one of the patients.

Of the remaining patients with a minimum 3-year follow-up, 17 remained alive and disease-free at the time of this writing, with a median follow-up of 44 months. Nineteen died of causes unrelated to their primary head and neck tumor, however, including 9 patients who died of other cancers. This includes one patient who died of a second head and neck primary, a left pyriform sinus lesion

TABLE II   CAUSES OF DEATH[a]

Cause	Number of patients
Head and neck cancer	10
Other cancers	9
Chronic obstructive pulmonary disease	5
Alcohol related	4
Cardiovascular disease	4

[a]Minimum 36-month follow-up.

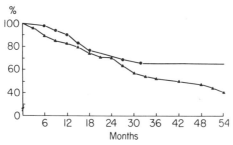

Fig. 2. Survival (minimum follow-up, 3 years) of patients dying of head and neck cancer only (●, determinant) and those dying of all causes (▲, indeterminant).

that developed 3 years after successful treatment of a right retromolar trigone lesion. The causes of death are shown in Table II. Figure 2 plots survival of those dying of all causes, compared with those who died of head and neck cancer only. At the time of this writing, 43% of patients treated prior to May 1981 were alive; however, when deaths due to other causes are excluded, more than 60% of the patients remained alive and disease free.

IV. DISCUSSION

Induction chemotherapy in head and neck cancer has a twofold purpose: to reduce the mass of local tumor and to improve the results of definitive surgery and radiotherapy. Such systemic treatment also means that any microscopic disease outside the head and neck area should be treated simultaneously. Earlier studies suggested that the response of head and neck cancer to chemotherapy was better when the drugs were administered prior to surgery or radiotherapy, since surgery can change the blood supply significantly and radiotherapy may cause vascular fibrosis, thus reducing drug delivery to the local tumor. Because local–regional recurrence has remained a major problem in the treatment of head and neck cancer despite aggressive surgery and radiation, control of the gross tumor mass is most important. In this study, almost 90% of the patients showed significant (>50%) tumor shrinkage prior to the use of definitive therapy. Nevertheless, those who ultimately died of head and neck cancer died with local–regional disease rather than distant metastases.

In developing our treatment plan of induction chemotherapy, we did not intend to change the extent of the local therapy but, rather, to add chemotherapy to what is already considered standard treatment. Throughout the study, great pains were taken to define the original tumor mass with tattoos and multiple photographs. A complete description of the appropriate surgery for the original tumor mass was written prior to the administration of any chemotherapy. Several of our patients with grossly normal-appearing mucosa following chemotherapy were found to have multiple islands of apparently viable tumor cells in the resected specimen. A lesser operation clearly would not have removed this disease. Whether the routine use of postoperative radiotherapy would have controlled this residual tumor, as suggested by others, remains to be determined in a controlled study. Although several pilot studies have suggested that response to chemotherapy also predicts for sensitivity to radiotherapy (Sheitz *et al.*, 1984; Ervin *et al.*, 1984), it is equally possible that resistance to chemotherapy (represented by islands of persistent tumor) predicts for radiotherapy resistance. In our study, five of the six patients treated with radiotherapy rather than surgery showed disease recurrence, although all had significant tumor shrinkage from the chemotherapy.

The high response rate seen with our combination is not unique. Weaver *et al.* (1980) administered cisplatin, vincristine, and bleomycin on a slightly different schedule to similar patients and observed an 80% response rate. Amrein *et al.* (1983) treated 37 patients with advanced disease with a modification of this combination and observed a slightly lower response rate. However, half of their patients presented with unresectable stage IV tumors. Our patients, although presenting with advanced disease, were all believed to be resectable and, therefore, probably had less tumor mass.

The toxicity of our combination was extremely limited. The mild renal impairment noted in six patients was reversible in all and did not require dialysis. Gastrointestinal symptoms, although initially significant, became minimal as we improved our antiemetic regimen. All patients at the time of this writing routinely received several doses of oral prochlorperazine and a bolus injection of dexamethasone prior to chemotherapy.

Although all of our patients were heavy smokers and many had physical signs and symptoms of obstructive pulmonary disease, we noted no pulmonary problems related to the bleomycin. The drug was given by infusion, a practice that might decrease the incidence of pulmonary toxicity (Sikic *et al.*, 1978). At the time of surgery, the anesthetic was combined with a fractional inspired oxygen (F_1O_2) of less than 50%.

The absence of myelotoxicity and stomatitis with this combination of chemotherapeutic agents means a shorter treatment period than required in other induction protocols. Our initial study design called for delaying definitive therapy until 2 weeks after completion of the second course of chemotherapy. We soon became comfortable with surgery taking place immediately following completion of chemotherapy. This may have avoided the problem of patient dropout or refusal of definitive therapy that other investigators have noted with induction regimens that are longer or have an obligatory break between completion of chemotherapy and surgery due to myelosuppression or stomatitis. In patients being treated primarily with radiotherapy rather than surgery, we did defer radiation therapy for 2 weeks to avoid severe mucositis.

At the time of this writing, only 19 of the 93 patients treated had developed disease recurrence. All but one recurrence in this group took place within the first 18 months of follow-up, similar to the pattern observed prior to the use of induction chemotherapy. Thus, it would appear that induction programs do not delay the onset of recurrence if it is to occur. Spaulding *et al.* (1982) reported that 70% of a similar group of patients with stage III and stage IV head and neck cancer treated by members of the Eastern Great Lakes Head and Neck network developed disease recurrence after 24 months of follow-up. Our treated patients appear to have done better, although follow-up is short. Patients with advanced head and neck cancer tend to be older, with histories of heavy alcohol ingestion and tobacco use. Consequently, their life span may be shortened by factors other than head and neck cancer. Although fewer than 20% of our patients died from head and neck cancer, many more died from causes related to aging and their alcohol and tobacco habits. Even if we only have changed the cause of death in these patients, however, this still would be a significant advance, since it is an improvement over death by starvation, asphyxiation, or hemorrhage from locally recurrent head and neck cancer. Nonetheless, if deaths due to other causes are excluded, more than 60% of our initial population remained alive and disease free.

V. CONCLUSION

Patients with advanced head and neck cancer can tolerate chemotherapy administered prior to definitive therapy, as has been shown by a number of investigators. Our bleomycin-containing regimen has been well tolerated, has a high response rate, and adds only 1 month to the total treatment plan. Although the decreased frequency of relapse and improved survival that we have observed are promising, results of this and comparable studies still need confirmation in controlled trials.

REFERENCES

Amrein, P. C., Fingert, H., and Weitzman, S. A. (1983). *J. Clin. Oncol.* **1,** 421–427.
Ervin, T. J., Weichselbaum, R. R., Fabian, R. L., Miller, D., Norris, C. M., Posner, M. R., Rose, C., Lockhart, P., Tuttle, S. A., MacIntyre, J. M., and Frei, E. (1984). *Arch. Otolaryngol.* **110,** 241–245.
Management Guidelines for Head and Neck Cancer. (1979). NIH Publ. No. 80-2037.
Sheitz, S., O'Donoghue, G., Bromer, R., Vaughn, C., Willett, B., Welch, J., and Fofonoff, S. (1984). *Proc. Am. Soc. Clin. Oncol.* **3,** 183.
Sikic, B. I., Collins, J. M., Mimnaugh, E. G., and Gram, T. E. (1978). *Cancer Treat. Rep.* **62,** 2011–2017.

Snow, J. B., Gelber, R. D., Kramer, S., Davis, L. W., Marcial, V. A., and Lowry, L. D. (1981). *Acta Otolaryngol.* **91,** 611–626.

Spaulding, M. B., Khan, A., De Los Santos, R., Klotch, B., and Lorè, J. (1982). *Am. J. Surg.* **144,** 432–436.

Weaver, A., Loh, J. J. K., Vandenberg, H., Powers, W., Fleming, S., Mathog, R., and Al-Sarraf, M. (1980). *Am. J. Surg.* **140,** 549–552.

Section IV
THE MALIGNANT LYMPHOMAS

.

Bleomycin Chemotherapy
(B. I. Sikic, M. Rozencweig, and S. K. Carter, eds.)

Chapter 10

HODGKIN'S DISEASE: AN OVERVIEW AND ABVD STUDIES IN MILAN

Valeria Bonfante
Armando Santoro
Emilio Bajetta
Pinuccia Valagussa
Simonetta Viviani
Roberto Buzzoni
Gianni Bonadonna
Division of Medical Oncology
Istituto Nazionale Tumori
Milan, Italy

I. INTRODUCTION

Since 1970, remarkable progress has been achieved in the treatment of advanced Hodgkin's disease (HD) by moving from single-agent to multiple-drug therapy. However, despite the increased incidences of complete response (CR), long-term remission, and cure, primary resistance to therapy and relapse following initial CR still represent problems in a considerable percentage of patients. Patients failing on chemotherapy often display pretreatment characteristics that indicate the presence of a high tumor-cell burden (e.g., bulky disease in a single lymph node–bearing region, multiple extranodal involvement, or systemic

127

symptoms). Moreover, the following findings have been frequently observed: the median time to CR is usually the fourth treatment cycle, and progressive disease during chemotherapy often occurs following initial tumor response after two to four treatment cycles. In addition, when the duration of first CR is less than 12 months, retreatment with the same drug combination is often ineffective. Finally, modification of one or more components of an active drug regimen, such as MOPP (mechlorethamine, vincristine, procarbazine, and prednisone), in treating Hodgkin's disease fails to improve clinical results substantially.

These clinical observations have been very instructive and useful in designing new treatment strategies. Furthermore, they largely can be explained according to the basic tenets of the somatic mutation theory, as recently adapted to the area of cancer chemotherapy by Goldie and Coldman (1979). Therefore, the lack of curative effect of combination chemotherapy can be attributed to the presence of drug-resistant neoplastic cells before starting treatment and to the overgrowth of these cells during therapy.

Successful results have been achieved at our institution with the evaluation of non–cross-resistant and combined-modality therapies. In particular, the overall prognosis of HD has improved with the development in 1973 of ABVD (doxorubicin, bleomycin, vincristine, and dacarbazine), designed to employ new, effective drugs that had been included in the original MOPP regimen but were equally effective and non–cross-resistant with MOPP (Bonadonna *et al.*, 1975). Moreover, the effective clinical results achieved with the cyclic delivery of ABVD alternated monthly with MOPP versus MOPP alone in patients with pathologic stage (PS) IV HD confirmed the superiority of alternating chemotherapy strategy and supported the new concepts in terms of drug resistance (Bonadonna, 1982). This chapter presents an overview of the current status of the clinical trials for HD that have been conducted since the mid-1970s at the Milan Cancer Institute.

II. MOPP VERSUS ABVD

MOPP chemotherapy, as developed by the National Cancer Institute (NCI) group, dramatically improved the prognosis of advanced HD. The consequence of this intensive polychemotherapy is cure in a large percentage of patients [80% CR and 63.4% 10-year relapse-free survival (RFS)] (De Vita, 1981). However, follow-up indicated that about 20% of all patients with advanced HD treated with MOPP chemotherapy failed to attain CR, and an additional 40% who achieved CR ultimately relapsed. Furthermore, when the duration of first CR was less than 12 months, retreatment with MOPP yielded second remission in less than 30% of patients (Fisher *et al.*, 1979).

In the mid-1970s, following the confirmation that none of the MOPP-derived combinations could induce higher CR and long-term remission rates than achieved by the original MOPP, the ABVD regimen was designed, employing new drugs, including bleomycin, that were effective individually in HD and non–cross-resistant with MOPP components. ABVD first was tested against MOPP in a prospective randomized study, which demonstrated that the two combinations were equally effective in terms of CR (Bonadonna *et al.*, 1975).

Subsequently, to compare iatrogenic morbidity of ABVD versus MOPP and to further assess the comparative efficacy of the two treatments, a second randomized study with combined chemotherapy and radiotherapy (RT) was started in patients with PS IIB, IIIA, or IIIB disease. As detailed in previous publications (Santoro *et al.*, 1981; Bonadonna *et al.*, 1982), patients were randomly allocated to receive three cycles of either MOPP or ABVD administered according to the classic dose schedule. In the absence of tumor progression, treatment was continued with high-energy irradiation at the doses of 3500 rad to involved lymphoid areas and 3000 rad to uninvolved areas. At 1 month from the end of RT, treatment was completed with three additional cycles of either regimen.

The 5-year results are summarized in Table I. The CR rate following ABVD combined with RT was significantly superior to that of MOPP plus RT, particularly in patients with B symptoms. The most interesting comparative results were observed in PS IIIA, where the 5-year RFS was 100% in the ABVD group and 74.2% in the MOPP group ($p < .02$). Analysis of total survival failed to show a significant difference between the two treatment groups, probably because of the efficacy of salvage treatment with ABVD in MOPP-resistant patients.

TABLE I   MOPP–RT–MOPP VERSUS ABVD–RT–ABVD IN STAGES
IIB AND STAGE III HD: COMPARATIVE 5-YEAR OVERALL
RESULTS[a]

Result	MOPP (113 cases) (%)	ABVD (116 cases) (%)	p
Complete remission	81.4	92.2	.03
A symptoms	96.6	96.9	
B symptoms	76.2	90.5	.03
5-Year relapse-free survival	80.9	90.7	.09
A symptoms	74.2	100.0	<.02
B symptoms	77.3	88.6	
5-Year total survival	69.9	84.9	.12
A symptoms	74.8	93.4	
B symptoms	68.1	81.3	

[a]From Bonadonna *et al.* (1984a).

In terms of acute toxicity, ABVD produced a comparatively higher incidence of vomiting and hair loss than did MOPP. There was no detectable difference between the two treatment groups for chronic toxicity (doxorubicin-induced cardiomyopathy and bleomycin-induced pulmonary fibrosis). ABVD chemotherapy also was associated with a significantly lower incidence of gonadal dysfunction and carcinogenesis. Gondal damage was evaluated in patients of both sexes less than 45 years of age who received subtotal nodal irradiation. Among a total of 29 and 24 male patients evaluable in the MOPP and in the ABVD groups, respectively, azoospermia and oligospermia developed in 97% treated with MOPP and in 54% with ABVD. More importantly, the recovery of spermatogenesis in the ABVD patients in whom the sperm count was repeated occurred in all instances within a median of 10 months, compared with 3 of 21 patients (14%) given MOPP. Similarly, prolonged amenorrhea (in excess of 6 months) was detected in 16% of 37 evaluable women treated with MOPP and in none of the patients who received ABVD chemotherapy.

The comparative incidence of treatment-induced second neoplasms in patients receiving drug regimens containing alkylating agents and/or procarbazine (e.g., MOPP) versus ABVD has been published previously (Valagussa *et al.*, 1982). An updated analysis confirmed the absence of iatrogenic leukemia following ABVD administered either alone or combined with radiotherapy (Bonadonna *et al.*, 1984a).

III. SALVAGE TREATMENT

The usefulness of non–cross-resistant regimens in patients resistant to primary chemotherapy became clearly evident from initial results achieved with ABVD in MOPP-resistant patients (Bonadonna, 1982; Santoro *et al.*, 1982). Resistant patients are considered those who have progressive disease during primary therapy administered at full or nearly full doses, and those relapsing within the first 12 months after achieving pathologic CR. As previously described, CR patients received ABVD, plus two additional cycles (minimum of six cycles), and consolidation with RT limited to nodal site(s) of initial bulky lymphoma was carried out in most patients. Patients were restaged pathologically if they showed extranodal involvement in liver and/or bone marrow, and they were considered evaluable if they completed the treatment program or if they showed disease progression while on primary therapy.

Table II summarizes the essential findings observed in 71 consecutive patients given ABVD as first salvage treatment, that is, as soon as they were considered to be MOPP-resistant (Santoro *et al.*, 1984). Present results confirm that ABVD induced a high frequency of CR, which was influenced by certain prognostic variables, such as systemic symptoms and extranodal extent. At 7 years, 50% of

TABLE II   SALVAGE ABVD IN 71 MOPP-RESISTANT
PATIENTS[a]

Result	%	p
Partial remission	14	
Complete remission (CR)	55	
Symptoms: A/B	79/36	.01
Extent: nodal/extranodal	69/42	<.05
Response to MOPP: CR/non-CR	77/33	<.01
7-Year results		
Relapse-free survival	46	
Survival of CRs	51	
Total survival	27	

[a]From Bonadonna et al. (1984a).

complete responders remained continuously disease-free, and total survival analysis indicates that ABVD can salvage 27% of all MOPP-resistant to ABVD yielded CR in only 25% of patients and partial remission (PR) in 6%. The median RFS was 10 months, and the survival of complete responders was less than 3 years.

Since February 1980, CEP chemotherapy was administered as third-line treatment to patients resistant to both MOPP and ABVD. As previously reported (Bonadonna, 1982), this new regimen consisted of CCNU 80 mg/m^2 on day 1, etoposide 100 mg/m^2 po on days 1 through 5, and prednimustine 60 mg/m^2 po on days 1 through 5. Treatment was recycled on day 29. Results achieved in 40 patients are illustrated in Table III. CEP was effective in patients resistant to MOPP and ABVD administered either sequentially (MOPP ⇆ ABVD) or concomitantly (MOPP/ABVD), and it induced only moderate and reversible toxicity.

Following the successful experience with primary cyclic chemotherapy, we currently are testing the efficacy of two alternating regimens as salvage chemo-

TABLE III   RESULTS OF SALVAGE THERAPY WITH CEP[a]

Result	Total (40 cases)	MOPP ⇄ ABVD (28 cases)	MOPP/ABVD (12 cases)
Partial remission	25%	21%	33%
Complete remission	35%	39%	25%
RFS, median (months)	17	17	6
Survival CRs, median (months)	>30	>30	>6
Survival, median (months)	30	16	>8

[a]From Bonadonna et al. (1984a).

therapy. Very preliminary findings indicate that among 18 MOPP-resistant patients, ABVD/CEP induced CR in 61%, with a median in excess of 20 months. Among 5 ABVD-resistant patients, MOPP/CEP achieved CR in 3 patients, with a median duration of 10 months (Santoro *et al.*, 1984).

IV. CYCLIC MOPP/ABVD

The rationale for alternating one cycle of MOPP with one cycle of ABVD in patients previously untreated with chemotherapy, as detailed elsewhere by Bonadonna (1982), was first based on the clinical observation that patients resistant to primary MOPP usually show either lack of further tumor response or disease progression by the third cycle. A second reason for the alternating program was also derived from clinical experience. In fact, MOPP and ABVD appeared to be equally effective non–cross-resistant combinations, and the median time to CR with either regimen was the third cycle. The first randomized study comparing MOPP alone versus MOPP/ABVD was carried out in adults with PS IV HD. From 1974 to 1982, a total of 88 patients were entered into the study. As outlined in Table IV, the distribution of primary preclinical characteristics was comparable between the two treatment groups. Updated 7-year results are summarized in Table V, as reported (Bonadonna *et al.*, 1984b). They confirmed the superiority of the MOPP/ABVD program versus MOPP alone in terms of CR rate, freedom from progression (FFP), and RFS, and also indicated that total survival was improved significantly by the alternating regimen. Cyclic MOPP/ABVD also yielded better results than MOPP alone in some unfavorable prognostic subgroups (i.e., age 40 years, systemic symptoms, and bulky lymphoma).

Marked vomiting occurred more frequently after ABVD than MOPP ex-

TABLE IV   MOPP VERSUS MOPP/ABVD IN STAGE IV HD:
PATIENT CHARACTERISTICS

Characteristic	MOPP (43 patients) (%)	MOPP/ABVD (45 patients) (%)
Male patients	63	49
Age >40 years	35	36
Nodular sclerosis histology	58	53
Bulky lymphoma	33	40
Systemic symptoms (B)	70	69
>3 Nodal sites	60	73
Multiple extranodal	23	16
Prior radiotherapy	28	29

[a]From Bonadonna *et al.* (1984a).

TABLE V   MOPP VERSUS MOPP/ABVD IN STAGE IV HD:
COMPARATIVE 7-YEAR OVERALL RESULTS[a]

Result	MOPP (%)	MOPP/ABVD (%)	p
Complete remission	74.4	88.9	.14
Freedom from progression	35.1	68.1	.001
Relapse-free survival	44.4	76.8	.004
Survival of CRs	73.2	90.3	.038
Total survival	61.1	82.3	.043

[a]From Bonadonna et al. (1984a).

posure, but myelosuppression was comparatively less severe in patients given alternating chemotherapy, and these patients were able to receive a higher percentage of the planned dose for all drugs compared with patients treated with MOPP alone. No patient developed symptoms and signs of doxorubicin-induced cardiomyopathy or bleomycin-induced pulmonary fibrosis, as already observed in patients treated with MOPP or ABVD combined with RT. One patient given MOPP alone following prior extensive irradiation developed fatal acute nonlymphoblastic leukemia 37 months from starting chemotherapy.

From the reported results, alternating chemotherapy appears to be a very effective strategy in the primary management of advanced HD (Bonadonna, 1982). We now are testing, through a prospective randomized study activated in July 1982, the efficacy of cyclic MOPP/ABVD given in two different sequences. The control arm consists of MOPP/ABVD alternating after each full monthly cycle of either chemotherapy, while in the experimental arm the half-cycle of MOPP (mechlorethamine and vincristine on day 1, procarbazine and prednisone on days 1 through 7) is alternated within a 1-month period with the half-cycle of ABVD given on day 15. Theoretically, by testing more appropriately the hypothesis of Goldie and Coldman (1979), this new alternating-sequence therapy should be able to improve further the RFS achieved in our previous study. This clinical trial requires a large series of patients, and it is being performed in high-risk groups, such as those with stage IA to stage IIA bulky disease and stage IIB, stage III (A and B), and stage IV (A and B) disease. According to the study design, CR is followed by two consolidation cycles and by low-dose radiotherapy (2500 rad) delivered only to the area(s) with bulky lymphoma at the start of chemotherapy. The CEP regimen, with or without irradiation, is reserved for patients not achieving CR following six cycles of either alternating sequence chemotherapy. Very preliminary comparative findings are summarized in Table VI and would suggest that MA/MA may be more efficacious than the MM/AA sequence (where M represents MOPP and A represents ABVD) (Bonadonna et al., 1984a).

TABLE VI   COMPARATIVE PRELIMINARY
RESULTS WITH TWO ALTERNATING
SEQUENCES IN PS II, III, AND IV HD[a]

Result	MM/AA[b]	MA/MA[b]
Total evaluable	36	40
Complete remission	89%	93%
"A" symptoms	90%	87%
"B" symptoms	89%	96%
Bulky disease	77%	88%
Nonbulky disease	100%	96%

[a]From Bonadonna *et al.* (1984a).
[b]M, MOPP; A, ABVD.

V. CONCLUSION

A major step in the control of Hodgkin's disease has been the development of non–cross-resistant regimens, particularly the introduction of alternating chemotherapy with MOPP/ABVD. Results obtained with the sequential delivery of MOPP, ABVD, CEP, as well as the superiority of the MOPP/ABVD program versus MOPP alone, confirmed that cell heterogeneity and the fluctuating ratios of drug-resistant to drug-sensitive neoplastic cells represent a crucial prognostic variable in many patients. Another important benefit reached through the ABVD regimen and its cyclic delivery with MOPP combination concerns acute and delayed toxicity. Patients treated with ABVD alone or combined with RT failed to develop second leukemia and experienced a lower incidence of reversible gonadal damage compared with patients given MOPP. Moreover, patients who received cyclic MOPP/ABVD had less frequent and severe myelosuppression than those treated with MOPP.

To confirm further the usefulness of the alternating strategy following the principles of the Goldie and Coldman hypothesis, we now are exploring the efficacy of a more frequent alternating sequence by delivering within 1 month the half-cycle of two non–cross-resistant combinations in HD.

Considering that a plateau has been reached in the management of malignant lymphomas with single-drug combinations, our findings stress the importance of new therapeutic strategies to improve the cure rate of patients with advanced HD.

REFERENCES

Bonadonna, G., Zucali, R., Monfardini, S., De Lena, M., and Uslenghi, C. (1975). *Cancer* **36.** 252–259.
Bonadonna, G. (1982). *Cancer Res.* **42,** 4309–4320.

Bonadonna, G., Santoro, A., Bonfante, V., and Valagussa, P. (1982). *Cancer Treat. Rep.* **66,** 881–887.

Bonadonna, G., Santoro, A., Valagussa, P., Viviani, S., Zucali, R., Bonfante, V., and Banfi, A. (1984a). *In* "Second International Conference on Malignant Lymphoma" Martinus Nijhoff Publishing, Boston, in press.

Bonadonna, G., Viviani, S., Bonfante, V., Valagussa, P., and Santoro, A. (1984b). *Proc. Am. Soc. Clin. Oncol.* **3,** 254.

De Vita, V. T., Jr. (1981). *Cancer* **47,** 1–13.

Fisher, R. I., De Vita, V. T., Jr., Hubbard, S. M., Simon, R., and Young, R. C. (1979). *Ann. Intern. Med.* **90,** 761–763.

Goldie, J. H., and Coldman, A. J. (1979). *Cancer Treat. Rep.* **63,** 1727–1733.

Santoro, A., Bonfante, V., Bonadonna, G., Zucali, R., Pagnoni, A. M., Recchioni, C., Valagussa, P., and Banfi, A. (1981). *In* "Adjuvant Therapy of Cancer" (S. E. Salmon and S. E. Jones, eds.), Vol. III, pp. 85–91. Grune & Stratton, New York.

Santoro, A., Bonfante, V., and Bonadonna, G. (1982). *Ann. Intern, Med.* **96,** 139–144.

Santoro, A., Bonfante, V., Viviani, S., Valagussa, P., and Bonadonna, G. (1984). *Proc. Am. Soc. Clin. Oncol.* **3,** 254.

Valagussa, P., Santoro, A., Fossati-Bellani, F., Franchi, F., Banfi, A., and Bonadonna, G. (1982). *Blood* **3,** 488–494.

Bleomycin Chemotherapy

(B. I. Sikic, M. Rozencweig, and S. K. Carter, eds.)

Chapter 11

BLEOMYCIN IN COMBINATION WITH MOPP IN THE MANAGEMENT OF ADVANCED HODGKIN'S DISEASE: A SOUTHWEST ONCOLOGY GROUP EXPERIENCE*

Charles A. Coltman, Jr.

Department of Medicine
Division of Oncology
University of Texas Health Sciences Center
San Antonio, Texas

Stephen E. Jones

University of Arizona Health Sciences Center
Tucson, Arizona

Petre N. Grozea

University of Oklahoma Health Sciences Center
and Presbyterian Hospital
Oklahoma City, Oklahoma

Edward J. De Persio

Wenatchee Valley Clinic
Wenatchee, Washington

Dennis O. Dixon

Southwest Oncology Group Biostatistical Center
Houston, Texas

I. INTRODUCTION

Following the definitive studies of DeVita *et al.* (1970) with MOPP chemotherapy, the Southwest Oncology Group (SWOG) participated in three sequential

*Supported, in part, by the following U.S. Public Health Service Cooperative Agreement grant numbers, awarded by the National Cancer Institute, Department of Health and Human Services: CA-26766, CA-03195, CA-13612, CA-03392, CA-22411, CA-04919, CA-03096, CA-04915, CA-12644, CA-27057, CA-16385, CA-12213, CA-04920, CA-16957, CA-21116, CA-22416, CA-22433, CA-28862, CA-20319, CA-03389, CA-13238, CA-14028, CA-12014, and CA-32102.

studies, beginning in 1969, using MOPP alone for remission induction of Hodgkin's disease (Frei *et al.*, 1973; Coltman *et al.*, 1978). A detailed analysis of the SWOG experience using MOPP alone in patients who received no major prior chemotherapy shows a 62% overall complete response rate for 294 patients, with a median survival of 7 years (Coltman, 1980).

In 1971, SWOG found that bleomycin alone (SWOG 440) was active in 37% of heavily pretreated patients with Hodgkin's disease (Haas *et al.*, 1976). The rationale for the initial study of MOPP plus bleomycin (SWOG 774) was based on the concept that this relatively nonmyelosuppressive antibiotic could be added to the intensively myelosuppressive MOPP regimen without significant added toxicity, but with a potential for improving the overall complete response rate and survival. There was suggestive, although not statistically significant, evidence that bleomycin added to MOPP in a low dose (2 U/m^2 on days 1 and 8) enhanced the complete response rate ($p = .076$) and survival ($p = .06$) when compared with MOPP alone (Coltman *et al.*, 1978). Of substantial interest was the observation that patients treated with MOPP plus bleomycin at a dose of 10 U/m^2 on days 1 and 8 developed unacceptable myelosuppression.

Between 1974 and 1978, SWOG compared the MOPP plus low-dose bleomycin regimen (MOPP LDB) with MOPP plus low-dose bleomycin plus doxorubicin, in an attempt to confirm the previous study and to improve the complete response rate and survival of patients with advanced Hodgkin's disease. Doxorubicin 30 mg/m^2 on day 8 replaced the nitrogen mustard of the MOPP plus low-dose bleomycin program (MOP BAP 1). This sequence was compared to a third arm in which 15 mg/m^2 of doxorubicin was added on days 1 and 8 to an attenuated dose of nitrogen mustard at 3 mg/m^2 (MOP BAP 2) (SWOG 7406). Results of the study favored the six-drug combination (MOP BAP), revealing a particularly improved complete response rate among favorable prognostic groups (Jones *et al.*, 1983). The study failed to show comparable complete response and survival rates of patients entered into the MOPP plus low-dose bleomycin arm when compared with the earlier study (SWOG 774).

From 1975 to 1980, SWOG developed a study to compare MOPP LDB for 10 cycles with the same regimen for three cycles followed by total nodal radiotherapy in laparotomy-staged patients with stage III Hodgkin's disease (SWOG 7518) (Grozea *et al.*, 1982).

This chapter updates the current status of three SWOG studies, which involve MOPP plus bleomycin in the management of advanced Hodgkin's disease.

II. PATIENT AND METHODS

A. All Studies

Each of the three studies was conducted by members of the Southwest Oncology Group. Tissues of patients with histologically proven Hodgkin's disease were submitted for review by the Pathology Panel and Repository for Lymphoma Clinical Studies. Patients in whom Hodgkin's disease was not found on review were considered ineligible for the study. Each patient in the study provided a complete medical history and underwent a physical examination, with appropriate laboratory studies. Preoperative clinical staging included isotope scans, metastatic bone survey, bipedal lymphography, full chest tomography (for those with hilar node enlargement), and a bone marrow biopsy.

Freedom from relapse was defined as the time from treatment initiation to the time of disease progression (relapse). Freedom from relapse and overall survival curves were plotted by the method of Kaplan and Meier (1958), and survival curves were compared by the Gehan modification of the generalized Wilcoxon test (Gehan, 1965), as well as by the logrank test (Peto *et al.*, 1977).

B. MOPP versus MOPP plus Bleomycin (SWOG 774)

Patients with advanced Hodgkin's disease, who had not previously received chemotherapy and who did not show significant compromise of pulmonary function, were assigned randomly to receive MOPP alone or MOPP plus bleomycin in two different dose levels (Fig. 1). A low dose of 2 U/m^2 bleomycin on days 1 and 8 of cycles 1 through 6 of MOPP represented the MOPP plus low-dose bleomycin arm. In the MOPP plus high-dose bleomycin arm, 10 U/m^2 of bleomycin was administered on days 1 and 8 of cycles 2 through 6, following administration of a 5-U dose on days 1 and 8 of the first cycle. Because of potential bleomycin pulmonary toxicity, patients considered to show significant compromise of pulmonary function were treated on a separate arm with MOPP alone. This determination of significant compromise of pulmonary function was made jointly in telephone conversation between the investigator and study coordinator.

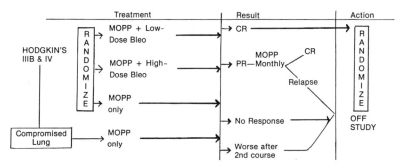

Fig. 1. MOPP versus MOPP plus bleomycin (SWOG 774).

The consolidation phase of this study (SWOG 775) (Fig. 2) was based on the prior Southwest Oncology Group experience of Frei *et al.* (1973) in which it appeared that administering MOPP every other month for 18 months after 6 months of MOPP remission induction was advantageous in terms of disease-free survival ($p = .025$). However, this observation was disproven after additional follow-up of the same study (Coltman *et al.*, 1976). A second consideration, which was important in the remission consolidation design of this study, was the observation from a previous study (Frei *et al.*, 1973) that the area of major involvement prior to the induction of MOPP was the most common site of relapse following complete remission, suggesting a role for radiotherapy to major bulk disease present prior to MOPP induction.

Patients who had achieved complete remission after induction were assigned randomly to three different arms. The first was remission consolidation with MOPP every other month for 18 months, followed by unmaintained remission. The second arm involved the administration of 4000 rad of radiotherapy to the areas of major lymph node involvement at the time of complete response, prior to instituting MOPP. This radiotherapy was followed by MOPP every other month for 18 months. The third arm of the study involved administration of MOPP every month for a total of 18 months. All patients were followed in unmaintained remission after their consolidation regimen.

C. MOPP plus Low-Dose Bleomycin versus MOPP plus Low-Dose Bleomycin plus Doxorubicin (SWOG 7406)

Patients who had not received previous chemotherapy were assigned randomly to receive treatment with MOPP LDB or MOP BAP 1. A third studied treatment included MOP BAP 2 (Fig. 3). This study differed significantly from the previous one (SWOG 774) because systematic restaging was required to determine the completeness of the patients' response. In a preliminary analysis by Herman

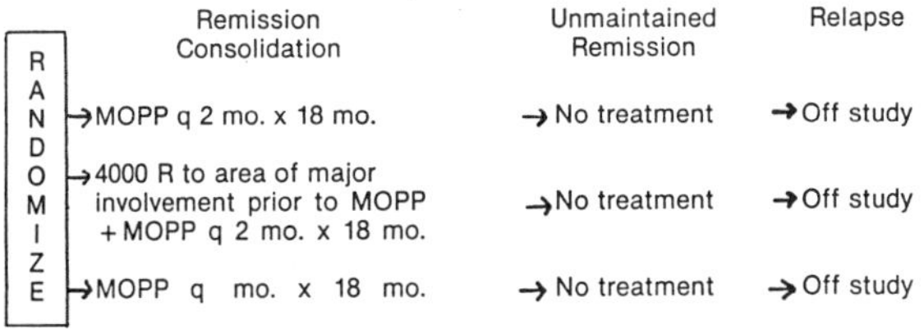

Fig. 2. MOPP versus MOPP plus bleomycin, consolidation (SWOG 775).

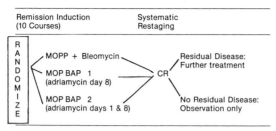

Fig. 3. MOPP plus low-dose bleomycin versus MOPP plus low-dose bleomycin plus doxorubicin (SWOG 7406).

and Jones (1978), Hodgkin's disease was identified in 12% of the patients thought to be in clinical complete remission who subsequently underwent systematic restaging. It also differed from all previous SWOG studies in that patients who were documented to have complete remission based on systematic restaging were followed in unmaintained remission until relapse. Finally, while the initial MOPP plus low-dose bleomycin study (SWOG 774) excluded patients with significant compromise of pulmonary function, that group was not excluded from this study (SWOG 7406), but patients with compromised cardiac function were.

D. MOPP plus Low-Dose Bleomycin versus MOPP plus Low-Dose Bleomycin plus Radiotherapy (SWOG 7518)

This study differed from the previous two studies in that all patients underwent an exploratory laparotomy to establish pathologic stage IIIA or stage IIIB Hodgkin's disease. Patients had not previously received chemotherapy or radiotherapy. Patients were treated with MOPP LDB for 10 cycles or MOPP LDB for three cycles followed by total nodal radiotherapy (Fig. 4). All complete

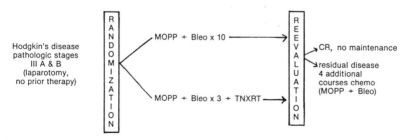

Fig. 4. MOPP plus low-dose bleomycin versus MOPP plus low-dose bleomycin plus radiotherapy (SWOG 7518).

remissions were documented by systematic restaging. Total nodal radiotherapy consisted of an upper mantle and inverted Y beginning 4 weeks after completion of the chemotherapy.

Radiotherapy requirements included (1) supervoltage radiation equipment of a minimum energy of 2.0 MeV, (2) central-axis and off-axis tumor measurements, (3) beam verification films, (4) tumor dosage of 150 to 200 rad/day and a total of 4000 to 4500 rad during 4 to 6 weeks, and (5) monitoring of each institution for individual dose measurements and calculations by the Radiological Physics Center.

The major or dominant involvement prior to chemotherapy was the first area to be treated with radiotherapy. The usual sequence was upper mantle, then inverted Y, designed as a single field or fractionated into an upper periaortic and splenic pedicle and a lower pelvic femoral area, if there had been poor tolerance to chemotherapy and slow hematologic recovery. Radiotherapy was interrupted if the white blood count was less than 2000/liter or the platelet count was less than 50,000/liter. Upon completion of treatment on both arms of the study, patients were followed in unmaintained remission at 3-month intervals for 2 years and 6-month intervals for 5 years, or until relapse or death.

III. RESULTS

A. MOPP versus MOPP plus Bleomycin (SWOG 774)

Between 1971 and 1974, a total of 215 evaluable patients were assigned randomly to treatment in this four-arm study (Fig. 1). After 42 case entries into each arm of study, we identified three successive patients on the high-dose bleomycin limb (10 U/m^2 on days 1 and 8) who developed irreversible myelosuppression. That arm of the study was discontinued immediately. At approximately the same time, because the complete response rate of the MOPP alone limb was comparable to previous experience in patients treated with MOPP alone (Frei *et al.*, 1973; Coltman *et al.*, 1973) and it was unlikely for the complete response rate to reach the level of MOPP plus low-dose bleomycin, the MOPP alone limb was discontinued. MOPP LDB was continued as a single arm, although patients who showed significant compromise of pulmonary function continued to receive MOPP alone. This was done in an attempt to firmly establish the complete response rate. Table I shows the complete response rate for the four arms of the study. MOPP LDB had a substantially higher complete response rate, but it was not statistically significantly higher than MOPP alone ($p = .06$). The complete response rate for patients treated on the compromised pulmonary function (CPF) limb of the study (MOPP CPF) was 70%.

Survival of patients treated with MOPP LDB was above the other three curves,

TABLE I RESPONSE RATE OF MOPP VERSUS MOPP
PLUS BLEOMYCIN COMBINATIONS (SWOG 774)

Regimen	Number of patients	Number of CRs (%)
MOPP	42	30 (71)
MOPP LDB	111	94 (85)
MOPP HDB	35	29 (82)
MOPP CPF	27	19 (70)

Comparison	p
MOPP versus MOPP LDB	.06
MOPP versus MOPP HDB	.24
MOPP versus MOPP CPF	.92
Overall	.16

but the differences were not statistically significant (Fig. 5). The median follow-up of surviving cases was 80 months.

Survival curves for the three arms of the remission consolidation portion of the study are shown in Fig. 6. They begin from the time of randomization to consolidation. There were no statistically significant differences among the three

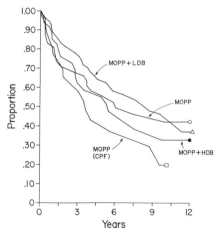

Fig. 5. Survival of MOPP versus MOPP plus bleomycin survival (SWOG 774). MOPP versus MOPP + HDB: $p = .986$.

Total	Fail	Median			
42	22	72	○	MOPP	} $p = .282$
111	54	100	△	MOPP + low BLEO	
35	19	64	●	MOPP + high BLEO	} $p = .436$
27	17	42	□	MOPP (CPF)	

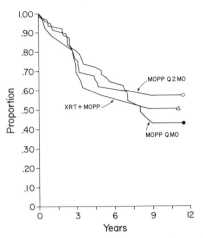

Fig. 6. Survival of MOPP versus MOPP plus bleomycin, consolidation survival (SWOG 775). MOPP q 2 mo. versus MOPP q mo.: $p_{\text{GEHAN}} = .464$.

Total	Fail	Median			
64	24	106+	○	MOPP q 2 mo.	$\Big\} p = .393$
26	12	104+	△	XRT + MOPP	
58	28	95	●	MOPP q mo.	$\Big\} p = .828$

arms of the study ($p = .614$). Second malignancy in this study occurred in 14 of 215 patients (6.5%), and all occurred during complete remission. Ten of the 14 patients died of acute nonlymphocytic leukemia.

B. MOPP plus Low-Dose Bleomycin versus MOPP plus Low-Dose Bleomycin plus Doxorubicin (SWOG 7406)

A total of 281 evaluable patients were randomized between the two arms of this study (Fig. 3). Between the two treatment groups, there were imbalances in various patient characteristics, with the MOPP LDB group containing fewer ambulatory and asymptomatic patients (19 versus 31%), fewer nodular sclerosis cases (48 versus 61%), more clinical stage IV cases (66 versus 49%), more pathologic stage IVB cases (59 versus 43%), and more patients with positive bone-marrow biopsies (35 versus 21%). These imbalances generally favor the MOP BAP group and make overall comparisons of induction treatment somewhat difficult to interpret.

Sixty-six percent of the MOPP-bleomycin cases and 77% of the MOP BAP cases achieved complete remission, which was a statistically significant difference ($p = .024$, one-sided test) (Table II). The difference between the two complete response rates is slightly exaggerated in terms of what might have

TABLE II   RESPONSE RATE OF MOPP PLUS LOW-DOSE
BLEOMYCIN VERSUS MOPP PLUS LOW-DOSE BLEOMYCIN
PLUS DOXORUBICIN (SWOG 7406)

Regimen	Number of patients	Number of CRs (%)
MOPP LDB	121	80 (66)
MOPP BAP	160	124 (77)

Comparison	p (One-sided)
MOPP LDB versus MOP BAP	.024

resulted had the two treatment groups been completely balanced in patient characteristics. However, none of the imbalances has caused a bias of more than 2% of the complete response rate, and the imbalances are not sufficient to change the basic conclusion that MOP BAP is associated with a higher complete response rate than is MOPP LDB.

In previous reports (Jones *et al.*, 1983), it has been noted that there is some tendency for the superiority of MOP BAP chemotherapy to be concentrated in subgroups of favorable prognosis. MOP BAP produced higher complete response rates than MOPP LDB among patients with a hemoglobin of greater than 12, performance status of 70 to 100, absence of bone-marrow involvement, those older than 40 years of age, those who were asymptomatic, and those without prior therapy. However, there are exceptions, and a recent analysis shows that the complete response rate for MOPP–bleomycin in patients who are pathologic stage IVB is 56% compared with 70% among MOP BAP patients.

There is no difference in complete remission duration between the two arms of the study ($p= .31$) (Fig. 7). Because of the higher complete response rate, the relapse-free survival favors MOP BAP ($p= .021$) (Fig. 8), but there is no significant difference in overall survival ($p= .073$) (Fig. 9).

Comparison of MOPP LDB in SWOG 774 and in SWOG 7406 is fraught with hazard because the former excluded patients with significant pulmonary function compromise and the latter excluded patients with significant heart disease. However, a comparison of survival of MOPP LDB patients from 774 and 7406 and MOP BAP patients shows no significant differences in survival ($p= .327$) (Fig. 10).

An analysis of the three successive SWOG studies involving MOPP or its variants (SWOG 772, SWOG 774, and SWOG 7406) has examined the impact of the treatment regimens on survival based on histologic disease types. This analysis combined the MOPP patients from 772 and 774 and the MOPP LDB patients from 774 and 7406, and compared them with the MOP BAP patients

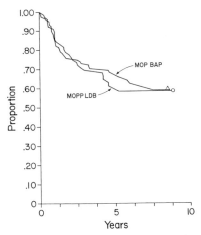

Fig. 7. Complete remission duration of MOPP plus low-dose bleomycin versus MOPP plus low-dose bleomycin plus doxorubicin (SWOG 7406).

5-Year rates (SE)		Total	Fail	75%			
61.1%	(5.9%)	80	29	26	○	MOPP BLEO	$p = .31$
68.4%	(4.3%)	124	42	30	△	MOP BAP	

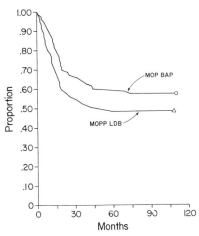

Fig. 8. Relapse-free survival of MOPP plus low-dose bleomycin versus MOPP plus low-dose bleomycin plus doxorubicin (SWOG 7406).

5-Year rates (SE)		Total	Fail	75%			
48.3%	(4.7%)	121	60	11	○	MOPP BLEO	$p = .021$
59.7%	(4.1%)	160	62	17	△	MOP BAP	

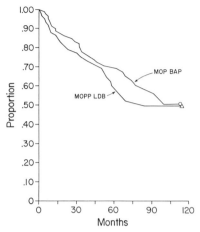

Fig. 9. Survival of MOPP plus low-dose bleomycin versus MOPP plus low-dose bleomycin plus doxorubicin (SWOG 7406).

5-Year rates (SE)	Total	Fail	75%			
58.7% (4.9%)	121	49	33	○	MOPP BLEO	$p = .073$
69.8% (3.8%)	160	57	40	△	MOP BAP	

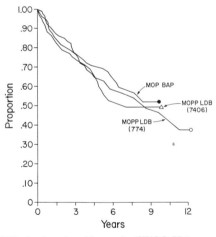

Fig. 10. Survival of MOPP plus low-dose bleomycin (SWOG 774) versus MOPP plus low-dose bleomycin (SWOG 7406) and MOPP plus low-dose bleomycin plus doxorubicin (SWOG 7406). p_{GEHAN} (all groups) = .327.

Total	Fail	Median		
111	54	100	○	MOPP + B (774)
121	50	78	△	MOPP + B (7406)
161	60	100+	●	MOP + BAP

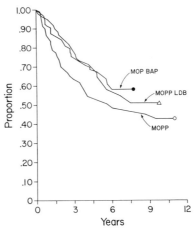

Fig. 11. Survival of MOPP, MOPP plus low-dose bleomycin, and MOPP plus low-dose bleomycin plus doxorubicin (nodular sclerosis cases) (SWOG 772, 774, 7406). MOPP versus MOP BAP: *p* = .013.

Total	Fail	Median			
129	63	68	○	MOPP	
133	50	91+	△	MOPP + LDB $\}$ *p* = .008	
101	34	72+	●	MOP + BAP $\}$ *p* > .05	

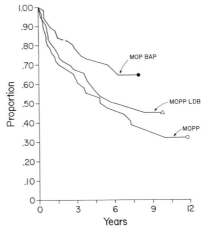

Fig. 12. Survival of MOPP, MOPP plus low-dose bleomycin, and MOPP plus low-dose bleomycin plus doxorubicin (mixed cellular cases) (SWOG 772, 774, 7406). MOPP versus MOP BAP: *p* = .004.

Total	Fail	Median			
105	54	58	○	MOPP	
109	49	71	△	MOPP + LDB $\}$ *p* = .17	
59	17	76+	●	MOP + BAP $\}$ *p* = .022	

from 7406. Because there were no substantial differences between the survival curves of MOPP alone and MOPP plus high-dose bleomycin, those curves were combined. In nodular sclerosis cases, MOPP LDB and MOP BAP are comparable in terms of patient survival ($p > .50$) and significantly superior to MOPP alone ($p = .013$) (Fig. 11).

For mixed cellular cases, the MOPP and MOPP LDB cases have similar survival curves ($p = .17$), and both are significantly worse than the MOP BAP curve ($p = .004$ and $p = .022$, respectively) (Fig. 12).

C. MOPP plus Low-Dose Bleomycin versus MOPP plus Low-Dose Bleomycin plus Radiotherapy (SWOG 7518)

Between 1975 and 1980, a total of 117 evaluable patients were randomized to the two arms of this study. As shown in Table III, the complete response rates were 89% for MOPP LDB and 96% for MOPP LDB + XRT ($p = .480$). Figure 13 shows relapse-free survival by treatment for all eligible patients. There is no significant trend ($p = .30$) for later relapses in the MOPP LDB + XRT group. In patients with nodular sclerosis histology (Fig. 14), there is a trend in favor of MOPP LDB + XRT ($p = .051$). However, no relapses have been reported among patients in the MOPP LDB group after 18 months, compared with 3 in the MOPP LDB + XRT group. There is no difference in survival between the two groups ($p = .48$) (Fig. 15).

IV. DISCUSSION

The Southwest Oncology Group has conducted a series of studies in patients with advanced Hodgkin's disease using MOPP alone for remission induction (Frei *et al.*, 1973; Coltman *et al.*, 1973; Coltman *et al.*, 1978). The complete

TABLE III RESPONSE RATE OF MOPP PLUS LOW-DOSE BLEOMYCIN VERSUS MOPP PLUS LOW-DOSE BLEOMYCIN PLUS XRT (SWOG 7518)

Regimen	Number of patients	Number of CR (%)
MOPP LDB × 10	64	57 (89)
MOPP LDB × 3 + XRT	53	51 (96)

Comparison	p (Two-sided)
MOPP LDB versus MOPP LDB + XRT	.480

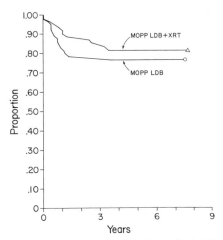

Fig. 13. Relapse-free survival of MOPP plus low-dose bleomycin (×10) versus MOPP plus low-dose bleomycin (×3) plus radiotherapy (SWOG 7518).

5-Year rate (SE)	Total	Fail	75%		
77% 5.1	68	15	43+	○	MOPP BLEO
81% 4.9	65	11	42+	△	MOPP BLEO RT

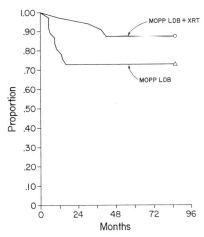

Fig. 14. Relapse-free survival (nodular sclerosis cases) of MOPP plus low-dose bleomycin (×10) versus MOPP plus low-dose bleomycin (×3) plus radiotherapy (SWOG 7518).

Total	Fail	75%		
37	10	14	○	MOPP BLEO
33	4	42+	△	MOPP BLEO RT

$\left.\begin{array}{c} \\ \end{array}\right\} p = .051$

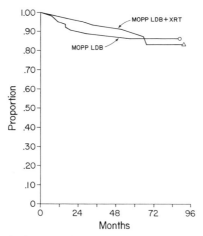

Fig. 15. Survival of MOPP plus low-dose bleomycin (×10) versus MOPP plus low-dose bleomycin (×3) plus radiotherapy (SWOG 7518).

5-Year rate (SE)		Total	Fail	75%			
86%	4.6%	68	8	57+	○	MOPP BLEO	$p = .48$
91%	3.8%	65	7	68+	△	MOPP BLEO RT	

response rate of 62% among 294 patients, with a median survival reached at 7 years, is of the same magnitude as results achieved by other cooperative groups. When bleomycin—a relatively nonmyelosuppressive compound—was identified as having activity alone in 37% of heavily pretreated patients with Hodgkin's disease, it seemed logical to add it to the myelosuppressive regimen of MOPP in an attempt to improve the overall complete response rate and survival. The initial study, which excluded patients with significant compromise of pulmonary function, demonstrated suggestive, but not statistically significant, evidence that low-dose bleomycin added to MOPP enhanced the complete response rate and survival when compared with MOPP alone. However, high-dose bleomycin combined with MOPP was associated with unacceptable myelosuppression that may or may not have been related to bleomycin. It is clear, though, that bleomycin is relatively nonmyelosuppressive.

Since the release of the preliminary data on MOPP plus low-dose bleomycin, two additional studies have employed the same regimen. The British National Lymphoma Trials Investigation compared MOPP alone with MOPP plus low-dose bleomycin in 139 patients, and while the MOPP plus low-dose bleomycin complete response rate was higher (65%) than MOPP (52%), the difference was not statistically significant (Goldman, 1981). Glick et al. (1984) employed MOPP plus low-dose bleomycin for six cycles of remission induction in a regimen that was followed by ABVD as an alternating non–cross-resistant combination chemotherapy. A complete response rate of 59% among 232 patients was achieved with the regimen.

The remission consolidation regimen of SWOG 774 was designed prior to the Southwest Oncology Group concluding, as others had, that maintenance therapy was of no value in the management of advanced Hodgkin's disease (Coltman et al., 1976). In addition, the role of radiotherapy in this consolidation regimen could not be measured satisfactorily because patients received maintenance MOPP following radiotherapy. Clearly, that part of the study was flawed, but because there were no differences in the three remission consolidation arms of the study, this does not have an impact on the overall message of this remission induction regimen.

The identification of 14 second malignancies, 10 of which were acute leukemia, is relatively high. Patients with these malignancies received excessive amounts of chemotherapy, but apparently that did not increase the risk of acute leukemia (Coltman and Dixon, 1982). The most important factor to increase the risk of acute leukemia development was the age of the patient at the initiation of treatment. Older patients (40 years or beyond) were at significantly increased actuarial risk to develop acute leukemia at 7 years (20.7 ± 6.2%). Bleomycin did not appear to be an important factor in enhancing the risk in this analysis.

SWOG attempted to confirm the low-dose bleomycin regimen by using it as a control arm in the subsequent study (SWOG 7406) and comparing it with the same combination to which doxorubicin was added. We were unable to confirm the high complete response rate of MOPP LDB. The significant imbalances in the potentially important pretreatment prognostic characteristics of the patients involved in the two arms of the study tend to cloud the interpretation, but it remains clear that the complete response rate for the doxorubicin-containing six-drug regimen (MOP BAP) is associated with a higher complete response rate. This is particularly important among patients who have better prognostic characteristics. The increased complete response rate, while translated into an improved relapse-free survival, is not associated with significant enhancement of overall survival ($p = .073$) (Fig. 9). It is not totally legitimate to compare the survival of patients treated with MOPP LDB in the initial study (SWOG 774) with the survival rate of patients in the subsequent study (SWOG 7406) because of the differing pretreatment characteristics and exclusions. However, Fig. 12 shows that there are no statistically significant differences in survival between the two arms of the study and MOP BAP.

While the third study (SWOG 7518) compares MOPP LDB for 10 cycles with MOPP LDB for three cycles plus total nodal radiotherapy, it does not address the role of bleomycin. The high complete response rate in patients with stage III disease on both regimens is impressive, and the observation that more patients with nodular sclerosis histology have relapsed on chemotherapy alone than on combined therapy is important. However, the late relapses among patients treated with the combined modality ultimately may negate that early advantage of the combined modality. This early relapse among patients with nodular sclerosis histology treated by chemotherapy has been reported elsewhere (DeVita *et al.*, 1972; Nissen *et al.*, 1979). Preliminary conclusions suggest that the value of combined modality treatment may be limited to nodular sclerosis histology. The comparison of MOPP, MOPP LDB, and MOP BAP in patients with nodular sclerosis and mixed histology does not tend to corroborate the findings relating to patients with stage III disease (SWOG 7518).

After extensive study of the MOPP plus low-dose bleomycin combination by the Southwest Oncology Group and others, it is not possible to conclude that bleomycin has added substantially to MOPP combination chemotherapy in terms of complete response and survival.

REFERENCES

Coltman, C. A., Jr., Frei, E., III, and Delaney, F. C. (1973). *Proc. Am. Soc. Clin. Oncol.* **9,** 78.

Coltman, C. A., Frei, E., III, and Moon, T. E. (1976). *Proc. Am. Soc. Clin. Oncol.* **17,** 300.

Coltman, C. A., Jr., Jones, S. E., Grozea, P. N., De Persio, E., and Moon, T. E. (1978). *In* "Bleomycin[:] Current Status and New Developments" (S. K. Carter, S. T. Crooke, and H. Umezawa, eds.), pp. 227–242. Academic Press, New York.

Coltman, C. A., Jr. (1980). *Sem. Oncol.* **7,** 155.

Coltman, C. A., Jr., and Dixon, D. O. (1982). *Cancer Treat. Rep.* **66,** 1023–1033.

DeVita, V. T., Serpick, A. A., and Carbone, P. P. (1970). *Ann. Intern. Med.* **73,** 881–895.

DeVita, V. T., Canellos, G. P., and Moxley, J. H. (1972). *Cancer* **30,** 1495–1504.

Frei, E., III, Luce, J. K., Gambie, J. F., Coltman, C. A., Jr., Constanzi, J. J., Talley, R. W., Monto, R. W., Wilson, H. E., Hewlett, J. S., Delaney, F. C., and Gehan, E. A. (1973). *Ann. Intern. Med.* **79,** 367–382.

Gehan, E. A. (1965). *Biometrika* **52,** 203.

Glick, J., Tsiatis, A., Prosnitz, L., Rubin, P., and Bennett, J. (1984). *Proc. Am. Soc. Clin. Oncol.* **3,** 237.

Goldman, J. M. (1981). *Clin. Radiol.* **32,** 531–536.

Grozea, P. N., De Persio, E. J., Coltman, C. A., Jr., Fabian, C. J., Morrison, F. S., Gehan, E. A., and Jones, S. E. (1982). *Recent Res. in Cancer Res.* **80,** 83–91.

Haas, C. D., Coltman, C. A., Jr., Gotlieb, J. A., Haut, A., Luce, J. K., Tally, R. W., Samal, B., Wilson, H. E., and Hoogstraten, B. (1976). *Cancer* **38,** 8–12.

Herman, T. S., and Jones, S. E. (1978). *Cancer* **42,** 1976–1981.

Jones, S. E., Haut, A. M., Weick, J. K., Wilson, H. E., Grozea, P., Fabian, C., McKelvey, E., Byrne, G. E., Hartsock, R., Dixon, D. O., and Coltman, C. A., Jr. (1983). *Cancer* **51,** 1339–1347.

Kaplan, E. L., and Meier, P. (1958). *J. Am. Stat. Assoc.* **53,** 456.

Nissen, N. I., Pajak, T. F., Glidewell, O., Pedersen-Bjergaard, J., Stutzman, L., Falkson, G., Cuttner, J., Blom, J., Leone, L., Sawitsky, A., Coleman, M., Haurani, F., Spurr, C. L., Harley, J. B., Seligman, B., Cornell, C., Jr., Henry, P., Senn, H., Brunner, K., Martz, G., Maurice, P., Bank, A., Shapiro, L., James, G. W., and Holland, J. F. (1979). *Cancer* **43,** 31–40.

Peto, R., Pike, M. C., Armitage, P., Breslow, N. E., Cox, D. R., Howard, S. V., Mantel, N., McPherson, K., Peto, J., and Smith, P. G. (1977). *Br. J. Cancer* **35,** 1.

Bleomycin Chemotherapy
(B. I. Sikic, M. Rozencweig, and S. K. Carter, eds.)

Chapter 12

COMBINED-MODALITY STUDIES IN THE TREATMENT OF HODGKIN'S DISEASE

Richard T. Hoppe

Department of Radiology
Division of Radiation Therapy
Stanford University School of Medicine
Stanford, California

I. BACKGROUND

The management of Hodgkin's disease provides an ideal opportunity to exploit the potential benefits of combined-modality therapy because both radiation therapy and chemotherapy are curative in this disease. The curative potential of radiation therapy in Hodgkin's disease was demonstrated more than two decades before this writing (Kaplan, 1980). The impact of chemotherapy was demonstrated by investigators from the National Cancer Institute in the late 1960s (DeVita *et al.*, 1970).

In addition, the pattern of failure for patients treated with each modality is different. Patients who relapse after radiation treatment for early-stage Hodgkin's disease most often fail in contiguous unirradiated lymph nodes or in unirradiated extralymphatic sites (Kaplan, 1980). In contrast, patients with advanced-stage disease treated with combination chemotherapy most often exhibit failure in sites of initial involvement, usually sites of bulky lymphadenopathy (Young *et al.*, 1978).

The potential benefit of combined-modality therapy was apparent to many investigators in the late 1960s and early 1970s. Combined-modality therapy could exploit the concept of "spatial cooperation," with radiation therapy providing the primary component of control for local disease and chemotherapy treating occult sites of involvement. In addition, improved local control of disease could be expected by combining these two effective modalities.

Some investigators began to use combined-modality therapy in the context of well-designed clinical trials, in an effort to prove the superiority of the combined-modality approach over the use of either modality alone. Initial enthusiasm was tempered with the identification of long-term complications of therapy, which occurred more frequently in combined-modality programs. Because of these complications, the significance of randomized clinical trials became even more important: only by analyzing data from these trials could accurate statements about the relative efficacy and toxicity of combined-modality versus single-modality treatment programs be made. Therefore, although numerous reports have appeared in the literature describing results of combined-modality therapy in all stages of Hodgkin's disease, this chapter will address primarily data reported from prospective, randomized clinical trials.

II. PROSPECTIVE CLINICAL TRIALS

A. Stage I to Stage II Disease

Several large studies have examined combined-modality therapy in stage I to stage II Hodgkin's disease, as summarized in Table I (Anderson et al., 1984; Jones et al., 1982; LYGRA, 1984; Wiernik et al., 1979). These trials share many design concepts. For example, patients treated with combined-modality therapy received the entire course of irradiation first and the drugs were used purely as adjuvant therapy. The drug combination in these trials was always MOPP (nitrogen mustard, vincristine, procarbazine, prednisone) or MVPP (vinblastine substituted for vincristine). However, the results are not strictly comparable to each other, since criteria for patient selection and the extent of the radiation fields varied.

Data from these trials are mature, with follow-up ranging from 7 to 15 years, and remarkably similar general conclusions can be drawn from each study. In every instance, there was an improved freedom from relapse in the combined-modality group. This improvement ranged from 9 to 25%, and in nearly every instance the difference was statistically significant. However, despite the improvement in freedom from relapse, no trial showed a significant survival benefit with combined-modality therapy. In fact, in some studies survival among patients treated with combined therapy was not superior to irradiation.

TABLE I COMBINED-MODALITY THERAPY TRIALS: STAGE I TO STAGE II HODGKIN'S DISEASE

Study	Treatment[a]	Number of patients	Freedom from relapse (%)[b]	Survival (%)[b]	Follow-up
Baltimore Cancer Research Program (Wiernik et al., 1979)	EFI	29	69 } p = .04	86 } p = .4	7-year data
	EFI + MOPP	17	94	100	
Danish National Study Group (LYGRA, 1984)	TNI	159	62 } p = .001	82 } p = .84	11-year data
	Mantle + MOPP	158	86	90	
Manchester Lymphoma Group (Anderson et al., 1984)	Mantle	55	69 } p = .002	94 } p = .54	8-year data
	Mantle + MVPP	59	93	91	
Southwest Oncology Group (SWOG) (Jones et al., 1982)	EFI	115	71 } p = .12	85	8-year data
	IFI + MOPP	120	80	82	
Stanford Adjuvant MOPP Trials	STLI, TLI	108	72 } p = .06	74 } p = .86	15-year data
	IFI, STLI, or TLI + MOPP	112	82	75	

[a]IFI, Involved-field irradiation; EFI, extended-field irradiation; STLI, subtotal lymphoid irradiation; TLI, total lymphoid irradiation; TNI, total nodal irradiation; MOPP, nitrogen mustard, vincristine, procarbazine, and prednisone; MVPP, nitrogen mustard, vinblastine, procarbazine, and prednisone.
[b]In some instances, data were estimated from published curves.

A more complete analysis of the Stanford data, which included 220 patients, is shown in Fig. 1. The primary explanation for the lack of a survival benefit among patients treated with combined-modality therapy is that patients who relapsed after initial treatment with irradiation alone had a 50–60% likelihood of salvage after subsequent management with MOPP. This is reflected in the freedom from second relapse. In addition, there were more deaths from treatment-related toxicity among patients treated with the combined modalities.

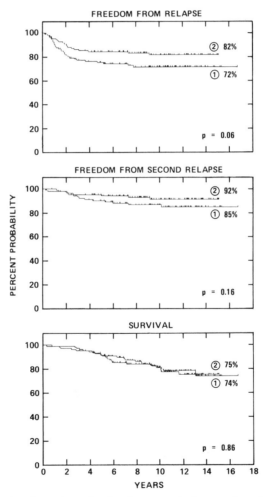

Fig. 1. Current freedom from relapse, freedom from second relapse, and survival of 220 patients with stage I to stage II Hodgkin's disease treated on the Stanford Adjuvant MOPP trials: 1, irradiation alone (108 patients); 2, irradiation plus adjuvant MOP(P) (112 patients).

TABLE II   COMBINED-MODALITY THERAPY AT STANFORD: STAGE I TO STAGE II
HODGKIN'S DISEASE

Mediastinal involvement	Treatment[a]	Number of patients	10-Year freedom from relapse (%)	10-Year survival (%)
Uninvolved	STLI or TLI	37	84	83
	XRT + CHX	37	89	93
$<\frac{1}{3}$	STLI or TLI	49	84	83
	XRT + CHX	50	84	85
$>\frac{1}{3}$	STLI or TLI	14	$\left.\begin{matrix}45\\81\end{matrix}\right\} p = .03$	84
	XRT + CHX	27		74

[a]XRT, Irradiation (involved-field, subtotal lymphoid, or total lymphoid irradiation); CHX, chemotherapy (MOPP or PAVe); STLI, subtotal lymphoid irradiation; TLI, total lymphoid irradiation.

In an effort to define more clearly those patients who might benefit from combined-modality therapy, we analyzed the pretreatment characteristics of patients treated in the Stanford clinical trials (Hoppe *et al.*, 1982). Many prognostic factors were examined, but the only one that had a substantial effect on outcome and helped to identify patients likely to benefit from combined-modality therapy was the presence of extensive mediastinal involvement (Table II). A large mediastinal mass was defined as one with a transverse diameter exceeding one-third of the maximum intrathoracic diameter. Patients with an uninvolved mediastinum or a small mediastinal mass achieved a similar survival and relapse-free rate, whether treated with irradiation alone or combined modality therapy. However, for patients with a large mediastinal mass, the freedom from relapse was significantly better for combined-modality therapy as compared with irradiation alone (81 versus 45% at 10 years, $p = .03$). Despite this substantial and significant difference in freedom from relapse, though, patients treated with combined-modality therapy did not have an improved survival (10-year survival: 74% for combined modality therapy, 84% for irradiation alone). Again, this was attributable to the efficacy of salvage chemotherapy if initial irradiation was unsuccessful.

B. Stage IIIA Disease

Several trials that have been reported for stage IIIA disease employed the same treatment options as for stage I to stage II (Table III). Both the Baltimore Cancer Research Program and the Stanford Adjuvant MOPP Trials compared treatment

TABLE III COMBINED-MODALITY THERAPY TRIALS: STAGE IIIA HODGKIN'S DISEASE

Study	Treatment[a]		Number of patients	Freedom of relapse (%)[b]	Survival (%)[b]	Follow-up
Baltimore Center Research Program (Wiernik et al., 1979)	EFI		12	58 } $p = .018$	57 } $p = .029$	6-year data
	EFI + MOPP		16	94	100	
Cancer and Leukemia Group B (CALGB) (Bloomfield et al., 1982)	TNI	(A)	29	39		
	BOPP	(B)	34	25 } $p = .03$		5-year data
	BOPP + TNI	(C)	26	46 } (A + B + C vs. D)		
	TNI + BOPP	(D)	25	84		
Manchester Lymphoma Group (Anderson et al., 1984)	MVPP		26	82	88	5-year data
	MVPP + IFI		30	80	85	
Stanford Adjuvant MOPP Trials	TLI		35	70 } $p = .08$	63 } $p = .05$	15-year data
	TLI + MOPP		24	87	82	

[a]MOPP, Nitrogen mustard, vincristine, procarbazine, and prednisone; MVPP, nitrogen mustard, vinblastine, procarbazine, and prednisone; BOPP, BCNU, vincristine, procarbazine, and prednisone; EFI, extended-field irradiation; TNI, total nodal irradiation; IFI, involved-field irradiation; TLI, total lymphoid irradiation.

[b]In some instances, data were estimated from published curves.

with irradiation alone (extended field or total lymphoid irradiation, respectively) and a similar extent of irradiation followed by adjuvant MOPP. Although the number of patients in these trials was smaller than in those for earlier stage disease, both trials showed a substantial improvement in freedom from relapse when using the combined-modality approach. Unlike the trials for stage I to stage II disease, a significant survival benefit also could be demonstrated for the combined-modality approach.

In the Stanford series, the 15-year freedom-from-relapse rate for patients treated with irradiation alone was 70%. In view of this outcome, it did not seem logical to treat all patients with combined-modality therapy. An analysis of pretreatment prognostic factors was undertaken. One clinical feature had a significant effect on outcome in the total lymphoid irradiation (TLI) group: the extent of splenic involvement (Table IV) (Hoppe et al., 1980). Extensive splenic involvement was defined as the presence of five or more nodules visible in the splenectomy specimen. Patients with minimal splenic involvement had a 10-year freedom-from-relapse rate of 80 or 85% after treatment with irradiation alone or combined-modality therapy. The corresponding 10-year survival rates were 82 and 83%. Therefore, no benefit of the combined-modality approach was apparent for those patients. On the other hand, patients with extensive splenic involvement had a 10-year freedom-from-relapse rate of 34 or 89% for the two different treatment approaches ($p = .001$) and a 10-year survival of 60 and 92%, respectively ($p = .1$), indicating a clear superiority of the combined-modality approach.

Other investigators have identified different prognostic factors that may be important in predicting outcome of stage IIIA disease. For example, the location of disease in the upper or lower abdomen (anatomic substage) may identify a group of patients likely to benefit from combined-modality therapy (Desser et al., 1977). Stage IIIA disease includes a broad spectrum of patients with Hodgkin's disease. Those with limited disease may enjoy a good prognosis with treatment similar to that used for patients with stage I to stage II disease. There-

TABLE IV   COMBINED-MODALITY THERAPY AT STANFORD: STAGE IIIA HODGKIN'S DISEASE

Splenic involvement	Treatment[a]	Number of patients	10-Year freedom from relapse	10-Year survival
Minimal	TLI	46	80	82
	TLI + CHX	46	85	83
Extensive	TLI	39	34 ⎱ $p = .0001$	60 ⎱ $p = .1$
	TLI + CHX	41	89 ⎰	92 ⎰

[a]CHX, MOPP or PAVe; TLI, total lymphoid irradiation.

fore, it is important to know the proportion of patients in each of these prognostic categories assigned to different treatment arms in the prospective trials. Unfortunately, when these studies were initiated, the important prognostic variables had not been identified, and stratified randomization was not employed. All of the trials summarized in Table III suffer from this deficiency.

Two more recent trials in stage IIIA disease have compared chemotherapy alone with combined-modality therapy. The Cancer and Leukemia Group B (CALGB) compared four different treatment programs: total nodal irradiation (TNI), BOPP chemotherapy (BCNU, vincristine, procarbazine, and prednisone), BOPP followed by TNI, and TNI followed by BOPP (Bloomfield *et al.*, 1982). In a previous trial, CALGB had shown that BOPP was equivalent to MOPP in the treatment of advanced-stage disease. The number of stage IIIA disease patients randomized into each arm of this study was not adequate to draw any definitive conclusion. Patients treated on three of the treatment arms had a disappointingly poor freedom-from-relapse rate, including a 5-year freedom-from-relapse in only 25% of those treated with BOPP alone. However, the group of patients treated with TNI followed by BOPP had a 5-year freedom-from-relapse rate of 84%. The freedom from relapse in this group was significantly better than in the other three treatment arms combined ($p = .03$).

A more encouraging result in the treatment of stage IIIA Hodgkin's disease with chemotherapy alone has been reported recently by the Manchester Lymphoma Group (Crowther *et al.*, 1984). In a group of 56 patients randomized to receive treatment with MVPP (nitrogen mustard, vinblastine, procarbazine, and prednisone) or MVPP followed by involved-field irradiation (IFI) (3000 rad), the 5-year freedom-from-relapse rates were 82 and 80%, respectively. Survivals were 88 and 85%, respectively.

C. Stage IIIB to Stage IV Disease

Combined-modality therapy trials in stage IIIB to stage IV disease have varied widely in terms of the types of drugs used, radiation fields and doses, and methods of data reporting. For example, the radiation employed in combined-modality trials has varied from low-dose involved-field irradiation (IFI) to high-dose total lymphoid irradiation (TLI). Freedom-from-relapse and survival rates are reported for some series only as a percentage of the patients who achieved a complete response, whereas in other series all patients are included. An early Stanford trial compared treatment of TLI with TLI followed by MOPP for stage IIIB disease (Horning *et al.*, 1984). In this trial, treatment with irradiation alone was inadequate in these patients: systemic therapy was required. More recent trials in stage IIIB to stage IV are summarized in Tables V and VI.

The details of an early CALBG study were described previously (Bloomfield

TABLE V   COMBINED-MODALITY THERAPY TRIALS: STAGE IIIB TO STAGE IV HODGKIN'S DISEASE (CALGB)

Disease stage	Treatment[b]		CR (%)	Freedom from relapse (%)	Death rate (%)
IIIB	TNI	(A)	60	29[c]	18
	BOPP	(B)	74	23	32
	TNI + BOPP	(C)	79	55	32
	BOPP + TNI	(D)	94	48	47
IIIB–IV	CVPP × 6	(A)	68	61 (% of CR)	26[d]
	CVPP × 12	(B)	59	56 (% of CR)	36
	CVPP × 6 + IFI	(C)	57	56 (% of CR)	34
	CVPP × 3 + IFI + CVPP × 3	(D)	65	65 (% of CR)	14

[a]From Bloomfield et al. (1982).
[b]TNI, Total nodal irradiation; IFI, involved-field irradiation; BOPP, BCNU, vincristine, procarbazine, and prednisone; CVPP CCNU, vincristine, procarbazine, and prednisone.
[c]Significant at $p = .02$ for A + B versus C + D.
[d]Significant at $p = .01$ for A + B + C versus D.

et al., 1982). Stage IIIB single-modality treatment with TNI or BOPP resulted in 5-year freedom-from-relapse rates of only 29 and 23%, respectively. In contrast, the two combined-modality approaches (TNI + BOPP or BOPP + TNI) resulted in freedom-from-relapse rates of 48 and 55%, respectively. The difference in freedom-from-relapse between combined-modality and single-modality therapy was significant ($p = .02$). However, the improved freedom-from-relapse in the combined-modality group did not result in an improved survival.

In a subsequent CALGB study (Bloomfield *et al.*, 1982), which included patients with stage IIIB and stage IV disease, patients were treated either with

TABLE VI   COMBINED MODALITY THERAPY TRIALS: STAGE IIIB TO STAGE IV HODGKIN'S DISEASE

Study	Treatment[a]	CR (%)	Freedom from relapse (% of CR)	Survival (% of CR)
ECOG	Bleo–MOPP + IFI	73	66	83
(Glick *et al.*, 1984)	Bleo–MOPP + ABVD	76	68	92
Stanford University	PAVe/TLI	94	87	92
	PAVe/ABVD	77	66	91

[a]IFI, Involved-field irradiation; TLI, total nodal irradiation; MOPP–Bleo, nitrogen mustard, vincristine, procarbazine, and prednisone; ABVD, doxorubicin, bleomycin, vinblastine, and DTIC; PAVe, procarbazine, melphalan, and vinblastine.

chemotherapy alone (six or 12 courses of CVPP–CCNU, vincristine, procarbazine, and prednisone), CVPP followed by adjuvant IFI (2500 rad), or CVPP sandwiched around IFI (2500 rad). Complete response rates and freedom from relapse for the different treatment modalities were similar. However, the survival rate for patients treated with chemotherapy sandwiched around irradiation was significantly better than the other three treatment programs combined ($p = .01$). The improved outcome in the split-course group compared with the adjuvant irradiation group suggests that the sequence of treatment in combined-modality therapy may be an important variable. A problem with the CALGB trials is that while BOPP and CVPP were reasonable choices of chemotherapy at the time these trials were initiated, these drug regimens do not represent the most effective chemotherapy combinations available today.

Alternating MOPP/ABVD (doxorubicin, bleomycin, vinblastine, and DTIC) chemotherapy has been shown to be superior to MOPP chemotherapy alone in a prospective randomized trial (Santoro et al., 1982). The Eastern Cooperative Oncology Group (ECOG) initiated a trial for advanced-stage disease that incorporates both MOPP and ABVD in its chemotherapy treatment arm (Table VI) (Glick et al., 1984). Patients with stage IIIB to stage IV Hodgkin's disease are treated with six cycles of Bleo–MOPP. If they achieve a partial or complete response, they then are randomized to consolidation therapy with either IFI (1500 to 2000 rad) or three cycles of ABVD chemotherapy. Complete response rates after consolidation therapy were 73 and 76%, respectively. Corresponding freedom-from-relapse rates for patients who achieved a complete response were 66 and 68%, respectively. The 5-year survival rate was 83% after irradiation consolidation and 92% after ABVD consolidation ($p = .01$). This difference was due primarily to late deaths in the radiation treatment group.

At Stanford, following completion of the adjuvant MOPP trials in which chemotherapy was shown to be essential for treating stage IIIB disease, combined-modality therapy was used routinely, and a comparison was made between two different chemotherapy regimens: MOPP and PAVe (procarbazine, melphalan, and vinblastine) (Wolin et al., 1979). As part of the combined-modality treatment program, a policy of alternating chemotherapy and irradiation evolved (Hoppe et al., 1979). Since the toxicities of the two treatment modalities differed and disease potentially resistant to one modality might be sensitive to the other, alternating chemotherapy and irradiation provided an attractive treatment program. A similar rationale was used later in the development of alternating non–cross-resistant chemotherapy programs. The alternating chemotherapy and irradiation program proved vastly superior to our previous experience and was adopted as our standard treatment for stage IIIB to stage IV disease in subsequent clinical trials. Current results for patients with stage IIIB to stage IV disease treated with alternating chemotherapy and irradiation in our prospective clinical trials are summarized in Fig. 2. Since our combined-modality programs for

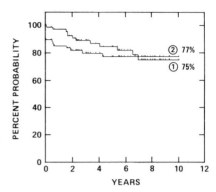

Fig. 2. Current survival (1) and freedom from relapse (2) of 67 patients with advanced-stage Hodgkin's disease (IIIAS++ = 5; IIIB = 49; IV = 13) treated on prospective clinical trials at Stanford with alternating chemotherapy and irradiation. All patients (67) are included in the analysis.

advanced stage disease using PAVe provided equivalent results but less toxicity than MOPP, PAVe was chosen later as our standard chemotherapy combination in this clinical setting.

In our first attempt to compare combined-modality therapy with chemotherapy alone in patients with stage IIIB to stage IV disease, we selected alternating PAVe/TLI as our combined-modality arm and alternating PAVe/ABVD (total of 12 cycles) as the chemotherapy arm (Table VI). Patients also were included who had stage IIIA disease with extensive splenic involvement. In our early experience, patients treated with PAVe/ABVD chemotherapy did poorly, and the study was terminated. In the most recent analysis of data, the 3-year freedom-from-relapse rate for PAVe/ABVD is only 51% and survival is only 75%. In contrast, patients treated with alternating PAVe/TLI achieved a 3-year freedom-from-relapse rate of 81% ($p= .08$) and a 3-year survival rate of 92% ($p= .1$).

III. COMBINED-MODALITY THERAPY IN PEDIATRIC HODGKIN'S DISEASE

An important consideration in the management of pediatric Hodgkin's disease that is not relevant in the adult population is the growth-inhibitory effect of radiation. The doses of radiation necessary to achieve local control will significantly impair growth. Therefore, several institutions have developed combined-modality therapy programs with only low doses of radiation for all stages of pediatric Hodgkin's disease. Results from two of these institutions, Princess Margaret Hospital (Jenkins *et al.*, 1982) and Stanford University, are summarized in Table VII.

At the Princess Margaret Hospital, the standard treatment program avoided laparotomy and used clinical staging only. Patients were treated with three cycles of MOPP, low-dose (2000–3000 rad) extended-field irradiation, and then three

TABLE VII COMBINED-MODALITY THERAPY: PEDIATRIC HODGKIN'S DISEASE

Study	Number of patients	Staging laparotomy	Radiation fields	5-Year freedom from relapse (%)	5-Year survival (%)
Princess Margaret Hospital (Jenkins *et al.*, 1982)	57	No	Extended	82	92
Stanford University	44	Yes	Involved	92	97

more cycles of MOPP. At Stanford, a policy evolved that included routine staging laparotomy followed by combined-modality treatment in which the irradiation was limited to the involved sites and a dose of only 1500 to 2500 rad was used. For patients with stage I to stage II disease, all of the irradiation was administered prior to chemotherapy; however, for patients with more advanced-stage disease, the chemotherapy and irradiation were administered in an alternating fashion, as discussed previously. The chemotherapy used was primarily MOPP, although more recent patients have been treated with alternating MOPP and ABVD. Overall results of the Stanford approach are displayed in Fig. 3. This combined-modality approach has less effect on bone growth than does the use of irradiation alone (Donaldson and Kaplan, 1982). However, other toxicities now have become more prevalent, including sterility problems and secondary acute leukemia.

IV. FUTURE DIRECTIONS

It is likely that the definitive role of combined-modality therapy in the management of Hodgkin's disease will have to be demonstrated in the context of prospective randomized clinical trials. In stage I to stage II disease, radiation therapy provides optimal treatment for the majority of patients, achieving excel-

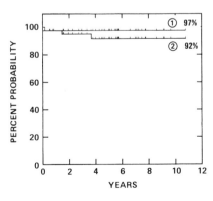

Fig. 3. Current survival (1) and freedom from relapse (2) of 44 children with Hodgkin's disease (all stages) treated with combined-modality therapy (including low-dose irradiation) at Stanford.

lent long-term survival and feedom from relapse. The addition of chemotherapy improves the freedom from relapse somewhat but has no impact on survival. Therefore, any future direction in the use of combined-modality therapy to manage these patients would have to test less toxic chemotherapy programs. At Stanford, for example, we are testing involved-field irradiation followed by VBM (vinblastine, bleomycin, and methotrexate) chemotherapy in patients who have stage I to stage IIA–B or stage IIIA disease without unfavorable prognostic signs and comparing this treatment to the use of irradiation alone. Thus far, the 3-year survival is 100% and the 3-year freedom-from-relapse rate is 91 and 89% for the irradiation and combined-modality groups, respectively. We are measuring treatment toxicities, including pulmonary function and fertility, in the two treatment groups.

In stage I to stage II patients who have large mediastinal masses, combined-modality therapy provides a significantly better freedom from relapse, although survival is not really improved over treatment with radiation alone. Thus, among these patients the least toxic combined-modality programs must be identified. Current Stanford clinical trials for these patients include staging limited to clinical studies plus bone-marrow biopsy (i.e., staging laparotomy is not performed routinely). Patients then are randomized to receive treatment with either PAVe or ABVD chemotherapy, in either instance combined with mantle-field irradiation. Among the patients randomized in this study, the 3-year survival thus far is 89%, and the 3-year freedom-from-relapse rate is 77%. There is no difference favoring either PAVe or ABVD chemotherapy, and studies are in progress to determine potential differences in toxicity, including effects on cardiac and pulmonary function and fertility. A similar approach is being used in clinical trials at the National Cancer Institute, where all patients with bulky stages I to II disease are treated with alternating MOPP/ABVD sandwiched around mantle-field irradiation.

In stage IIIB to stage IV disease, previous trials have suffered largely from failure to use what is currently considered to be the most effective chemotherapy program for advanced-stage disease—alternating MOPP/ABVD. A current Stanford trial, initiated in 1983, was designed to address this issue. Patients with stage IIIB to stage IV disease are randomized to receive treatment with either alternating PAVe/TLI or alternating MOPP/ABVD. In addition to outcome, these patients will be followed closely for toxicity, including effects on pulmonary and cardiac function, fertility, and secondary malignancy.

REFERENCES

Anderson, H., Deakin, D. P., Wagstaff, J., Jones, J. M., Todd, I. D. H., Wilkinson, P. M., James, R. D., Steward, W. P., Blackledge, G., Scarffe, J. H., and Crowther, D. (1984). *Br. J. Cancer* **49,** 695–702.

Bloomfield, C. D., Pajak, T. F., Glicksman, A. S., Gottlieb, A. J., Coleman, M., Nissen, N. I., Rafla, S., Stutzman, L., Vinciguerra, V., Glidewell, O. J., and Holland, J. F. (1982). *Cancer Treat. Rep.* **66,** 835–846.

Crowther, D., Wagstaff, J., Deakin, D., Todd, I., Wilkinson, P., Anderson, H., Blackledge, G., Jones, M., and Scarffe, J. H. (1984). *J. Clin. Oncol.* **2** 892–897.

Desser, R. K., Golomb, H. M., Ultmann, J. E., Ferguson, D. J., Moran, E. M., Griem, M. L., Kinzie, J. J., and Blough, R. (1977). *Blood* **49,** 883–893.

DeVita, V. T., Serpick, A. A., and Carbone, P. P. (1970). *Ann. Intern. Med.* **73,** 881–895.

Donaldson, S. S., and Kaplan, H. S. (1982). *Cancer Treat. Rep.* **66,** 977–989.

Glick, J., Tsiatis, A., Prosnitz, L., Rubin, P., and Bennett, J. (1984). *Proc. Am. Soc. Clin. Oncol.* **3,** 237.

Hoppe, R. T., Portlack, C. S., Glatstein, E., Rosenberg, S. A., and Kaplan, H. S. (1979). *Cancer* **43,** 472–481.

Hoppe, R. T., Rosenberg, S. A., Kaplan, H. S., and Cox, R. S. (1980). *Cancer* **46,** 1240–1246.

Hoppe, R. T., Coleman, C. N., Cox, R. S., Rosenberg, S. A., and Kaplan, H. S. (1982). *Blood* **59,** 455–465.

Horning, S. J., Hoppe, R. T., and Rosenberg, S. A. (1984). *In* "Adjuvant Therapy of Cancer" (S. E. Jones, and S. E. Salmon, eds.), Vol. IV. Grune & Stratton, Orlando.

Jenkins, D., Chan, H., Freedman, M., Greenberg, M., Gribbin, M., McClure, P., Saunders, F., and Sonley, M. (1982). *Cancer Treat. Rep.* **66,** 949–959.

Jones, S. E., Coltman, C. A., Grozea, P. N., DePersio, E. J., and Dixon, D. O. (1982). *Cancer Treat. Rep.* **66,** 847–853.

Kaplan, H. S. (1980). "Hodgkin's Disease" 2nd. Ed. Harvard University Press, Cambridge Massachusetts.

"LYGRA Report 17" (1984). Denmark.

Santoro, A., Bonadonna, G., Bonfante, V., and Valagussa, P. (1982). *N. Engl. J. Med.* **306,** 770–775.

Wiernik, P. H., Gustafson, J., Schimpff, S. C., and Diggs, C. (1979). *Am. J. Med.* **67,** 183–192.

Wolin, E. M., Rosenberg, S. A., and Kaplan, H. S. (1979). *In* "Adjuvant Therapy of Cancer" (S. E. Jones, and S. E. Salmon, eds.), Vol. II. pp. 119–127. Grune & Stratton, New York.

Young, R. C., Canellos, G. P., Chabner, B. A., Hubbard, S. M., and DeVita, V. T. (1978). *Cancer* **42,** 1001–1007.

Bleomycin Chemotherapy
(B. I. Sikic, M. Rozencweig, and S. K. Carter, eds.)

Chapter 13

THE NON-HODGKIN'S LYMPHOMAS: AN OVERVIEW

Sandra J. Horning

Department of Medicine
Division of Oncology
Stanford University School of Medicine
Stanford, California

The non-Hodgkin's lymphomas (NHLs) are a group of lymphoid neoplasms with diverse morphologic, clinical, and immunologic features. The morphologic diversity of the NHL has been appreciated by pathologists for many years, leading to multiple classification systems. The Rappaport classification gained wide acceptance because of its reproducibility and clinical relevance (Rappaport, 1966). In this system, the lymphomas are classified by architectural pattern as nodular or diffuse, and the cytologic characteristics are described as well or poorly differentiated lymphocytic, histiocytic, mixed histiocytic, and lymphocytic or undifferentiated. The Rappaport system required subsequent revision to acknowledge two new clinicopathologic entities, Burkitt's tumor and lymphoblastic lymphoma. In addition, recognition that most of the "histiocytic" malignancies were composed of large, transformed lymphocytes and that all nodular lymphomas originated in follicular or germinal centers challenged the scientific accuracy of the classification. These considerations, together with modern concepts of the immune system that characterize the NHL as neoplasms of T, B, or monocyte–histiocyte lineage, led to the development of multiple pathologic classifications. The major classifications include the Lukes and Collins, Kiel,

Dorfman, British National Lymphoma Group, and the World Health Organization, in addition to that of Rappaport.

In 1979, the National Cancer Institute (NCI) sponsored a project to devise a working formulation to facilitate translation among these six major histopathologic classifications (The Non-Hodgkin's Lymphoma Pathologic Classification Project, 1982). An international group of six expert pathologists agreed on a Working Formulation based on morphology alone (Table I). Ten major categories are recognized and grouped prognostically, based upon survival, as low, intermediate, or high grade. This overview discusses the clinical features of the NHLs according to histologic grade.

I. LOW-GRADE LYMPHOMAS

The low-grade lymphomas include small lymphocytic, follicular small cleaved cell, and follicular mixed small cleaved and large cell (diffuse well-differentiated lymphocytic, nodular poorly differentiated lymphocytic, and nodular mixed in the Rappaport classification). The low-grade lymphomas characteristically are advanced in stage at diagnosis. Following pathologic staging, ~80% or more are

TABLE I   A WORKING FORMULATION OF NON-HODGKIN'S LYMPHOMA

Working formulation	Rappaport equivalents
Low grade	
Small lymphocytic	Well-differentiated lymphocytic
Follicular, predominantly small cleaved cell	Nodular poorly differentiated lymphocytic
Follicular, mixed small cleaved and large cell	Nodular mixed lymphocytic–histiocytic
Intermediate grade	
Follicular, predominantly large cell	Nodular histiocytic
Diffuse small cleaved cell	Diffuse poorly differentiated lymphocytic
Diffuse mixed small and large cell	Diffuse mixed lymphocytic–histiocytic
Diffuse large cell (cleaved/noncleaved)	Diffuse histiocytic
High grade	
Diffuse large-cell immunoblastic	Diffuse histiocytic
Lymphoblastic (conv/nonconv)[a]	Lymphoblastic (conv/nonconv)[a]
Small noncleaved cell	Diffuse undifferentiated
(Burkitt's/non-Burkitt's)	(Burkitt's/non-Burkitt's)

[a]conv, Convoluted; nonconv, nonconvoluted.

stage III or IV, according to the Ann Arbor criteria. Low-grade lymphomas occur in middle-aged patients, 55–65 years old. At diagnosis, the disease typically involves lymph nodes, spleen, and bone marrow. As the name implies, the low-grade lymphomas have an indolent natural history, with a median survival of 6 to 10 years. They characteristically express B-lymphocyte markers.

The low-grade lymphomas are responsive to a variety of therapeutic approaches. In consecutive randomized trials at Stanford University, 114 stage III and stage IV patients have been treated with either CVP (cyclophosphamide, vincristine, prednisone) combination chemotherapy, CVP and total nodal irradiation (TNI), single-agent cyclophosphamide or chlorambucil, or whole-body irradiation with boosts to involved areas (Hoppe *et al.*, 1981). No significant differences among the various treatment arms were appreciated for either freedom from relapse (FFR) or survival. Histologic type did not affect FFR, although patients with the small lymphocytic subtype survived longer than those in the other two groups, despite a high relapse rate. The combined results in this group of stage III and stage IV patients demonstrated a 5-year survival rate of 76% and a 10-year survival of 55%, with a median survival of 10 to 11 years (Rosenberg, 1985) (Fig. 1). Although the complete remission rate was 65–80%, half of the patients relapsed after 3.5 years of follow-up.

The indolent natural history of recurrent low-grade lymphoma is evident by the low likelihood of cure and good survival. Because patients over 65 years of age were excluded from the Stanford trials and the conservative treatment group did so well, a group of 44 asymptomatic patients gradually accumulated who were managed with no initial therapy (Portlock and Rosenberg, 1979). Given the

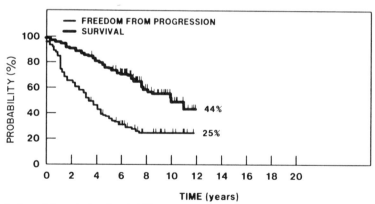

Fig. 1. Actuarial survival and probability of freedom from relapse in 114 patients with advanced-stage, low-grade non-Hodgkin's lymphomas. These are the combined results (as of March 1984) of patients receiving four treatment programs at Stanford University. 5-Year survival, 76%; 10-year survival, 55%; median survival, 10–11 years; relapses, 50% at 3.5 years.

failure to define curative therapy and the indolent nature of the low-grade lymphomas, we now have 83 patients who have been managed with no initial therapy (Horning and Rosenberg, 1984). The overall survival of these selected patients is excellent, with a projected median of 11 years. Patients with the follicular small cleaved subtype have done especially well, with 80% surviving actuarially more than 10 years. However, the majority of these patients will require therapy. Half of the patients in the group had received treatment at 3 years. The three histologic subtypes differ in this regard, with half of the follicular mixed patients requiring therapy by 18 months and the others enjoying significantly longer periods without treatment.

It is difficult to conduct a randomized trial to compare the no-initial-therapy approach with immediate therapy, but we and others are attempting to do so. In retrospective comparisons of our concurrent protocol patients, we see no differences in survival between the no-initial-therapy and protocol groups, even when comparing the 60% of protocol patients who would have been considered eligible for the no-initial-treatment approach (Fig. 2). Series in the literature providing 5-year results of therapy in advanced-stage patients indicate that no reported approach is more curative and none is superior in survival to our group of patients managed without initial therapy (Portlock, 1980).

Radiation therapy may be acceptable treatment for selected patients with low-grade lymphoma. A recent retrospective analysis by Paryani et al. (1984) at Stanford University indicates that selected patients with stage III disease treated with TLI may enjoy extended FFR and good survival. This was especially true among patients with limited disease extent and bulk. Asymptomatic patients with stage III disease also enjoy excellent survival if their treatment is delayed until required, with 80% survival at 10 years. Radiotherapy can be very effective for

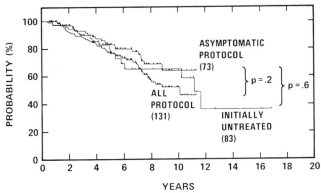

Fig. 2. Actuarial survival and freedom from relapse in the total group of patients with advanced-stage, low-grade lymphoma treated on clinical protocols and the group of "asymptomatic" patients treated on these protocols compared with the initially untreated patients.

the minority of patients with stage I and stage II disease, especially for those under age 40 (Paryani *et al.*, 1983). The extent of radiotherapy required and the role of laparotomy staging have not been resolved in these patients.

The availability of a group of patients observed without initial therapy has allowed us to estimate the incidence of spontaneous regression in the low-grade lymphomas. In untreated patients, more than 20% will enjoy a spontaneous regression (Horning and Rosenberg, 1984). Almost one-third of patients with the follicular small cleaved subtype will have a spontaneous regression. Regressions also occur in patients who have relapsed after initial therapies, but this has yet to be quantitated. Histologic transformation of a low-grade NHL to a higher-grade lymphoma is another important clinical observation. The actuarial risk and time to histologic transformation appears to be very similar among our patients, approximately 40–50% actuarially by 8 to 10 years after diagnosis, whether receiving primary treatment or no initial therapy (Horning and Rosenberg, 1984).

II. INTERMEDIATE-GRADE LYMPHOMAS

The intermediate-grade lymphomas include follicular large cell, diffuse large cell (cleaved or noncleaved), diffuse mixed small cleaved and large cell, and diffuse small cleaved cell. Of these, diffuse large cell (DLC) (or diffuse histiocytic) is the most common subtype, and discussion of the intermediate lymphomas is based primarily on the DLC subtype. In contrast to the low-grade lymphomas, about half of the intermediate grade lymphomas are localized, stage I or stage II, at diagnosis. Laparotomy staging at Stanford has revealed occult disease in only 4 to 10% of the diffuse NHLs (Goffinet *et al.*, 1977). Systemic symptoms are more common in these lymphomas, and extranodal sites of involvement occur in as many as one-third of patients. Overall, the intermediate-grade lymphomas are characterized by more rapid growth and the propensity for early dissemination. While the majority of intermediate-grade lymphomas are B-cell neoplasms, some of the DLC lymphomas express T-cell markers (Horning *et al.*, 1984). Finally, disease-free survival correlates well with overall survival, particularly in DLC, and approximately 90% of recurrences are manifest within the first 2 years following treatment.

Historically, radiation therapy has been the standard treatment for stage I and stage II diffuse lymphoma. Data from a recent retrospective analysis of patients with stage I and stage II disease that was treated with radiation therapy at Stanford University, half of whom were pathologically staged, indicate a 5-year survival rate of 49% for the entire group, with 53% for stage I and 47% for stage II disease (Kaminski *et al.*, 1983). Results were significantly better with radiation therapy to both sides of the diaphragm, while laparotomy staging was not a significant variable. These figures are in general agreement with those in the literature that indicate a 5-year FFR of 20 to 40% for stage II and 40 to 60% for stage I disease (Horwich and Peckham, 1983). The exceptions to these results are two reports of 100% disease-free survival in a small number of pathologic stage I patients (Sweet, et al., 1981; Levitt et al., 1980). Analyses at Stanford and several other centers have defined prognostic factors for limited-stage disease, including bulk, site, age, and at Stanford, the extent of radiotherapy (Kaminski et al., 1983; Gospodarowicz et al., 1984; Lester et al., 1982). Dissatisfaction with the results of radiotherapy alone led to the use of adjuvant chemotherapy, from which variable results were achieved (Monfardini et al., 1980).

Initial chemotherapy in stage I and stage II disease has been explored by Miller and Jones (1983). Forty-four patients received initial CHOP (cyclophosphamide, doxorubicin, vincristine, and prednisone) chemotherapy with or without irradiation in a nonrandomized study. With a median follow-up of 41 months, these authors project 89% FFR at 5 years in stage I patients and 75% in stage II patients. The FFR rate is 75% for those receiving chemotherapy only and 82% for those treated with combined modality. A retrospective analysis of primary chemotherapy in stage I and stage II from M. D. Anderson confirms these data (Cabanillas et al., 1980).

The morbidity of staging laparotomy in this group of usually older patients, the finding that 10% or less of patients with diffuse lymphoma were upstaged by laparotomy at Stanford (prior to the use of computed tomography), and the tendency for rapid dissemination of these tumors would suggest that laparotomy rarely is warranted. Even in stage I disease it is appropriate to consider initial chemotherapy. The contribution of radiation therapy to initial chemotherapy is the subject of a current randomized trial at Stanford.

New therapeutic strategies have been developed in the treatment of advanced-stage intermediate-grade lymphomas to meet the objectives of increasing the complete remission (CR) rate and improving the durability of those complete remissions. Intensive multidrug regimens have been designed that, in addition to including the standard agents of cyclophosphamide, doxorubicin, vincristine and prednisone, also have included bleomycin, procarbazine, methotrexate, cytosine arabinoside, and the new drugs etoposide and ifosfamide (Laurence et al., 1982; Skarin et al., 1983; Fisher et al., 1983; Cabanillas et al., 1983). Midcycle therapy with high-dose methotrexate and leucovorin rescue, as in the M-BACOD regimen, has been employed. Results of these treatment programs and others are discussed by Skarin in this volume. Sequential chemotherapy with a different drug combination is used in the ProMACE–MOPP regimen. Late intensification therapy similar to the approach in acute leukemia also has been employed. These new approaches have resulted in higher CR rates and suggest that greater than 50% of patients will have durable remissions (Table II).

TABLE II 2-YEAR TREATMENT RESULTS IN ADVANCED-STAGE INTERMEDIATE-GRADE LYMPHOMAS[a]

Reference	Treatment program[b]	Number of patients	Complete response rate (%)	Actuarial survival at 2 years (%)	Median follow-up (months)
Skarin et al. (1983)	M-BACOD	101	72[c]	65	38
Fisher et al. (1983)	ProMACE–MOPP	79	74[c]	73	31
Laurence et al. (1982)	COP–BLAM	33	73	70	23
Cabanillas et al. (1983)	Sequential chemotherapy	56	82[d]	—	22

[a]Including 23 patients with small noncleaved (high-grade) lymphoma.
[b]M-BACOD, methotrexate, bleomycin, doxorubicin, cyclophosphamide, vincristine, dexamethasone; ProMACE–MOPP, prednisone, methotrexate, doxorubicin, cyclophosphamide, etoposide and mechlorethamine, vincristine, procarbazine, prednisone; COP–BLAM, cyclophosphamide, vincristine, prednisone, bleomycin, doxorubicin, procarbazine.
[c]Results include some patients with stage II disease.
[d]Results include some patients with stage I and stage II disease.

While these results are better than historical controls, it is often difficult to compare published reports because of the influence of multiple prognostic factors and the heterogeneous clinical presentations of these patients. Therapeutic challenges still remain for many patients, especially those with bulky disease and/or those with high tumor burden, central nervous system (CNS) or marrow involvement, those with relapsed or intermediate-grade lymphoma occurring in the setting of histologic transformation, and the elderly. New treatment strategies, such as marrow transplantation in selected young patients, are needed.

III. HIGH-GRADE LYMPHOMAS

The high-grade lymphomas, considered to be the least favorable on the basis of survival, include large-cell immunoblastic, lymphoblastic, and small noncleaved cell (Burkitt's and non-Burkitt's). Immunoblastic lymphomas may be subdivided further into plasmacytoid and clear cell types (based on cytoplasmic characteristics) and polymorphous immunoblastic lymphoma, which includes a wide spectrum of T-cell lymphomas. The immunoblastic lymphomas may express either T- or B-cell markers, and some authors have defined distinct clinical features that correlate with their immunopathology (Levine *et al.*, 1981). In the NHL Classification Project, a small but statistically significant survival difference could be demonstrated that separated the immunoblastic lymphomas from the diffuse large cell, follicular center lymphomas (cleaved and noncleaved). However, these distinctions have not been made routinely in the literature, since these histologic subtypes have been combined as "diffuse histiocytic" lymphoma. It is unclear whether the immunoblastic lymphomas require unique therapeutic approaches.

Lymphoblastic lymphoma is a unique clinicopathologic entity characterized by a male predominance. It occurs in older children and young adults with mediastinal masses and supradiaphragmatic adenopathy. The lymphoblastic lymphomas routinely express T-cell markers. Although apparently limited at diagnosis, the disease consistently evolves rapidly, with early marrow and CNS involvement. Remarkable improvement in prognosis has resulted from intensive multidrug therapy, incorporating more aggressive and continuous induction therapy (Levine *et al.*, 1983; Coleman *et al.*, 1981; Weinstein *et al.*, 1983; Magrath *et al.*, 1984). These protocols have incorporated early CNS prophylaxis using intrathecal drugs, cranial irradiation, and/or high doses of systemic methotrexate. Complete response rates range from 75 to 100%, and 40 to 60% of adult patients are disease-free at 2 years. Bone-marrow involvement and markedly elevated lactate dehydrogenase (LDH) confer a poor prognosis, probably as a reflection of total tumor burden. Potential treatment strategies for these patients with poor prognosis might include the use of new drugs for induction or, possibly, the use of consolidative marrow transplantation.

Small noncleaved-cell lymphoma encompasses both Burkitt's tumor and lymphomas that have been described previously as undifferentiated, non-Burkitt's type. The term "small noncleaved" may be confusing, since the nuclei of these cells clearly are larger than small lymphocytes but small relative to large noncleaved cells. The pathologic distinction is based on degree of nuclear variation and pleomorphism not acceptable for Burkitt's tumor. Both are characterized by rapid proliferation. Nonendemic Burkitt's tumors most often occur within the abdomen, particularly in the ileocecal region and mesenteric nodes. Curative therapy has centered around the use of high-dose cyclophosphamide in combination with other drugs (Ziegler, 1981). Dramatic tumor reduction may be accompanied by the tumor lysis syndrome. Careful monitoring of metabolic characteristics during the first 48 hr after treatment is essential; isolated central nervous system relapses occur frequently. Magrath *et al.* (1984) at the NCI reported results of a protocol employing combination chemotherapy with high-dose methotrexate and both intrathecal methotrexate and cytosine arabinoside. Disease-free survival at 12 months is 50 and 60% for non-Burkitt's and Burkitt's, respectively. A high tumor burden (extensive intraabdominal or bone marrow disease) confers a poor prognosis in these patients.

IV. FUTURE DIRECTIONS

Recent developments in many fields promise to advance our understanding of the nature of lymphoproliferation. Techniques employing monoclonal antibodies for surface marker analyses of the NHLs are allowing clinical correlation of immunophenotype (Horning *et al.*, 1984). The new technique of identifying immunoglobulin gene rearrangements as sensitive and specific markers for B-cell neoplasms already is providing important new information about the clonal populations of the NHLs (Cleary *et al.*, 1984). Lymphomas occurring after organ transplantation and in the acquired immunodeficiency syndrome provide interesting models for study, particularly in regard to the question of multiclonality (Ziegler *et al.*, 1984). Characteristic chromosomal aberrations have been described for the NHLs, and great excitement has developed over the link between the c-*myc* oncogene and the 8;14 translocation in Burkitt's tumor (Rowley, 1983). Finally, the human T-cell leukemia/lymphoma virus is the first retrovirus considered to be an etiologic agent for human lymphoma (Broder *et al.*, 1984). Advances such as these stimulate interest in the further study of the diverse and fascinating NHLs.

REFERENCES

Broder, S., Bunn Jr., P. A., Jaffe, E. S., Blattner, W., Gallo, R. C., Wong-Staal, F., Waldmann, T. A., and DeVita V. T., Jr. (1984). *Ann. Intern. Med.* **100**, 543–557.

Cabanillas, F., Bodey, G., and Freireich, F. J. (1980). *Cancer* **46**, 2356–2359.

Cabanillas, F., Burger, M. A., Bodey, G. P., and Freireich, F. J. *et al.* (1983). *Am. J. Med.* **74**, 382–388.

Cleary, M. L., Chao, J., Warnke, R., and Sklar, J. (1984). *PNAS* **81**, 593–597.

Coleman, C. N., Cohen, J. R., Burke, J. S., and Rosenberg, S. A. (1981). *Blood* **57**, 679–684.

Fisher, R. I., DeVita Jr., V. T., Hubbard, S. M., Longo, D. L., Wesley, R., Chabner, B. A., and Young, R. C. (1983). *Ann. Intern. Med.* **98**, 304–309.

Goffinet, D. R., Warnke, R. A., Dunnick, N. R., Castellino, R., Glatstein, E., Nelsen, T. S., Dorfman, R. F., Rosenberg, S. A., and Kaplan, H. S. (1977). *Cancer Treat. Rep.* **61**, 981–992.

Gospodarowicz, M. K., Bush, R. S., and Brown, T. C. (1984). *Proc. Am. Soc. Clin. Oncol.* **3**, 236.

Hoppe, R. T., Kushlan, P., Kaplan, H. S., Rosenberg, S. A., and Brown, B. W. (1981). *Blood* **58**, 592–598.

Horning, S. J., and Rosenberg, S. A. (1984) *N. Engl. J. Med.* **311**, 1471–1475.

Horning, S. J., Doggett, R. S., Warnke, R. A., Dorfman, R. F., Cox, R. S., and Levy, R. (1984). *Blood* **63**, 1209–1215.

Horwich, A., and Peckham, M. (1983). *Semin. Hematol.* **20**, 35–56.

Kaminski, M. S., Coleman, C. N., Cox, R. S., Colby, T., Suey, L., Kushlan, P., Rosenberg, S. A., and Kaplan, H. S. (1983). *Proc. Am. Soc. Clin. Oncol.* **2**, 214.

Laurence, J., Coleman, M., Allen, S. L., Silver, R. T., and Pasmantier, M. (1982). *Ann. Intern. Med.* **97**, 190–195.

Lester, J. N., Fuller, L. M., Conrad, F. G., Sullivan, J. A., Velasquez, W. S., Butler, J. J., and Shullenberger, C. C. (1982). *Cancer* **49**, 1746–1753.

Levine, A. M., Taylor, C. R., Schneider, D. R., Koehler, S. C., Forman, S. J., Lichtenstein, A., Lukes, R. J., and Feinstein, D. I. (1981). *Blood* **58**, 52–61.

Levine, A. M., Forman, S. J., Meyer, P. R., Koehler, S. C., Liebman, H., Paganini-Hill, A., Pockros, A., Lukes, R. J., and Feinstein, D. I. (1983) *Blood* **61**, 92–98.

Levitt, S. H., Bloomfield, C. D., Frizzera, G., and Lee, C. K. K. (1980). *Cancer Treat. Rep.* **64**, 175–177.

Magrath, I. T., Janus, C., Edwards, B. K., Spiegel, R., Jaffe, E. S., Berard, C. W., Miliauskas, J., Morris, K., and Barnwell, R. (1984). *Blood* **63**, 1102–1110.

Miller, T. P., and Jones, S. E. (1983). *Blood* **62**, 413–418.

Monfardini, S., Banfi, A., Bonadonna, G., Rilke, F., Milani, F., Valagussa, P., and Lattuada, A. (1980). *Int. J. Radiat. Oncol. Biol. Phys.* **6**, 125–134.

Paryani, S. B., Hoppe, R. T., Cox, R. S., Colby, T. V., Rosenberg, S. A., and Kaplan, H. S. (1983). *Cancer* **52**, 2300–2307.

Paryani, S. B., Hoppe, R. T., Cox, R. S., Colby, T. V., and Kaplan, H. S. (1984). *J. Clin. Oncol.* **2**, 841–848.

Portlock, C. S. (1980). *Semin. Oncol.* **7**, 292–299.

Portlock, C. S., and Rosenberg, S. A. (1979). *Ann. Intern. Med.* **90**, 10–13.

Rappaport, H. (1966). "Tumors of the Hematopoietic System." Armed Forces Institute of Pathology, Washington, D.C.

Rosenberg, S. A. (1985). *J. Clin. Oncol.* **3,** 299–310.

Rowley, J. D. (1983). *Nature* **301,** 290–291.

Skarin, A. T., Canellos, G. P., Rosenthal, D. S., Case Jr., D. C., MacIntyre, J. M., Pinkus, G. S., Moloney, W. C., and Frei E., III (1983). *J. Clin. Oncol.* **1,** 91–97.

Sweet, D. L., Kinzie, J., Gaeke, M. E., Golomb, H. M., Ferguson D. L., and Ultmann, J. E. (1981). *Blood* **58,** 1218–1223.

Bleomycin Chemotherapy
(B. I. Sikic, M. Rozencweig, and S. K. Carter, eds.)

Chapter 14

NON-HODGKIN'S LYMPHOMAS: MILAN STUDIES

Valeria Bonfante
Armando Santoro
Emilio Bajetta
Pinuccia Valagussa
Simonetta Viviani
Roberto Buzzoni
Gianni Bonadonna

Division of Medical Oncology
Istituto Nazionale Tumori
Milan, Italy

I. INTRODUCTION

Since the early 1970s, remarkable progress has been achieved in the treatment of high-grade non-Hodgkin's lymphomas (NHLs) by moving from single-agent to multiple-drug therapy. Despite the increased incidence of complete response (CR), long-term remission, and cure, however, primary resistance to therapy and relapse following initial CR still represent problems in a considerable percentage of patients. Patients failing on chemotherapy often display pretreatment characteristics that indicate the presence of a high tumor cell burden (e.g., bulky disease in a single lymph node-bearing region, multiple extranodal involvement, and systemic symptoms). Moreover, the following findings have been frequently observed: the median time to CR is usually the fourth treatment cycle, and progressive disease during chemotherapy often occurs following initial tumor response after two to four treatment cycles. In addition, when the duration of first

CR is less than 12 months, retreatment with the same drug combination is often ineffective. Finally, modification of one or more components of an active drug regimen, such as CHOP (cyclophosphamide, adriamycin, vincristine, and prednisone), in treating NHLs fails to improve clinical results substantially.

These clinical observations have been very instructive and useful in designing new treatment strategies. Furthermore, they largely can be explained according to the basic tenets of the somatic mutation theory, as adapted to the area of cancer chemotherapy by Goldie and Coldman (1979). Therefore, the lack of curative effect of combination chemotherapy can be attributed to the presence of drug-resistant neoplastic cells before starting treatment and to the overgrowth of these cells during therapy. Successful results have been achieved at our institution with the evaluation of non–cross-resistant and combined modality therapies. This chapter presents an overview of the current status of the clinical trials for NHLs that have been conducted since the mid-1970s at the Milan Cancer Institute.

II. COMBINED-MODALITY THERAPY FOR STAGE I TO STAGE II DISEASE

Since the mid-1970s our trials for localized NHL have been aimed primarily at evaluating combined modality therapies. The principal reasons for this program were the failure of radiotherapy (RT) alone to cure a considerable percentage of patients with stage I to stage II disease, as well as the remarkable progress achieved with intensive chemotherapy in advanced disease. In fact, among patients with stage I to stage II NHLs, only a large proportion of patients with pathologic stage (PS) I diffuse histiocytic lymphoma (DHL) staged with laparotomy can be cured by optimal irradiation. In all other cases, the 5-year relapse-free survival (RFS) ranges from 35 to 55% in patients clinically staged, and from 45 to 65% in those pathologically staged with bone marrow biopsies and laparoscopy (Bush *et al.*, 1977; Fuller *et al.*, 1977; Glatstein *et al.*, 1977; Hellman *et al.*, 1977; Timothy *et al.*, 1980). Moreover, our first randomized study (Bonadonna *et al.*, 1982) comparing RT alone versus RT combined with CVP (cyclophosphamide, vincristine, prednisone) chemotherapy showed an improvement in RFS and total survival in the group that underwent combined treatment modality. In addition, other authors (Landberg *et al.*, 1979; Nissen *et al.*, 1983) demonstrated that multimodality treatment was superior to irradiation alone in stage I to stage II patients with unfavorable histology.

In 1976 we began a new, prospective, combined trial with two purposes in mind: to compare the efficacy of CVP versus an adriamycin- and bleomycin-containing regimen (BACOP), and to reduce disease progression during RT by starting treatment with chemotherapy. After pathologic staging, patients were randomized to receive three cycles of either CVP or BACOP (bleomycin, adriamycin, cyclophosphamide, vincristine, prednisone), administered according to the classic dose schedules. In the absence of tumor progression, the treatment was continued with high-energy irradiation to the involved areas (4000–5000 rad) as well as to proximal clinically uninvolved lymph node-bearing region(s) (3500–4000 rad), with a schedule of 800 to 1000 rad/week. Approximately 3 weeks from the end of RT, treatment was completed with three additional cycles of either chemotherapy.

As detailed by Bonadonna et al. (1982, 1984), from 1976 to 1983 a total of 148 patients were entered into the study, and the distribution of primary patient characteristics was comparable between the two treatment groups (Table I). Prophylactic irradiation to the immediately adjacent lymphoid area(s) was not carried out in patients with primary involvement of skin (11 cases), maxilla (2 cases), bone (2 cases), and upper cervical nodes (2 cases).

The 5-year results are presented in Table II. The CR rate was similar between the two treatment groups. It is important to point out that 63 patients (CVP, 33; BACOP, 30) started treatment while they already were in CR following excisional biopsy or surgical removal of primary disease. The comparative 5-year freedom from progression (FFP) was significantly superior in the BACOP group. Among complete responders, the recurrence rate within 5 years was 26.4% (19 of 72 patients) in the CVP group and 13% (9 of 69 patients) in the BACOP group. True recurrence in irradiated sites was documented in 2 patients (one in each treatment group) and marginal recurrence in 1 patient of the CVP group. All other recurrences occurred in distant sites.

TABLE I   CVP–RT–CVP VERSUS BACOP–RT–BACOP IN STAGE I
TO STAGE II DIFFUSE NON-HODGKIN'S LYMPHOMAS:
PATIENT CHARACTERISTICS[a]

	CVP (77 patients) (%)	BACOP (71 patients) (%)
Stage I	34	35
IE	30	20
II	30	28
IIE	6	17
Age, ≤40 years	73	62
Bulky disease (>10 cm)	9	10
B symptoms	3	6
Extranodal ± nodal	36	37
Histiocytic	43	51
Lymphocytic	36	31
Other high grade	21	18

[a]From Bonadonna et al. (1984).

TABLE II   CVP–RT–CVP VERSUS BACOP–RT–BACOP IN STAGE I
TO STAGE II DIFFUSE NON-HODGKIN'S LYMPHOMAS:
COMPARATIVE 5-YEAR OVERALL RESULTS

	CVP group (77 cases) (%)	BACOP group (71 cases) (%)	p
Complete remission	93.5	97.2	
5-Year freedom from progression	67.8	83.9	.013
5-Year relapse-free survival	72.6	86.4	.03
5-Year total survival	72.9	88.8	.16

Analysis of the relapse-free survival shows the superiority of BACOP versus CVP, with a marked trend in patients with stage II disease [CVP (59.9%) versus BACOP (83.3%), $p = .09$]. Salvage therapy achieved CR in 80% of patients failing in the CVP group, and in 62.5% of patients started on BACOP. The median duration of second CR was 18 months (range, 9–63 months) for the CVP group and 8 months for the BACOP group. At present, comparative analysis of the 5-year total survival has failed to indicate a significant difference between the two treatments, although the trend in favor of patients given BACOP combined with radiotherapy is considerable.

Toxicity was moderate with either treatment. One patient died because of radiation necrosis of the brain stem following 4500 rad. Other radiation sequelae were due exclusively to fibrosis.

Altogether, results of the present trial indicated the superiority of the BACOP regimen in preventing early disease progression and show that the role of RT remained important because first manifestation of recurrent disease in irradiated areas was documented in only 3 of 28 relapses.

III. ALTERNATING CHEMOTHERAPY IN STAGE III TO STAGE IV DISEASE

In recent years, considerable progress has been achieved in the overall prognosis of patients with high-grade histology NHLs through the use of intensive combination programs. In adults with advanced stages of diffuse aggressive lymphomas, two prospective trials using non–cross-resistant polydrug regimens were started in 1977 (Fisher *et al.*, 1983; Skarin *et al.*, 1983). Preliminary results indicate that this strategic approach is very effective in producing a high percentage of CRs and relapse-free survivors. However, a comparison between the two series is difficult because of differences in patient selection. Therefore, the contribution of alternating chemotherapy as well as the role of high-dose methotrexate with leucovorin cannot be evaluated properly.

With the intent of determining whether the earlier introduction of alternating non–cross-resistant regimens will increase the cure rate of aggressive advanced NHLs, we started a randomized study in 1982 for patients with stage III to stage IV high-grade NHLs previously untreated with chemotherapy. Patients have been prospectively randomized to receive either the classical CHOP (cyclophosphamide, adriamycin, vincristine, prednisone) as a single combination regimen, or ProMACE (without high-dose methotrexate with leucovorin) alternated with MOP combination. ProMACE/MOP is delivered by alternating within a period of 1 month the half-cycle of either combination (ProMACE: prednisone on days 1 through 14, and adriamycin, cyclophosphamide, and vincristine on day 1; MOP: mechlorethamine and vincristine on day 15, and procarbazine on days 15 through 21). Therapy will be administered for a minimum of six cycles. Complete recovery will be followed by two additional cycles as consolidation chemotherapy. The CEP regimen will be used in patients showing progressive disease while on therapy or not achieving CR within six cycles. The study is ongoing, and findings are premature.

IV. CONCLUSION

Various degrees of response to combination chemotherapy were reported for non-Hodgkin's lymphoma (NHL) in adults, particularly in the presence of a high-growth fraction and tumor cell burden. Considering the tumor cell heterogeneity that will be associated with the emergence of cells resistant to one or more antineoplastic drugs, chemotherapy using non–cross-resistant combinations appears to be the logical strategy to apply in this complex group of diseases. Preliminary results achieved by Fisher *et al.* (1978) and by Skarin *et al.* (1983) with alternating chemotherapy would indicate that this strategic approach is very effective, but its superiority over a single multidrug regimen remains to be documented. To confirm further the usefulness of the alternating strategy following the principles of the Goldie and Coldman hypothesis, we now are exploring the efficacy of a more frequent alternating sequence by delivering within 1 month the half-cycle of two non–cross-resistant combinations in treating NHLs.

Considering that a plateau has been reached in the management of malignant lymphomas with single-drug combinations, our findings stress the importance of ɩew therapeutic strategies to improve the cure rate of patients with advanced NHLs.

REFERENCES

Bonadonna, G., Lattuada, A., Monfardini, S., Bajetta, E., Buzzoni, R., Canetta, R., Valagussa, P., and Banfi, A. (1982). *In* "Malignant Lymphomas" (S. A. Rosenberg and H. S. Kaplan, eds.), pp. 537–551, Academic Press, New York.

Bonadonna, G., Bajetta, E., Lattuada, A., Buzzoni, R., Valagussa, P., Rilke, F., and Banfi, A. (1984). *In* "Adjuvant Therapy of Cancer" (S. E. Salmon and S. E. Jones, eds.), Vol. IV. Grune & Stratton, Orlando.

Bush, R. S., Gospodarowicz, M., Sturgeon, J., and Alison, R. (1977). *Cancer Treat Rep.* **61,** 1129–1136.

Fisher, R. I., DeVita, V. T., Jr., Hubbard, S. M., Longo, D. L., Wesley, R., Chabner, B. A., and Young, R. C. (1983). *Ann. Intern. Med.* **98,** 304–309.

Fuller, L. M., Gamble, J. F., Butler, J. J., Sinkovics, J. G., Wallace, S., Martin, R. G., Gehan, E. A., and Shullenberger, C. C. (1977). *Cancer Treat. Rep.* **61,** 1137–1148.

Glatstein, E., Donaldson, S. S., Rosenberg, S. A., and Kaplan, H. S. (1977). *Cancer Treat. Rep.* **61,** 1199–1207.

Goldie, J. H., and Coldman, A. J. (1979). *Cancer Treat. Rep.* **63,** 1727–1733.

Hellman, S., Chaffey, J. T., Rosenthal, D. S., Moloney, W. C., Canellos, G. P., and Skarin, A. T. (1977). *Cancer* **39,** 843–851.

Landberg, T. G., Håkansson, L. G., Möller, T. R., Mattsson, W. K. I., Landys, K. E., Johansson, B. G., Killander, D. C. F., Björn, F. M., Westling, P. F., Lenner, P. H., and Dahl, O. G. (1979). *Cancer* **44,** 831–838.

Nissen, N. I., Ersboll, J., Hansen, H. S., Walbøm-Jorgensen, S., Pedersen-Bjergaard, J., Hansen, M. M., and Rygård, J. (1983). *Cancer,* pp. 1–7.

Skarin, A. T., Canellos, G. R., Rosenthal, D. S., Case, D. R., Jr., MacIntyre, J. M., Pinkus, G. S., Moloney, W. C., and Frei, E., III. (1983). *J. Clin. Oncol.* **1,** 91–98.

Timothy, A. R., Lister, T. A., Katz, D., and Jones, A. E. (1980). *Eur. J. Cancer* **16,** 799–807.

Bleomycin Chemotherapy
(B. I. Sikic, M. Rozencweig, and S. K. Carter, eds.)

Chapter 15

BACOP AND RELATED STUDIES IN NON-HODGKIN'S LYMPHOMA

Arthur T. Skarin
George P. Canellos
Department of Medicine
Harvard Medical School
and Dana–Farber Cancer Institute
Boston, Massachusetts

I. SINGLE-AGENT BLEOMYCIN

The activity of bleomycin as a single agent in the treatment of non-Hodgkin's lymphoma (NHL) has been reviewed by several investigators (Yagoda *et al.*, 1972; Blum *et al.*, 1973; Carter and Blum, 1974; Smith *et al.*, 1978; Bennett and Reich, 1979). A summary of the majority of studies is noted in Table I. These studies (Yagoda *et al.*, 1972; Blum *et al.*, 1973; Shastri *et al.*, 1971; Kimura *et al.*, 1972; Rudders, 1972; Haas *et al.*, 1976; Bonadonna *et al.*, 1976) were carried out in the early 1970s, when histopathologic terminology was not uniform. In the lymphocytic lymphomas (nodular and diffuse cell types), the response rates varied from 20 to 100%, while the range was 15–88% in the histiocytic lymphomas (diffuse large-cell types). The average response rates from most large series are generally 30–40% in previously treated patients. Almost no data exist in previously untreated patients. In all of the studies, the complete remission (CR) rate is low, less than 10%. In addition, the response durations

TABLE I   ACTIVITY OF BLEOMYCIN IN NON-HODGKIN'S LYMPHOMAS[a]

Study	Lymphocytic lymphomas[b]		Histiocytic lymphomas[c]	
	Number of patients	Overall response rate (%)	Number of patients	Overall response rate (%)
Shastri et al. (1971)	5	20	—	—
Kimura et al. (1982)	1	100	5	60
Rudders (1972)	13	31	5	20
Yagoda et al. (1972)	17	83	35	88
Blum et al. (1973)	43	35	59	29
Haas et al. (1976)	15	40	13	15
Bonadonna et al. (1976)	6	66	11	73

[a]Modified from Smith et al. (1978). Response durations range from 1 to 4 months.
[b]Mainly nodular poorly differentiated lymphocytic, but also diffuse well-differentiated lymphocytic, diffuse poorly differentiated lymphocytic, diffuse mixed, nodular mixed.
[c]Mainly diffuse histiocytic lymphoma.

generally have been short, ranging from 1 to 4 months and averaging 2 months. These results are not surprising for single-agent therapy in previously treated patients, generally with widespread disease.

The variability of results reflects data that are uncontrolled for disease stage, previous therapy, and other prognostic indicators. However, more important is the variable dose, route, and frequency of administration of bleomycin, ranging from a higher dose of 25 U/m² daily × 5 down to 0.1 U/kg daily.

It is of interest that a phase II study conducted by the Southwest Oncology Group (SWOG) in 1976 (Haas et al., 1976) used bleomycin at a dose and schedule of 10 U/m² twice a week for 3 months, employing both intravenous (iv) and intramuscular (im) routes of administration. When the results in the treatment of both Hodgkin's disease and NHL were analyzed together, the response rate for im bleomycin was 46% compared with 29% for the iv route. The difference was not statistically significant. While a decrease in the severity of pulmonary toxicity was noted in patients receiving im versus iv bleomycin, the overall incidence of the toxicity (10%) was identical for both routes.

High-dose bleomycin was evaluated by the National Cancer Institute (NCI) in 1975 (Hubbard et al., 1975) using a dose and schedule of 25 U/m²/day iv for 5 consecutive days, with repeat courses every month. Of 10 previously treated patients, 3 showed a transient response. Pulmonary toxicity occurred in 2 patients at total doses of 100 U/m² and 125 U/m² (204 and 245 U, respectively). It was concluded that there was no therapeutic advantage to the high-dose schedule.

In the prospectively randomized study of the Eastern Cooperative Group (Bennett et al., 1977), low-dose bleomycin (5 U/m²) was compared with high-dose

TABLE II   BACOP SCHEMA USED BY NCI[a]

Drug	Dose		Day				
		1	8	15	21	28	
Cyclophosphamide	650 mg/m^2	↓	↓				Repeat cycle
Doxorubicin	25 mg/m^2	↓	↓				
Vincristine	1.4 mg/m^2	↓	↓				
Bleomycin	5 U/m^2			↓	↓		
Prednisone	60 mg/m^2						→

[a]From Schein et al. (1976)

low total doses of 45 U/m^2, 45 U/m^2, 160 U/m^2, and 165 U/m^2. With accrual of further patients, CR was achieved in 25 of 32 patients (47%), and a 40% overall survival was projected beyond 3 years (Fisher et al., 1977). The results with BACOP showed no major differences when compared with the earlier NCI C-MOPP program. In both regimens, survival was affected adversely by stage IV disease, marrow involvement, gastrointestinal involvement, and a tumor mass greater than 10 cm in diameter. However, of interest was that patients receiving BACOP showed a slightly higher incidence of stage IV disease, including bone-marrow involvement (Fisher et al., 1977).

The BACOP (NCI schema) and C-MOPP programs were compared in a prospective randomized cooperative trial (Dupont et al., 1984). Both programs resulted in similar CR rates (Table III). Patients receiving BACOP had a better relapse-free survival at 48 months (60 versus 35%), primarily due to a higher

TABLE III   RANDOMIZED TRIAL OF C-MOPP VERSUS BACOP IN DM AND DHL[a]

	C-MOPP	BACOP	p
Evaluable patients	40	48	
CR patients	19 (48%)	25 (52%)	NS[b]
Relapse-free at 48 months			
Stage I and stage II	66%	71%	NS
Stage III and stage IV	24%	58%	.05
All stages	35%	60%	.05
Alive at 48 months	25%	32%	NS

[a]From Dupont et al. (1984).
[b]NS, Not significant.

relapse rate in stage III and stage IV patients on C-MOPP. However, overall survival of both groups was not significantly different. Also, the toxicity of both programs to date has been similar. Further follow-up of this study, with analysis of histologic subgroups (DM versus DHL) and other prognostic factors, will be important.

Several groups have used the same five drugs as in BACOP, with slight modifications of the dose and schedule (CHOP–Bleo) (Table IV). The experience of CHOP was published in 1976 (McKelvey *et al.*, 1976) and CHOP–Bleo in 1977 (Rodriguez *et al.*, 1977). The bleomycin dose was 15 U/day iv for 5 days, with reduction to 4 U/m^2 for patients over age 60 years (Table V). The dose subsequently was changed in all patients to 4 U/m^2 iv on day 1 only (Jones *et al.*, 1979) (Table VI). Results from the M. D. Anderson Hospital with the original bleomycin schedule in 1977 (Rodriguez *et al.*, 1977) are noted in Tables IV and VII. In 26 patients with DHL, 69% achieved a CR, with only three relapses at the time of the report. An equally high CR rate was noted for patients with NPDL, DPDL, and NM. While both groups of patients had prolonged survivals, the overall results were not better than with the use of CHOP alone (McKelvey *et al.*, 1976). However, it should be noted that the studies were conducted at different institutions (Table VII).

Early results of CHOP–Bleo from SWOG studies were published in 1979 (Jones *et al.*, 1979) and updated in 1983 (Jones *et al.*, 1983). In a prospective

TABLE IV   BACOP AND SIMILAR REGIMENS IN NHL[a]

Study	Regimen	NPDL, number of patients (% CR)	DPDL, number of patients (% CR)	DHL, number of patients (% CR)
Skarin *et al.* (1977)	BACOP	9 (89%)	22 (73%)	22[b](59%)
Schein *et al.* (1976)	BACOP	— —	25[c](48%)	
Dupont *et al.* (1984)	BACOP	— —	25[c](52%)	
Rodriguez *et al.* (1977)	CHOP–Bleo	13 (62%)	3 (67%)	26 (69%)
Jones *et al.* (1983)	CHOP–Bleo	48 (75%)	17 (47%)	61[d](48%)
Newcomer *et al.*(1982)	CHOP–Bleo	— —	15 (87%)	
Ginsberg *et al.* (1982)	CAVPB (CHOP–Bleo infusion)	24[e](37%)	11[c](45%)	17 (59%)

[a]NPDL, Nodular poorly differentiated lymphoma; DPDL, diffuse poorly differentiated lymphoma; DHL, diffuse histiocytic lymphoma.
[b]Includes diffuse undifferentiated.
[c]Includes diffuse mixed.
[d]Includes nodular histiocytic.
[e]Includes nodular mixed.

TABLE V   INITIAL CHOP–BLEO REGIMEN
USED BY M. D. ANDERSON HOSPITAL[a]

Drug	Dosage and schedule
Cyclophosphamide[b]	750 mg/m^2/day, day 1
Doxorubicin[b]	50 mg/m^2/day, day 1
Vincristine	2 mg/day, days 1 and 5
Prednisone	100 mg/day, days 1–5
Bleomycin[c]	15 U/day, days 1 and 5

[a]From Rodriguez et al. (1977).

[b]Starting dose reduced by 20% for patients with prior extensive radiotherapy or hypocellular bone marrow (< 20%).

[c]Dose reduced to 4 U/m^2 on days 1 and 5 for patients older than 60 years. Subsequently reduced to 4 U/m^2/day in all patients

randomized study, two doxorubicin-containing regimens, CHOP plus BCG and CHOP plus Bleo, proved superior to COP plus Bleo. The result of CHOP plus Bleo in DHL are noted in Tables IV and VII. The CR rate was slightly higher in patients receiving CHOP plus BCG (68%) compared with CHOP plus Bleo (48%, $p = 0.02$). Survival of the former group of patients, estimated at 50%, also was superior to the latter group of patients, estimated at 35% (Jones et al., 1983). Results of CHOP–Bleo in DHL from the cooperative group study (SWOG) are compared with CHOP as conducted by a single institution in Table VIII. While the overall prognosis appears to be similar in the two programs, firm conclusions cannot be made because of differences in age, stage, B symptoms, and other important factors.

At the M. D. Anderson Hospital, dose escalation of the CHOP–Bleo regimen in conjunction with the use of a protected environment–prophylactic antibiotic

TABLE VI   CHOP–BLEO REGIMEN SWOG[a]

Drug	Dose		Day 1	Day 5	Day 21	
Cyclophosphamide	750	mg/m^2	↓			
Doxorubicin	50	mg/m^2	↓			
						Repeat
Vincristine	1.4	mg/m^2	↓			cycle
Prednisone	100	mg, q.i.d.	→			
Bleomycin	4	U/m^2	↓			

[a]From Jones et al. (1979).

TABLE VII   RESPONSE TO CHOP AND CHOP–BLEO IN NHL

Histologic subgroup	CHOP,[a] number of patients (% CR)	CHOP–Bleo,[b] number of patients (% CR)	CHOP–Bleo,[c] number of patients (% CR)
Nodular poorly differentiated lymphocytic	34 (76%)	48 (75%)	13 (62%)
Nodular mixed	9 (78%)	19 (74%)	3 (67%)
Diffuse well-differentiated lymphocytic	23 (61%)	18 (50%)	—
Diffuse poorly differentiated lymphocytic	38 (68%)	17 (47%)	3 (67%)
Diffuse mixed	14 (71%)	4 (100%)	—
Diffuse histiocytic	53 (68%)	53 (49%)	26 (69%)

[a]SWOG, 1976; from McKelvey et al. (1976).
[b]SWOG, 1983; from Jones et al. (1983).
[c]Houston, 1977; from Rodriguez et al. (1977).

program resulted in prolonged survival in patients with NPDL and DHL, estimated at 70 to 85% beyond 104 weeks (Bodey et al., 1979). The latter was achieved by reducing the CR relapse rate and fatality rate from infectious complications. Longer follow-up will be required before definitive conclusions can be made.

The Yale results of CHOP–Bleo in patients with DHL are noted in Table III. A modified schema was employed, with the dose of cyclophosphamide increased to 1 g/m^2, doxorubicin reduced to 40 mg/m^2, and bleomycin at 15 U on days 1

TABLE VIII   COMPARISON OF CHOP AND CHOP–BLEO
IN DHL

Number of patients	CHOP[a] 75	CHOP–Bleo[b] 61
% CR	51	48
% Stage I and stage II	19	—
% Stage II and stage IV	81	100
% CR duration (5-year estimate)	65	55
% Survival of all patients	30 (disease-free)	35 (overall)

[a]Armitage et al. (1984).
[b]Smith et al. (1978).

and 5. The frequency of the cycles was extended to every 4 weeks for a total of nine cycles (Newcomer *et al.*, 1982). Patients were randomized to receive either CHOP–Bleo or ACOMLA [doxorubicin + COMLA (cyclophosphamide, vincristine, methotrexate, leucovorin, ara-C)]. While the CR rate with CHOP–Bleo was higher (87 versus 64%) and the actuarial freedom from relapse at 2 years was better (93 versus 50%, $p = .04$), prognostic factors varied between the two regimens, most likely accounting for the differences. Toxicity from both programs was substantial, although less nausea and emesis occurred with CHOP–Bleo.

IV. THERAPEUTIC PROGRAMS USING CONTINUOUS-INFUSION BLEOMYCIN

Other therapeutic programs have used continuous-infusion bleomycin. The CALGB evaluated low-dose continuous infusion bleomycin (2 U/day for 5 days) combined with the CHOP agents (CAVPB) in 58 evaluable patients (Ginsberg *et al.*, 1982). The results, noted in Table IV, are quite similar to the other five-drug programs. Pharmacokinetic data confirmed a steady-state plasma concentration of bleomycin at the low dose of 2 U/day. Also, no clinical or subclinical pulmonary changes occurred, suggesting a better therapeutic index compared to bolus injection of bleomycin.

The New York Hospital–Cornell Medical Center (Hollister *et al.*, 1982) evaluated continuous infusion vincristine ($1–2$ mg/m^2 daily $\times$ 2 days) and bleomycin (0.25 U/kg bolus followed by 0.25 U/kg daily $\times$ 5 days). Weekly high-dose methotrexate (1500 mg/m^2) with leucovorin rescue was added to the program in responding patients, repeating cycles every 6 weeks. The regimen was administered to 16 patients (9 DHL) failing standard chemotherapy programs. A total of 8 patients (50%) responded, 2 with complete remissions and 3 with partial remissions, including 3 with DHL, but the median response duration was only 29 weeks. The initial response to infusion vincristine and bleomycin occurred in patients previously resistant to bolus injection of each of the drugs. However, interpretation of the study is limited because of the critically ill status of the patients and the major toxicities of stomatitis (63%) and leukopenia (44%). Only 1 patient had possible pulmonary toxicity due to bleomycin.

Another bleomycin-containing regimen employed in treating refractory NHL contains cisplatin, vinblastine, and bleomycin (CVB), reported recently from Ann Arbor (Liepman *et al.*, 1982). Continuous 24-h infusion of cisplatin (80 mg/m^2) followed by vinblastine (0.1 mg/kg, days 1 and 2) every 4 weeks and bleomycin (10 U iv weekly) were administered to 14 patients. A CR was achieved in 3 of 7 DHL patients. lasting from 6 to 10 months. Of 7 patients with other histologies, PR occurred in two. Toxicities include severe myelosuppression, increase in serum creatinine (41%), and one case of fatal pulmonary fibrosis.

V. NEW INTENSIVE-TREATMENT MULTIDRUG REGIMENS

While major improvement in the prognosis of patients with untreated, advanced DHL has occurred with many of the mentioned regimens, more than half of all patients eventually fail. Thus, since the late 1970s, several new intensive multidrug programs were designed in an effort to increase the cure rate. Three of the five regimens contained bleomycin (Table IX).

In 1976, our institution incorporated high-dose methotrexate with leucovorin (citrovorum) factor rescue (MTX/CF) into a modification of the previous BACOP program. In the resulting M-BACOD regimen, MTX/CF was administered on days 14 and 15 in an effort to increase tumor cell kill and reduce relapse between cycles of standard agents (Table X). A CR was achieved in 73 of 101 study patients (72%) or 77% of evaluable patients with DHL and DU (Skarin et al., 1983). Overall and disease-free survivals of CR patients reached plateaus at 80 and 65%, respectively, with overall survival for all patients approaching 60% at 5 years.

We also used the M-BACOD regimen in 44 patients with advanced favorable and intermediate-grade NHL who showed poor prognostic features (B symptoms, bulky lesions, and rapidly progressive disease). A CR was achieved in 15 of 26 patients (57%) with DM and DPDL and 10 of 16 patients (63%) with NPDL and NH (Anderson et al., 1984). The median remission durations were 9 and 25 months, respectively. Projected overall survival for all 44 patients approached a plateau of 40% out to 5 years.

TABLE IX   INTENSIVE TREATMENT PROGRAMS IN DHL AND DUL

Study	Regimen	Number of patients	CR (%)	% Survival of all patients at 2 years	Median follow-up
Skarin et al. (1983)	M-BACOD	101[a]	73 (72%)	76	>3 years
		95	73 (77%)		
Laurence et al. (1982)	COP–BLAM	33[b]	24 (73%)	70	NA
		15	2 (13%)	—	
Connors and Klimo (1984)	MACOP-B	47	39 (83%)	NA	19 months
Sweet and Lesky (1983)	COMLA	52	29 (56%)	63	>4 years
Fisher et al. (1983)	ProMACE–MOPP	74	55 (74%)	72	>25 years

[a]Total patients 101, 95 evaluable patients.
[b]Previously untreated 33, 15 previously treated patients.

TABLE X   M-BACOD SCHEMA, DANA–FARBER CANCER INSTITUTE/BRIGHAM
AND WOMEN'S HOSPITAL[a]

Drug	Dose	Day				
		1	7	14	21	
Methotrexate	3.0 g/m²	—	—	↓	—	
Bleomycin	4.0 U/m²	↓	—	—	↓	
Adriamycin	45 mg/m²	↓	—	—	↓	Repeat cycles q 3
Cyclophosphamide	600 mg/m²	↓	—	—	↓	weeks × 10
Oncovin	1.0 mg/m²	↓	—	—	↓	
Dexamethasone	6 mg/m²	☐			☐	
		1 5			21 25	

[a]From Skarin et al. (1983).

In 1981, moderate-dose MTX/LF (200 mg/m²) was substituted for high-dose MTX, with doses administered on days 7 and 14 of each cycle. Of the 98 patients with DHL and DU entered into the study, 71 have completed the program to date. CR was achieved in 56 of 74 patients (76%), with a subsequent relapse rate of 18% (Skarin et al., 1984). Projected disease-free survival of CR patients is more than 90% for those achieving CR within 1 to 2 months versus 45% for those developing a CR within 3 or more months. Overall survival for all patients projected out to 30+ months is 65%. A comparison of side effects of the high-dose (M-) and moderate-dose (m-) BACOD programs is noted in Table XI.

Another six-drug program (COP–BLAM) has been developed at the New York Hospital. It uses bleomycin (BL), 15 U iv on day 14 with procarbazine (M) for 10 consecutive days of each 3-week cycle together with doxorubicin (A) and

TABLE XI   MAJOR TOXICITY RELATED TO PROGRAM[a]

Toxicity	Moderate-dose m-BACOD, 74 patients	High-dose M-BACOD, 101 patients
Mucositis	29 (39%)	10 (10%)
	6% of courses	1% of courses
Increase in creatinine	2 (3%)	10 (10%)
Skin rash	1 (2%)	3(3%)
Acute CNS syndrome	0	1 (1%)
Leukopenia with fever	19 (26%)	8 (8%)
fatal	2 (3%)	3 (3%)
Pulmonary infiltrates related to bleomycin	11 (15%)	12 (12%)
Doxorubicin cardiotoxicity	3 (4%)	2 (2%)

[a]From Skarin et al. (1983, 1984).

COP (Laurence *et al.*, 1982). Dose escalation of cyclophosphamide and doxorubicin was carried out. Results show in Table VI, indicate a CR rate of 73% in untreated patients and markedly lower CR rate in 15 previously treated patients. A durable CR was reported. The regimen subsequently was modified to a 2-day constant infusion of vincristine (1 mg/m^2) and 5-day infusion of bleomycin (7.5 U/m^2/day) given at 6–7 week intervals. Bleomycin toxicity occurred in 7 of 23 patients (30%) over age 60 (Coleman *et al.*, 1984).

An innovative 12-week intensive program called MACOP-B was devised by the Vancouver group and recently reported (Connors and Klimo, 1984). The program used moderate-dose MTX/LF (400 mg/m^2), doxorubicin (50 mg/m^2), and cyclophosphamide (350 mg/m^2) every other week along with bleomycin (10 U/m^2) every three weeks for three courses. While a high CR rate of 83% was achieved, median follow-up is quite short (Table IX).

Other intensive treatment multidrug regimens not containing bleomycin are noted in Table IX. The initial results of COMLA were published by the University of Chicago group in 1980 (Sweet *et al.*, 1980), with an update in 1983 (Sweet and Lesky, 1983). The NCI proMACE–MOPP regimen (Fisher *et al.*, 1983) subsequently was compared with proMACE–cytaBOM in a randomized study (Fisher *et al.*, 1984). The cytaBOM regimen used cytarabine at 300 mg/m^2, bleomycin at 5 U/m^2, vincristine at 1.4 mg/m^2, and moderate-dose MTX/LF at 120 mg/m^2 on day 8. In the randomized study, both arms achieved high CR rates, but proMACE–cytaBOM resulted in excessive toxicity due to *Pneumocystis carinii*, leading to use of prophylactic trimethoprim–sulfamethoxazole.

The longer-term results in DHL using intensive non-bleomycin-containing regimens, such as COMLA and proMACE–MOPP, have shown improved disease-free survival or possible cure comparable with the M-BACOD or m-BACOD and CHOP–Bleo programs. It would appear that the inherent sensitivity of DHL to the cytotoxic drugs included in CHOP represents the standard chemotherapeutic program for treatment of that disorder. It is unclear whether any additions to CHOP have increased the cure rate, since there have been few randomized trials. In fact, the few random studies to date show no advantage of bleomycin added to CHOP. Unfortunately, intensification of bleomycin is impossible because of toxicity, noted at low doses as well as higher "standard" doses (Bauer *et al.*, 1983; Comis, 1978). Longer follow-up of the intensive drug regimens, with analysis of prognostic variables, will be required to clarify these issues.

REFERENCES

Anderson, K. C., Skarin, A. T., and Rosenthal, D. S. *Cancer Treat. Rep.* (in press).
Armitage, J. O., Fyfe, M. A. E., and Lewis, J. (1984). *J. Clin. Oncol.* **2**, 898–902.
Bauer, K. A., Skarin, A. T., and Balikian, J. P. (1983). *Am. J. Med.* **74**, 557–563.

Bennett, J. M., Lenhard, R. E., Ezdinli, E., et al. (1977). Cancer Treat. Rep. **61**, 1079–1083.
Bennett, J. M., and Reich, S. D. (1979). Ann. Intern. Med. **90**, 945–948.
Blum, R. H., Carter, S. K., and Agre, K. (1973). Cancer **31**, 903–914.
Bodey, G. P., Rodriguez, V., Cabanillas F., and Freireich, E. J. (1979). Am. J. Med. **66**, 74–81.
Bonadonna, G., Tancini, G., and Bajetta, E. (1976). Prog. Biochem. Pharmacol. **11**, 172.
Carter, S. K., and Blum, R. H. (1974). Cancer **24**, 322–331.
Coleman, M., Boyd, D. B., Bernhardt, B., et al. (1984). Proc. Am. Soc. Clin. Oncol. **3**, 246.
Coltman, C. A., Luce, J. K., and McKelvey, E. M. (1977). Cancer Treat. Rep. **61**, 1067–1078.
Comis, R. L., (1978). In "Bleomycin: Current Status and New Developments" (S. K. Carter, S. T. Crooke, and H. Umezana, eds.), pp. 279–291. Academic Press, New York.
Connors, J. M., and Klimo, P. (1984). Proc. Am. Soc. Clin. Oncol. **3**, 238.
Dupont, J., Pavolvsky, S., and Woolley, P. (1984). In "Second International Conference on Malignant Lymphoma, Lugano, Switzerland," p. 83.
Fisher, R. I., DeVita, V. T., Johnson, B. L., et al. (1977). Am. J. Med. **63**, 177–182.
Fisher, R. I., DeVita V. T., and Hubbard, S. M. (1983). Ann. Intern. Med. **98**, 304–309.
Fisher, R. I., DeVita, V. T., Hubbard, S. M., et al., (1984). Proc. Am. Soc. Clin. Oncol. **3**, 242.
Ginsberg, S. J., Crooke, S. T., and Bloomfield, C. (1982). Cancer **49**, 1346–1352.
Haas, C. D., Coltman, C. A., and Gottlieb, J. A. (1976). Cancer **38**, 8–12.
Hollister, D., Silver, R. T., Gordon, B., and Coleman, M. (1982). Cancer **50**, 1690–1694.
Hubbard, S. P., Chabner, B. A., Canellos, G. P., et al. (1975). Eur. J. Cancer **11**, 623–626.
Jones, S. E., Grozea, P. M., and Metz, E. N. (1979). Cancer **43**, 417–425.
Jones, S. E., Grozea, P. N., Metz, E. N., et al. (1983). Cancer **51**, 1083–1090.
Kimura, I., Onoshi, T., and Kunimosa, I. (1972). Cancer **29**, 58–60.
Laurence, J., Coleman, M., Allen, S. L., et al. (1982). Ann. Intern. Med. **97**, 190–195.
Liepman, M. K., Wheeler, R. H., Zuckerman, K. S., and Lobuglio, A. F. (1982). Cancer **50**, 2736–2739.
McKelvey, E. M., Gottlieb, J. A., Wilson, H. E., et al. (1976). Cancer **38**, 1484–1493.
Newcomer, L. N., Cadman, E. C., and Nerenberg, M. I. (1982). Cancer Treat. Rep. **66**, 1279–1284.
Rodriguez, V., Cabanillas, F., Burgess, M. A., et al. (1977). Blood **49**, 325–333.
Rudders, R. A. (1972). Blood **40**, 317–332.
Schein, P. S., DeVita, V. T., Hubbard, S., et al. (1976). Ann. Intern. Med. **85**, 417–422.
Shastri, S., Slayton, R. E., Wolter, J., et al. (1971). Cancer **28**, 1142–1146.
Skarin, A. T., Rosenthal, D. S., Moloney, W. C., and Frei, E. III. (1977). Blood 49, 759–770.
Skarin, A. T., Canellos, G. P., Rosenthal, D. S., et al. (1983). J. Clin. Oncol. **1**, 91–98.
Skarin, A. T., Canellos, G. P., Rosenthal, D. S., et al. (1984). In "Second International Conference of Malignant Lymphoma, Lugano, Switzerland." Abstract 31.
Smith, F. P., Hoth, D., and Schein, P. (1978). In "Bleomycin: Current Status and New Developments" (S. K. Carter, ed.), pp. 243–253. Academic Press, New York.
Sweet, D. L., Golomb, H. M., and Ultmann, J. E. (1980). Ann. Intern. Med. **92**, 785–790.
Sweet, D. L., and Lesky, L. (1983). In "A Comprehensive Guide to the Therapeutic Use of Methotrexate in Poor-Prognosis Non-Hodgkin's Lymphoma" (A. Skarin, ed.), pp. 50–58. Pharma Libri Pharmanual, New York.
Yagoda, A., Mukherji, B., Young, C., et al. (1972). Ann. Intern. Med. **77**, 861–870

Section V
NON–SMALL-CELL LUNG CANCER

Bleomycin Chemotherapy
(B. I. Sikic, M. Rozencweig, and S. K. Carter, eds.)

Chapter 16

A REASSESSMENT OF BLEOMYCIN IN LUNG CANCER AND OTHER INTRATHORACIC NEOPLASMS*

Franco M. Muggia

Division of Oncology
Rita and Stanley H. Kaplan Center
New York University School of Medicine
New York, New York

Daniel D. Von Hoff

Department of Medicine
Division of Oncology
University of Texas Health Sciences Center
San Antonio, Texas

This chapter addresses the role of bleomycin in the management of squamous-cell carcinoma of the lung, pleural effusions, and mesothelioma. Adenocarcinoma and large-cell carcinomas of the lung fall within the scope of this review and are referred to within the non–small-cell lung cancer (NSCLC) group, but fewer data are available for these histologic types.

A reassessment is timely for the following reasons: (1) factors leading to dose-limiting pulmonary toxicity have been increasingly delineated (Muggia *et al.*, 1983), (2) there is increasing interest in chemotherapy of NSCLC because of some success with cisplatin combinations (Muggia *et al.*, 1984), (3) the usefulness of bleomycin for intracavitary treatment of malignant effusions has been reported (Ostrowski and Halsall, 1982), and (4) the potential use of the clonogenic assay in neoplasms with accessible tumors for sampling is evident.

*Supported in part by grant CA-27733 from the Department of Health and Human Services and grant CH162C from the American Cancer Society.

I. SYSTEMIC THERAPY OF LUNG CANCER

Critical variables in determining the role of bleomycin in the treatment of lung cancer are likely to be patient characteristics, histology, dose, and scheduling. Unfortunately, early single-agent studies yielded little information on these variables. Therefore, subsequent combination studies are difficult to interpret. Disappointing single-agent results coupled with the dose-limiting pulmonary toxicity have acted as a deterrent against the use of bleomycin in treating NSCLC. On the other hand, activity against other squamous-cell carcinomas and relative lack of myelosuppression are powerful rationales for its incorporation into trials.

A. Single-Agent Bleomycin

Reviews by Blum *et al.* (1972), Selawry (1973), and Cohen and Perevodchikova (1979) summarize several studies from Japan, Europe, and the United States (Table I). Blum *et al.* (1972) described four studies in squamous lung cancer: the European Organization for Research and Treatment of Cancer (EORTC), which attained no responses in 7 evaluable patients among a total of 13; U. S. studies, which attained 5 responses among 62 evaluable patients and a total of 82 entered; Scandinavian studies, which achieved 6 responses among 22 evaluable patients; and Japanese studies, which reported 5 responses among 6 evaluable patients. In his review, Selawry (1973) reported an overall response rate of 8% among 130 patients, and a similar response rate emerged from the review of Cohen and Perevodchikova (1979).

When squamous cancer was specified, only 9% of 75 patients achieved objective responses; among patients with adenocarcinoma, 2 of 9 showed objective responses, with insufficient observations in large-cell undifferentiated lung can-

TABLE I   BLEOMYCIN SINGLE-AGENT ACTIVITY LUNG CANCER: ALL CELL TYPES[a]

Trial	Histology	Response/total	Comment
Memorial	Not stated	0/14	Broad phase II, daily
EORTC	Squamous	0/13	Daily or b.i.w.
Japan–Oka	2/3 Squamous	9/52	Untreated, 15–30 U b.i.w.
Milan	2/3 Squamous	1/15	Phase I
SWOG	1/2 Squamous	2/76	10 U/m^2 b.i.w. $\times$ 12
ECOG	Not stated	1/10	Phase I/II trial im

[a]From Cohen and Perevodchikova (1979).

cer. Japanese data focused from the outset on squamous cancer because of bleomycin's success in treating penile and other squamous-cell cancers; a 17% response rate is quoted by Ota *et al.* (1978).

Most of the U.S. data are derived from the M. D. Anderson–Southwest Oncology Group study, which are included in the results cited above, and quickly incorporated the drug into combination in a "kinetic scheduling" with vincristine (Bodey *et al.*, 1973), despite only one partial response among 22 patients with squamous lung cancer and no partial responses among 14 patients with small-cell cancer. The rationale for this scheduling was the enhanced cytoxicity of bleomycin for G_2, M cells, as well as the synchronizing effect of vincristine achieved by inducing a mitotic arrest.

Experience with the analog peplomycin is limited; however, in 13 patients with previously untreated squamous lung cancer, no responses were observed after administering a weekly 20-U im dose (Depierre *et al.*, 1981). Nevertheless, peplomycin does form part of the combinations that are judged active against NSCLC by Japanese investigators.

Results of clonogenic assay using standard techniques (Von Hoff *et al.*, 1980) indicate modest bleomycin activity at concentrations of 1 µg and 0.2 µg/ml at 1-hr exposures in a small number of samples (Table II). A steady-state concentration of 0.2 µg/ml is readily achieved by 30-U bleomycin infusions (Broughton *et al.*, 1978). Greater than 50% inhibition was achieved at the highest concentrations in 4 of 16 lung cancers exclusive of adenocarcinoma.

B. Drug Combination Studies

Rather than attempting to review all drug combination experiences, only selected studies of interest will be discussed here. They are reviewed in chronologic order (Tables III–V), since many of the rationales are derived historically.

TABLE II   BLEOMYCIN *IN VITRO* RESPONSE: LUNG CANCER

Histology	Number of *in vitro* responses[a]	Number attempted
Adenocarcinoma	0	6
Small cell	2	5
Large cell	1	1
Squamous cell	1	9

[a]Survival of tumor colony-forming units ≤50%.

TABLE III EARLY CLINICAL TRIALS OF BLEOMYCIN COMBINATIONS
IN LUNG CANCER

Reference	Regimen	Number of responses	Number of patients	Comment
Bodey et al. (1973)	Bleomycin plus vincristine	3	12	Kinetic scheduling
Bodey et al. (1973)	COMB	5	12	Pilot study
Bodey et al. (1977)	COMB	1	37	Random versus cyclophosphamide
Livingston et al. (1977)	BACON	16	38	Pilot
Livingston et al. (1977)	BACON	24	116	Squamous random versus NAC regimen (18/115)

Kinetic scheduling (Bodey et al., 1973) led to the combining of vincristine (O) and bleomycin (B) to form a nonmyelosuppressive combination, and then to incorporating vincristine and bleomycin into combinations with the myelosuppressive drugs methyl CCNU (M) and cyclophosphamide (C). This gave rise to COMB, which was heralded as possessing unprecedented activity, achieving responses in 5 of 12 patients. Selawry's review (1973) stimulated a revival of interest in nitrogen mustard (N) instead of cyclophosphamide for squamous-cell carcinoma and led to the BACON combination, which also included doxorubicin (A) and substituted CCNU (C) for methyl CCNU. Disappointing assessments of these regimens emanated from randomized trials: COMB versus cyclophosphamide (Bodey et al., 1977) resulted in equivalent response rates of 7% for the combination and single drug, and BACON versus NAC yielded nearly equivalent low response rates and survival (Livingston et al., 1977) (Table III).

The outcome of these randomized studies discouraged combinations including bleomycin, even though other pilot studies indicated some activity (Table IV). Livingston et al. (1981) reported 2 complete responses (CR) and 3 partial responses (PR) in 45 patients treated with doxorubicin, bleomycin (5 U on days 2, 3, 4), cyclophosphamide, and mitomycin. The overall median survival was 13 weeks, and 1 patient developed pulmonary fibrosis. Eagan et al. (1975) reported no activity in 12 patients with squamous-cell carcinoma (7 previously untreated and 5 crossed over from ICRF-159 treatment), but 3 PR in 8 patients with large-cell cancer and 2 PR in 18 patients with adenocarcinomas were seen with bleomycin, vincristine, and doxorubicin. In Japan, the FOBEM (5-fluorouracil, vincristine, bleomycin, cyclophosphamide, and mitomycin) combination showed considerable activity (Ota et al., 1978). A 7-day bleomycin infusion with mitomycin also was strikingly active in a Japanese study (Kakusaki et al., 1982). However, a recently published study using the combination of bleomycin and CCNU with or without a retinoid reported no responses in 58 patients with

TABLE IV   CLINICAL TRIALS OF BLEOMYCIN REGIMENS IN LUNG CANCER[a]

Reference	Regimen[b]	Number of responses	Number of patients	Comments
Eagan et al. (1976)	Dox–Bleo–VCR	5	36	No responses in squamous
Livingston et al. (1981)	Dox–Bleo–Cy–Mi	5	45	SWOG study
Weber and Obrecht (1983)	Bleo–CCNU	0	58	Squamous, half with retinoid
Veronesi et al. (1982)	Bleo–BCNU–VCR	0	27	Squamous CAMP failures
Kakusaki et al. (1982)	Bleo–Mi	23	37	Squamous only, bleomycin infusion
Ota et al. (1978)	5-FU–Bleo–VCR–Cy–Mi	19	56	39 versus 25 versus 33% in squamous, adenocarcinoma, small cell (Japan)

[a]Exclusive of cisplatin.
[b]Dox, Doxorubicin; Bleo, bleomycin; VCR, vincristine; Cy, cyclophosphamide; Mi, mitomycin; 5-FU, 5-fluorouracil.

TABLE V CLINICAL TRIALS OF BLEOMYCIN (B) PLUS CISPLATIN (P) IN LUNG CANCER[a]

Reference	Regimen[b]	Number of responses	Number of patients	Comments
Israel et al. (1981)	B_I–$P_{20×6}$	14	20	Squamous, many CR; iv infusion
Israel et al. (1982)	B_I–$P_{20×5}$–Mito	28	38	As above, sequential study
Ruckdeschel et al. (1981)	$B_{1.8}$–P_{50}–Cy	6	26	ECOG squamous
Vogl et al. (1980)	B_W–P_{50}–A–M	12	31	Severe myelosuppression
Rosenthal et al. (1982)	B_I–$P_{20×5}$–VCR–M	19	28	Squamous and adenocarcinoma
Itri et al. (1983)	B_I–P_{120}–VDS	20	52	Squamous, 5/14 responses
Cohen et al. (1984)	B_W–P_{20}–VCR–M–5-FU	16	20	Squamous, rbc deformability study

[a]Exclusive of etoposide.
[b]I, Infusion; w, weekly; Mito, mitomycin; Cy, cyclophosphamide; A, doxorubicin; M, methotrexate; VCR, vincristine; VDS, vindesine; 5-FU, 5-fluorouracil; rbc, red blood cell.

advanced squamous lung cancer (Weber and Obrecht, 1983). Also inactive was a bleomycin, vincristine, and BCNU combination used second-line (Veronesi *et al.*, 1982).

Considerably greater activity recently has been reported as cisplatin was included in NSCLC combinations. Studies by the Eastern Cooperative Oncology Group (ECOG) indicate a regimen of cyclophosphamide, cisplatin, and bleomycin is significantly superior for treating squamous-cell carcinoma than the combination of CCNU and cyclophosphamide (Ruckdeschel *et al.*, 1981). The bleomycin in this regimen was administered at 20 U/m^2 iv on days 1 and 8 every 4 weeks. The estimated median survival of 18.1 weeks was the longest of six regimens (also superior to MACC and mitomycin), and this regimen achieved the highest number of responses (6 of 25 patients). One patient died of pulmonary toxicity. It was not tested in the other cell types; another cisplatin-containing regimen (5-fluorouracil, doxorubicin, cisplatin) was favored in the treatment of adenocarcinoma and large-cell types. The result with cyclophosphamide, cisplatin, and bleomycin is noteworthy, since 72% of patients were above 60 years of age and 41% had received prior radiation. The results of this combination were confirmed in a subsequent study, but trends favored a mitomycin, vinblastine, and cisplatin regimen, which was selected by ECOG for subsequent trials.

The role of bleomycin added to cisplatin also was explored by Israel *et al.* (1981) in treating a wide variety of squamous cancers. Both drugs were administered daily for 6 days, with bleomycin given by continuous iv infusion at dose of 6 $U/m^2/day$. Excellent responses were achieved in 14 of 20 patients, with 4 complete responses. Encouraging results also were reported by another group (Elson *et al.*, 1982). A similar 5-day regimen that also included vincristine and methotrexate has shown high degrees of activity (Rosenthal *et al.*, 1982). In another combination using bleomycin weekly, BAMP (bleomycin, doxorubicin, methotrexate, and cisplatin), activity was shown, but considerable myelosuppression also occurred (Vogl *et al.*, 1980) (Table V).

More recently, efforts have been directed toward improving the apparent synergism of cisplatin–etoposide and cisplatin–vinca combinations. In this volume, Osaba and associates review their experience in adding bleomycin to cisplatin–etoposide. One other group also has reported favorable results with this combination (Goodman *et al.*, 1983). Itri *et al.* (1983) followed their encouraging cisplatin–vindesine trial by including bleomycin in the combination. Bleomycin was administered only in the first two cycles by 4-day constant infusion of 10 $U/m^2/day$. Results for the 52 patients treated were no different from those treated without bleomycin: of the 14 patients with squamous cancers, 5 achieved partial responses. Another regimen including cisplatin, vinblastine, bleomycin (15 U iv weekly), 5-fluorouracil, and methotrexate was described by Cohen *et al.* (1984). Results included 3 CRs and 14 PRs among 20 patients. The role of bleomycin in these combinations is difficult to assess.

II. LOCALLY DIRECTED THERAPY

Radionuclide-labeled bleomycin (generally cobalt-57) localizes preferentially in malignant lung tumors to a greater extent than gallium (Nieweg et al., 1983). Therefore, bleomycin can be considered a form of targeted therapy. Intraarterial therapy of lung tumors has been used in Scandinavia, but there appear to be no persuasive advantages over iv therapy. Clonogenic assay information might help exploit this approach in the future. Radiation with simultaneous bleomycin has been evaluated in Japan through controlled trials, but no advantage was demonstrated in lung cancer (Ichikawa, 1978).

Intracavitary therapy is a locally directed form of treatment that may be important in the treatment of lung cancer, since the majority of malignant pleural effusions relate to this disease. Bleomycin has been evaluated in several series, but trials of intracavitary therapy are quite difficult to assess because of patient heterogeneity and variable treatment conditions. Nevertheless, such treatment may constitute an important palliative modality.

Use of intracavitary bleomycin has advantages over several other proposed therapies because of its very low morbidity confirmed by many authors, as reviewed by Ostrowski and Halsall (1982). These authors analyzed the results of a trial in the United Kingdom including 200 patients from 44 centers. Responses were assessed as initially proposed in the Albany experience with bleomcyin (Paladine et al., 1976). CR was defined as no fluid after 30 days, and PR was defined as minimal recurrence not requiring repeat aspiration within 30 days. The method consisted of drainage as completely as possible via a needle confirmed by chest X-ray, then followed by instillation of bleomycin in 100 ml of saline. The doses of bleomycin ranged between 30 and 180 U. The response rate in all patients with lung cancer was 37%, but the response was dependent upon cell type, with 8 of 10 patients (80%) with squamous cancer responding. Patients with breast cancer and miscellaneous tumor types were generally more responsive than those with lung cancer, with rates exceeding 60%. Peritoneal effusions from ovarian cancer were more refractory, showing a response rate of 39%. Toxicity was absent in 29.5% of patients. The most common side effect was pain and fever occurring in 10% of patients. The incidence of pain was 21% in patients with peritoneal effusions versus 5% in patients with pleural effusions. Only 2 patients developed symptoms of respiratory distress, but under circumstances that could not incriminate bleomycin.

Systemic absorption from intracavitary administration has been studied by Alberts et al. (1979). As predicted from its high molecular weight (1400), the absorption rate of bleomycin is likely to be low. Alberts et al. (1979) indicated that the systemic concentration × time was 44% after intraperitoneal administration compared with the same dose given iv. Absorption is likely to be highly variable in accordance with pathologic processes in the cavity involved and the amount of residual fluid.

If cytotoxicity is considered an important mediator of therapeutic effect on neoplastic effusions, then the results of the clonogenic assay may be relevant both in the selection of patients for this treatment and in providing a further rationale for its use. We examined responses to the assay according to whether samples were obtained from solid tumors or effusions. The overall sensitivity to bleomycin was similar (33 of 225 solid tumor specimens versus 36 of 240 effusion specimens). However, in lung cancer, using the criterion of at least 50% inhibition at the highest dose level, only effusions were sensitive to bleomycin (5 of 14 versus 0 of 13 in solid specimens; $p = .04$, Fisher's exact test). The dichotomy is not explained by histology and needs to be examined further.

Leads for intracavitary use of bleomycin for other tumors might be obtained from the cloning assay. As noted in Table VI, the drug does show activity against bladder, colon, ovary, and stomach cancer when the cells are exposed directly to bleomycin. Perhaps these would be areas worthy of futher exploration.

III. ROLE IN TREATING MESOTHELIOMA

In light of the rising interest in the role of bleomycin for neoplastic effusions, it is worth examining bleomycin's potential efficacy as an antineoplastic in the treatment of mesothelioma. Although this neoplasm is confused with adenocar-

TABLE VI   BLEOMYCIN *IN VITRO* RESPONSE: OTHER TUMORS[a]

Tumor type	Number of *in vitro* responses	Number evaluable
Bladder	1	2
Breast	1	9 (11%)
Cervix	1	6 (16%)
Colon	1	5 (20%)
Endometrial	0	4
Head and neck	0	2
Kidney	0	1
Liver	1	1
Lymphoma	1	4
Melanoma	2	9 (22%)
Neuroblastoma	1	3
Ovary	47	260 (18%)
Mesothelioma	0	3
Sarcoma	0	2
Stomach	1	3
Testis	0	11 (0%)
Thyroid	0	1

[a]With 1 hr exposure, 0.2 μg/ml.

cinomas of lung and ovarian origins, cytologic diagnosis is the exception in mesothelioma. Its plaque-like growth, with extensive sclerosis, is probably an obstacle to response to an intracavitary drug. Nevertheless, interest in bleomycin has been generated by the lack of otherwise generally effective drug therapy and by some experimental findings.

In this disease, the clonogenic assay identified one drug with activity—vinblastine—that led to a useful response (Von Hoff et al., 1981), and this finding is being pursued further in a trial by the Southwest Oncology Group. However, the closely related drug vindesine was found to be ineffective in a clinical trial of 17 patients; only 1 patient showed improvement for 5 months (Kelsen et al., 1983).

Data on bleomycin for mesothelioma in the clonogenic assay are confined to three samples (activity not present); there are no clinical data at present, but a study to be published by ECOG includes mesothelioma in their study of bleomycin in sarcomas. However, in studies of mesothelioma cell lines growing in nude mice, bleomycin was among the three active drugs, the others being cisplatin and cyclophosphamide. Bleomycin induced one CR and one PR among nine trials, whereas cisplatin yielded three PR and cyclophosphamide only two stabilizations (Chahinian et al., 1980). This finding encourages exploration of bleomycin in mesothelioma, taking into account the usual precautions related to pulmonary toxicity (i.e., age, prior radiation, and comorbid pulmonary disease).

IV. FUTURE DIRECTIONS

Although clinical single-agent activity of bleomycin in the treatment of NSCLC is in question, a role for this drug must be explored further, based on the results from cisplatin-containing regimens, coupled with renewed guidance from other preliminary findings from clonogenic assay specimens. Several questions and directions emerge from this experience:

1. Is there a greater sensitivity of squamous-cell cancer to bleomycin, and should trials be confined to this cell type of NSCLC?
2. Is the continuous infusion schedule superior in antitumor efficacy and/or toxicity sparing?
3. Is there synergy between cisplatin and bleomycin? Is this synergy dependent upon bleomycin schedule?
4. What accounts for a differential sensitivity to bleomycin between malignant cells in NSCLC effusions versus solid tumors? Is this an important clinical lead?

Other areas of future investigation with bleomycin in intrathoracic neoplasms include the mechanism of benefit from intracavitary administration and its clinical application in the treatment of mesothelioma. With regard to the pulmonary toxicity, the development of protectors of the normal lung by oxygen pretreatment, low oxygen concentrations during and after treatment, and proline hydroxylase inhibitors should be explored to improve the therapeutic index of the drug. This potential, together with the excellent localization of bleomycin in lung tumors, should be a stimulus for pursuing these studies further.

REFERENCES

Alberts, D. S., Cheng, H. S. G., Cheng, H. S. G., Mayersohn, M., Perrior, D., Moon, T. E., and Gross, J. F. (1979). *Cancer Chemother. Pharm.* **2,** 127–132.

Blum, R. H., Carter, S. K., and Agre, K. (1972). *Cancer* **31,** 903–914.

Bodey, G., Gottlieb, J. A., Livingston, R., and Frei, E., III. (1973). *Cancer Chemother. Rep.* **4**(3)-227–229.

Bodey, G. P., Lagakos, S. W., Gutierrez, A. C., Wilson, H. E., Selawry, O. S. (1977). *Cancer* **39,** 1026–1031.

Broughton, A., Strong, J. E., Crooke, S. T., and Prestayko, A. W. (1978). *In* "Advances in Cancer Chemotherapy" (S. K. Carter, A. Goldin, K. Kuretani, G. Mathe, Y. Sakurai, S. Tsukagoshi, and H. Umezawa, eds.), pp. 469–480. Japan Science Society Press, Tokyo/University Park Press, Baltimore.

Chahinian, A. P., Szrajer, L., Beranck, J. T., and Holland, J. F. (1980). *Proc. Am. Assoc. Clin. Res.* **21,** 289.

Cohen, M. H., and Perevodchikova, N. I. (1979). *In* "Lung Cancer: Progress in Therapeutic Research" (F. Muggia and M. Rozencweig, eds.), pp. 343–374. Raven, New York.

Cohen, M. H., Johnston-Early, A., Citron, M. L., Krashow, S. H., and Fossieck, B. E., Jr. (1984). *Cancer Treat. Rep.* **68,** 475–479.

Depierre, A., Clavel, M., Fournial, F., Carriere, J. C., Weber, B., Planting, A., Kirkpatrick, A., Rozencweig, M., and Kenis, Y. (1981). *Proc. Am. Assoc. Cancer Res./Proc. Am. Soc. Clin. Oncol.* **22,** 493.

Eagan, R. T., Carr, D. T., Coles, D. T., Rubin, J., and Frytak, S. (1976). *Cancer Treat. Rep.* **60,** 949–951.

Elson, D. L., Holm, M. E., and Reed, R. C. (1982). *Proc. Am. Soc. Clin. Oncol.* **1,** 147.

Goodman, G. E., Rivkin, S. E., Wasserman, P. B., and Kaplan, H. G. (1983). *Proc. Am. Soc. Clin. Oncol.* **2,** 185.

Ichikawa, T. (1978). *In* "Advances in Cancer Chemotherapy" (S. K. Carter, A. Goldin, K. Kiretani, G. Mathe, Y. Sakurai, S. Tsukagoshi, and H. Umezawa, eds.), pp. 469–480. Japan Science Society Press, Tokyo/University Park Press, Baltimore.

Israel, L., Breau, J. L., and Aguilera, J. (1981). *Proc. Am. Assoc. Clin. Res./Proc. Am. Soc. Clin. Oncol.* **22,** 508.

Israel, L., Breau, J. L., Kerbrat, G., Depierre, A., Morere, P., and Clavier, J. (1982). In "Abstracts, III World Conference on Lung Cancer," p. 186. Tokyo, Japan, May 17–20.

Itri, L. M., Gralla, R. J., Kelsen, D. P., Chapman, R. A., Casper, E. S., Braun, D. W., Jr., Howard, J. E., Golbey, R., and Heelan, R. T. (1983). *Cancer* **51,** 1050–1055.

Kakusaki, I., Takizawa, H., Watanabe, S., and Miyamoto, T. (1982). *In* "The III World Conference on Lung Cancer—Abstracts" (S. Ishikawa, Conference President), p. 183. National Cancer Center, Tsukiji, Tokyo.

Kelsen, D., Gralla, R., Cheng, E., and Martini, N. (1983). *Cancer Treat. Rep.* **67,** 821–822.

Livingston, R. B., Heilbrun, L., Lehane, D., Costanzi, J. J., Bottomley, R., Palmer, R. L., Stuckey, W. J., and Hoogstraten, B. (1977). *Cancer Treat. Rep.* **61**, 1623–1627.

Livingston, R. B., Mira, J., and O'Bryan, R. M. (1981). *Cancer Treat. Rep.* **65**, 143–144.

Muggia, F. M., Louie, A. C., and Sikic, B. I. (1983). *Cancer Treat Rev.* **10**, 221–243.

Muggia, F. M., Blum, R. H., and Foreman, J. D. (1984). *Int. J. Radiation Oncology Biol. Phys.* **10**, 137–145.

Nieweg, O. E., Beckhuis, H., and Piers, D. A. (1983). *Thorax* **38**, 16–21.

Ostrowski, M. J., and Halsall, G. M. (1982). *Cancer Treat. Rep.* **66**, 1903–1907.

Ota, K., Nishimura, M., Sugiura, T., Morishita, M., Morita, K., Karasawa, K., and Yamanaka, N. (1978). *In* "Advances in Cancer Chemotherapy" (S. K. Carter, A. Goldin, K. Kuretani, G. Mathe, Y. Sakurai, S. Tsukagoshi, and H. Umezawa, eds.), pp. 469–480. Japan Science Society Press, Tokyo/University Park Press, Baltimore.

Paladine, W., Cunningham, T. J., Sponzo, R., Donavan, M., Olson, K., and Horton, J. (1976). *Cancer* **38**, 1903–1908.

Rosenthal, C. J., Ritter, S., and Platica, O. (1982). *Cancer Treat. Rep.* **66**, 205–206.

Ruckdeschel, J. C., Mehta, C. R., Salazar, O. M., Cohen, M., Vogl, S., Koons, L. S., and Lerner, H. (1981). *Cancer Treat. Rep.* **65**, 965–972.

Selawry, O. S. (1973). *Cancer Chemother. Rep.* **4**(3), 177–189.

Veronesi, A., Magri, M. D., Trovo, M. G., Tirelli, U., Galligioni, E., Tumoto, S., and Grigoletto, E. (1982). *Cancer Treat. Rep.* **66**, 1877–1878.

Vogl, S. E., Wollner, D., Kaplan, B. H., and Berenzweig, M. S. (1980). *Cancer Treat. Rep.* **64**, 717–718.

Von Hoff, D. D. (1980). *In* "Therapeutic Progress in Ovarian Cancer, Testicular Cancer, and the Sarcomas" (A. T. van Oosterom, F. M. Muggia, and F. J. Cleton, eds.), pp. 225–234. Martinus Nijhoff, The Hague, Boston and London.

Von Hoff, D. D., Casper, J., Bradley, E., Sandbach, J., Jones, D., and Makuch, R. (1981). *Am. J. Med.* **70**, 1027–1032.

Weber, W., and Obrecht, J. P. (1983). *Cancer Treat. Rep.* **67**, 847–849.

Bleomycin Chemotherapy
(B. I. Sikic, M. Rozencweig, and S. K. Carter, eds.)

Chapter 17

NON–SMALL-CELL LUNG CANCER: BLEOMYCIN PLUS ETOPOSIDE AND CISPLATIN

David Osoba
James J. Rusthoven
Kathryn Turnbull
Ida Ackerman
Martin P. Berry
Pamela A. Catton
Geoffrey M. Davies
Hensley A. B. Miller
Glen A. Taylor
Peter M. Webster

Toronto–Bayview Regional Cancer Centre
Ontario Cancer Treatment and Research Foundation
and Sunnybrook Medical Centre
University of Toronto
Toronto, Ontario, Canada

William K. Evans   Martin E. Blackstein
Frances A. Shepherd   *Mount Sinai Hospital*
Toronto General Hospital   *Toronto, Ontario, Canada*
Toronto, Ontario, Canada

Martin Levitt
University of Manitoba Faculty of Medicine
Manitoba Cancer Foundation
Winnipeg, Manitoba, Canada

I. INTRODUCTION

Bleomycin (B), etoposide (E), and cisplatin (P) were combined (BEP) for the treatment of non–small-cell lung cancer (NSCLC) for a number of reasons. Stage IV squamous-cell carcinoma of the upper aerodigestive tract and the squamous-cell variety of NSCLC respond to bleomycin and cisplatin (Randolph *et al.*, 1978; Israel *et al.*, 1981). In cell culture, there is synergy between these two agents (Drewinko *et al.*, 1976). Etoposide was included because of its additive effect with cisplatin in cell culture (Drewinko *et al.*, 1976), as well as the success of etoposide plus cisplatin as second-line therapy in small-cell lung cancer (Osoba *et al.*, 1981; Evans *et al.*, 1984) and the preliminary results in the European Organization with Research and Treatment of Cancer (EORTC) trial of these agents in NSCLC (Klastersky *et al.*, 1982).

II. PATIENTS AND METHODS

BEP (Table I) was administered to 75 patients with biopsy-proven NSCLC, 45 with squamous-cell carcinoma, 9 with large-cell carcinoma, and 21 with adenocarcinoma. The patients form three subgroups with respect to previous treatment and extent of disease (Table II):

1. A subgroup of 31 patients with recurrent regional (primary site ± mediastinal or hilar or supraclavicular nodes) and/or disseminated NSCLC of all three histologic varieties. Of these, 28 had received previous radiation therapy to the primary tumor and regional nodes, and 3 had received previous chemotherapy containing not more than one of the drugs in the BEP regimen.

2. A subgroup of 29 patients with disseminated (M1) squamous, large-cell, or adenocarcinoma. None had received previous treatment other than surgery.

3. A subgroup of 15 patients with regional (TX-3, N1–2, ± supraclavicular nodes) squamous-cell lung cancer who had not received any previous treatment. (This subgroup is part of a separate study of combined modality therapy in which, after a maximum of two cycles of BEP, all patients receive radiation therapy to the primary tumor and involved regional lymph nodes. The chemo-

TABLE I   SCHEDULE OF BEP CHEMOTHERAPY

B (bleomycin):	10 U/m^2 iv push day 1, them 10 U/m^2/24 hr as infusion on days 1, 2, and 3
E (etoposide):	100 mg/m^2 iv over 30–60 min daily on days 1, 2, and 3
P (cisplatin):	25 mg/m^2 iv push daily on days 1, 2, and 3
Repeat every 28 days	

TABLE II   PATIENT DISTRIBUTION

	Not treated previously		Treated previously, recurrent disseminated disease	Total number
Histology	Regional disease	Disseminated disease		
Adenocarcinoma	0	7	14	21
Squamous cell	15	16	14	45
Large cell	0	6	3	9
	15	29	31	75

therapy schedule for this subgroup of patients differed from that of the first two subgroups only in that the B was given as 10 U/m^2 as a slow iv push daily on days 1, 2, and 3.)

There were 50 males and 25 females, ranging in age from 35 to 77 years (median = 61 years). They were treated at four institutions: the Toronto–Bayview Regional Cancer Centre (61 patients), the Toronto General Hospital (10 patients), the Manitoba Cancer Foundation in Winnipeg (3 patients), and Mount Sinai Hospital in Toronto (1 patient). Response and survival data are available from all four centers, toxicity data from the first two centers, and effect of treatment on symptoms from the Toronto–Bayview Centre.

Complete response (CR) and partial response (PR) in measurable disease were defined by the usual criteria (Eagan et al., 1979), except that the required duration of a response was at least 8 weeks. In this study, improvement (I) is a category used for patients with evaluable but nonmeasurable disease, in which the response seemed to be equivalent to at least a PR in the judgment of two investigators. Stable (S) disease is less than a PR or I, and progressive disease (PD) is as usually defined by others (Eagan et al., 1979).

Any patient showing progression of disease (PD) after one cycle of chemotherapy did not receive further treatment with BEP. Those with stable (S) disease after one cycle were given the option either to continue with a second cycle or to stop treatment with BEP. To be assessable for response and survival, each patient needed only to complete the first 3-day cycle of drug administration.

Survival curves were calculated by the Kaplan–Meier method.

III. RESULTS

A. Overall Response Rates and Survival

All 75 patients, including 4 who died (within 4 weeks of the first treatment with BEP) and 1 with inevaluable disease, were included in the analysis of response rates and survival. These latter 5 patients were placed in the PD category.

The mean number of cycles of BEP administered to the entire group was 2.2, with a mean of 2.0 cycles to each of the 15 patients with previously untreated regional disease and 2.3 cycles to the other 60 patients (range, one to seven cycles).

The overall response rate, consisting of the sum of CR, PR, and I, was 43% (Table III). Among the 21 patients with adenocarcinoma, the response rate was 19% (2 PRs and 2 Is), while among the 9 patients with large-cell carcinoma, 78% achieved a response (4 PRs, 3 Is), and among the 45 patients with squamous-cell carcinoma, 47% achieved a response (3 CRs, 16 PRs, 2 Is). The response rate achieved by the large-cell subgroup and squamous-cell subgroups combined was 52%, which is significantly higher than the response rate in adenocarcinoma (*p* = .01).

The overall survival of patients with squamous-cell and large-cell cancer showing recurrent and/or disseminated disease was somewhat better than that of patients with adenocarcinoma (*p* = .10), as shown in Fig. 1, with median survival times (MST) of 24 and 19 weeks, respectively. The MST in patients with regional squamous-cell disease has not yet been reached (>53 weeks).

We conclude that BEP is not likely to be effective therapy for adenocarcinoma of the lung. Therefore, this subgroup will not be considered further, except to indicate that there were no responses among the 6 previously untreated patients, who fared no better than the 13 previously treated patients.

Survival of patients with recurrent and/or disseminated squamous-cell and large-cell lung cancer is included in the analysis of whether the disease was responsive to therapy (Fig. 2). The MST in patients with responses (CR, PR, and

TABLE III   RESPONSE RATES AND MEDIAN SURVIVAL TIMES (MST) ACCORDING TO HISTOLOGY

Histology	Number of patients	Number of CRs	Number of PRs and Is	Response rate (%)	MST (weeks)
Squamous cell					
Regional	15	1	7	53	>53
Disseminated	30	2	11	43	24
Large cell	9	0	7	78	24
Squamous cell and large cell combined	54	3	25	52 ⎤	24[a]
				⎬ *p* = .01	
Adenocarcinoma	21	0	4	19 ⎦	19
	75	3	29	43	22[b]

[a]Applies only to patients with recurrent or disseminated disease.

[b]Does not include patients with regional squamous cell carcinoma.

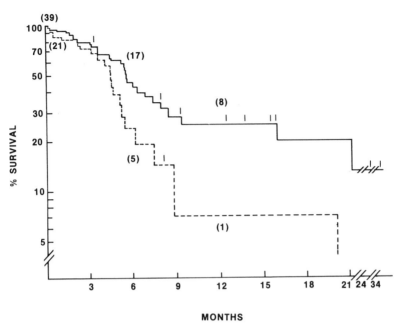

Fig. 1. Kaplan–Meier survival curves for all patients with recurrent regional and/or disseminated squamous-cell and large-cell carcinoma (——) and adenocarcinoma (– – –) of the lung. The numbers in parentheses represent patients at risk. $p = .10$.

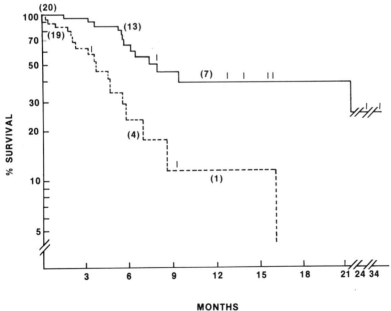

Fig. 2. Kaplan–Meier survival curves for patients with recurrent regional and/or disseminated squamous-cell or large-cell lung cancer achieving either a CR, PR, or I (——), or having no response or disease progression (– – –). The numbers in parentheses represent patients at risk. $p = .002$.

I) was 34 weeks, as compared with 16 weeks in patients with unresponsive disease (S and PD) ($p = .002$).

B. Previous Treatment

In the subgroups of patients with squamous-cell and large-cell carcinoma, only 6 of 17 previously treated patients with recurrent and/or disseminated disease achieved a response (1 CR, 2 PRs, 3 Is) for a response rate of 35% (Table IV). However, among 22 previously untreated patients with disseminated disease, the response rate was 64% (1 CR, 11 PRs, and 2 Is), while among 15 patients with regional disease also not previously treated the response rate was 53% (1 CR and 7 PRs). The combined response rate for the two groups of 37 previously untreated patients was 59%. The probability that the difference in the response rates in previously treated and previously untreated patients is due to chance is less than 1 in 14 ($p = .07$). However, overall survival and MST in these two groups (22 and 29 weeks, respectively) are not different ($p = .44$).

C. Extent of Disease

Response rates appear not to be related to extent of disease, since they were not different in previously untreated patients with regional squamous-cell disease as compared with disseminated squamous-cell disease (53 versus 64%). However, survival time is influenced by extent of disease. Patients with regional disease have a much longer survival (MST = 53 weeks) than patients with disseminated disease (MST = 24 weeks), as shown in Fig. 3.

D. Performance Status

Of all the patients with squamous-cell or large-cell carcinoma, 81% showed an Eastern Cooperative Oncology Group (ECOG) performance status of 0 or 1, and the remainder were at level 2 or 3 (Table V). The response in 44 patients with a level of 0 or 1 was 48%, while in 10 patients with a level of 2 or 3, it was apparently higher at 70%. However, this difference is not statistically significant

TABLE IV   RESPONSE RATES IN RECURRENT/DISSEMINATED SQUAMOUS-CELL AND LARGE-CELL CANCER ACCORDING TO PREVIOUS TREATMENT

Previous treatment	Number of patients	Number of CRs	Number of PRs and Is	Response rate (%)	MST (weeks)
No	22	1	13	64 ⎱ $p = .07$	29 ⎱ $p = .44$
Yes	17	1	5	35 ⎰	22 ⎰

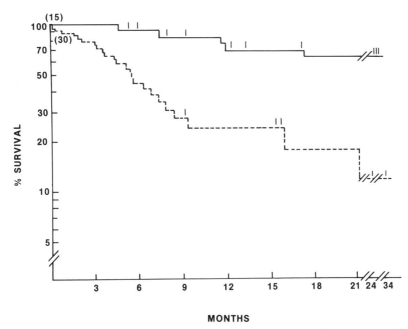

MONTHS

Fig. 3. Kaplan–Meier survival curves for previously untreated patients with squamous cell lung cancer whose disease was regional in extent (———) as compared with those whose disease was recurrent or disseminated (– – –). The numbers in parentheses represent patients at risk.

(p = .20). Similarly, the MST of the two groups did not differ significantly (p = .43), being 26 weeks in patients with an ECOG level of 0 or 1 and 23 weeks in those with an ECOG level of 2 or 3.

E. Palliation of Symptoms

Cough, hemoptysis, and pain were completely controlled or markedly improved in more than two-thirds of patients with these symptoms, often after a single cycle of BEP. Fatigue was improved in more than one-half of the patients, weight loss was reversed in two-fifths, and dyspnea was relieved in one-third of the patients. One patient with superior vena cava obstruction experienced complete relief of the obstruction, with chemotherapy being the only treatment given.

F. Toxicity

There were two treatment-related deaths, one from septicemia secondary to neutropenia and one secondary to acute nephrotoxicity. Both of these occurred during the first year of this study, and there have been no further treatment-related deaths.

TABLE V   PATIENT DISTRIBUTION WITH SQUAMOUS-CELL AND LARGE-CELL
CANCER ACCORDING TO (ECOG) PERFORMANCE STATUS, PREVIOUS TREATMENT,
AND EXTENT OF DISEASE

	Not treated previously		Treated previously recurrent/ disseminated disease	Total number
Performance status	Regional disease	Disseminated disease		
0	2	1	1	4
1	13	17	10	40
2	0	3	6	9
3	0	1	0	1
4	0	0	0	0
	15	22	17	54

Alopecia was universal, the degree being dependent on the number of cycles
of BEP. Four patients experienced clinical evidence of pulmonary toxicity, but
this was not life-threatening nor functionally debilitating in any of them. Skin
toxicity attributable to bleomycin was seen in 2 patients. Four patients refused
further treatment after one cycle of BEP.

Neutropenia was the most frequent form of myelosuppression observed (Table
VI). Even though 21% of treatment cycles given to patients with recurrent and/or
extensive disease were followed by neutropenia of less than 500/mm^3, very few
infective episodes resulted. All but one of these were treated successfully.
Thrombocytopenia was infrequent, being present after only 3% of treatment
cycles.

TABLE VI   TOXICITY AFTER BEP IN PATIENTS WITH RECURRENT
OR DISSEMINATED NSCLC

Effect	Extent	% Cycles affected
Hemoglobin	>3-g drop	18
Neutropenia	<1,000/mm^3	47
	<500/mm^3	21
Thrombocytopenia	<50,000/mm^3	6
	<25,000/mm^3	3
Creatinine	>2.1 mg/dl	3
	>3.0 mg/dl	1
Mucositis		1
Hypotension		1
Nausea and vomiting, controllable		26
Nausea and vomiting, intractable		1
Fever (38–40°C)		3

IV. DISCUSSION

Results of this study show that the major histologic types of NSCLC may respond differently to BEP. The response is significantly higher in squamous cell and large cell cancer than in adenocarcinoma ($p = .01$). The extent of disease and responsiveness to treatment were important factors in determining length of survival, but survival was not associated with previous treatment or performance status. This latter result is in contradistinction to the demonstration in previous studies that survival is related to performance status (Stanley, 1980). A possible explanation is that the 10 patients in our study with a performance status of 2 or 3 comprised too small a number to show a statistically significant difference when compared with the 44 patients with a performance status of 0 or 1.

Data conflict regarding whether bleomycin, used as single agent, is effective in treating NSCLC (Oka and Sato, 1970; Bonadonna et al., 1973; Blum et al., 1973), but in general it would seem to have little activity. Therefore, on the basis of the principles of chemotherapy, it would not be expected to be active in combination with other drugs. Yet, in instances when bleomycin was combined with cisplatin and given as a 5-day infusion, a 65–75% objective response rate in epidermoid lung cancer has been claimed (Israel et al., 1981, 1982). Bleomycin also is effective in combination with cisplatin in the treatment of squamous-cell carcinoma arising in the upper aerodigestive tract (Randolph et al., 1978; Pennacchio et al., 1982). Perhaps the explanation lies in the results of cell-culture studies with a human lymphoma cell line, in which bleomycin and cisplatin have been shown to act synergistically as compared with the cytotoxicity produced by cisplatin alone (Drewinko et al., 1976). On the other hand, the results of our study and of the EORTC study (Klastersky et al., 1982), in which only etoposide and cisplatin were used, are generally similar. This raises the question of whether the addition of bleomycin to the regimen of etoposide plus cisplatin was beneficial. A prospective, randomized, phase III study comparing BEP with EP in patients with squamous-cell and large-cell cancer would answer this question.

Our study suggests that chemotherapy with BEP for regional squamous-cell lung cancer prior to radiation therapy is feasible. Whether this combined modality approach would produce better results than that of radiation therapy alone needs to be tested in a prospective, randomized, phase III trial.

REFERENCES

Blum, R., Carter, S., and Agre, K. (1973). *Cancer* **31**, 903–914.
Bonadonna, G., Tancini, G., and Bajetta, E. (1973). *Cancer Chemotherapy Rep.* **4**, 231–237.
Drewinko, B., Green, C., and Loo, T. L. (1976). *Cancer Treat. Rep.* **60**, 1619–1625.
Eagan, R. T., Fleming, T. R., and Schoonover, V. (1979). *Cancer* **44**, 1125–1128.

Evans, W. K., Feld, R., Osoba, D., Shepherd, F. A., Dill, J. and DeBoer, G. (1984). *Cancer* **53,** 1461–1466.

Israel, L., Aguilera, J., and Breau, J. L. (1981). *Nouv. Presse Medicale* **10,** 1817–1824.

Israel, L., Breau, J. L., Kerbrat, G., De Pierre, A., Morere, P., Clavier, J., and Le Marie, E. (1982). *Bull Cancer* **69,** 355.

Klastersky, J., Longeval, E., Nicaise, C., and Weerts, D. (1982). *Cancer Treat. Rev.* **9**(suppl. A), 133–138.

Oka, S., and Sato, K. (1970). *Progress Antimicrob. Anticancer Chemother.* **2,** 712–714.

Osoba, D., Evans, W. K., and Feld, R. (1981). *Proc. Amer. Soc. Clin. Oncol.* **22,** 495.

Pnnacchio, J. L., Hong, W. K., Shapshay, S., Gillis, T., Vaughn, C., Bhutani, R., Ucmakli, A., Katz, A. E., Bromer, R., Willet, B., and Strong, S. M. (1982). *Cancer* **50,** 2795–2801.

Randolph, V. L., Vallejo, A., Spiro, R. H., Shah, J., Strong, E. W., Huvos, A. G., and Wittes, R. E. (1978). *Cancer* **41,** 460–467.

Stanley, K. E. (1980). *J. Natl. Cancer Inst.* **65,** 25–32.

Section VI
CERVICAL CANCER

Chapter 18

CERVICAL CANCER:
BLEOMYCIN STUDIES—AN OVERVIEW*

David S. Alberts
Silvio Aristizabal
Sheldon Weiner
Earl A. Surwit

The Cancer Center
College of Medicine
University of Arizona
Tucson, Arizona

I. INTRODUCTION

Although carcinoma of the cervix accounts for only ~7500 deaths annually in the United States, it is the leading cause of cancer deaths in women throughout Mexico, Central America, and South America. Aggressive Papanicolaou smear screening programs in the United States, as well as a higher socioeconomic status, which results in better access to the health care system and a greater knowledge of the importance of personal hygiene, are the primary reasons for the relatively low death rate in the United States from this disease. Because of the high cure rates of patients with stage I and stage II disease using either radiation therapy or primary surgery, the focus for new therapeutic approaches has been placed on patients with stage III and stage IV disease.

*Supported by U.S. Public Health Service grants CA 17094 and CA23074 from the National Cancer Institute, Bethesda, Maryland.

With the advent of iridium needle implant techniques, pelvic tumor masses now can be sterilized in the majority of patients; however, the high incidence of micrometastases outside radiation therapy portals in this patient population leads to treatment failure and ultimate death. Thus, chemotherapy is the only rational approach to the eradication of micrometastatic disease and may enhance the chances of controlling bulky, stage IIIB pelvic masses.

Unfortunately, the chemotherapy used in the treatment of advanced, recurrent cervical cancer to date has been relatively ineffective. Overall response rates are observed in less than 50% of patients, complete responses occur in less than 25% of patients, and long-term cures are rare. Clearly, improvement in the cure rate of stage III and stage IV cervical cancer will require both the development of more active cytotoxic agents and the use of more efficacious dosing schedules, administration routes, and drug combinations.

This chapter reviews published data concerning single- and multiple-agent chemotherapy used in the treatment of advanced, recurrent cervical cancers and discusses recent studies of drug administration prior to definitive radiation therapy in patients with metastatic lymph node or stage III and stage IV disease. The primary focus is on the role of bleomycin in the development of improved chemotherapy.

II. SINGLE-AGENT CHEMOTHERAPY

A. Active Agents Other than Bleomycin

Single-agent chemotherapy of squamous-cell cancers of the cervix has been associated with objective response rates of generally less than 30%, and no one anticancer drug has proven clearly more effective than the others. Complete response is unusual, and response durations are relatively short (i.e., <6 months). The most commonly used agents are listed in Table I. It should be noted that the largest number of trials have involved bleomycin, cisplatin, cyclophosphamide, 5-fluorouracil, doxorubicin, and methotrexate (Wasserman and Carter, 1977). Cisplatin appears to possess the most consistent activity, with overall response rates ranging from 23 to 27%. On the basis of the findings of a Gynecologic Oncology Group trial, a cisplatin dose of 50 mg/m^2 every 3 weeks is preferred over doses of 100 mg/m^2 every 3 weeks or 20 mg/m^2 daily for 5 days every 3 weeks (Bonomi *et al.*, 1982). Of the less frequently tested single agents, vincristine and mitomycin have shown considerable activity, with response rates of 23 and 22%, respectively (Wasserman and Carter, 1977).

TABLE I   SINGLE-AGENT ACTIVITY IN THE TREATMENT OF SQUAMOUS-CELL
CARCINOMA OF THE CERVIX

Reference	Number of patients	% Response	Agent
Bonomi *et al.* (1982)	138	27	Cisplatin (100 mg/m^2)
Bonomi *et al.* (1982)	122	23	Cisplatin (50 mg/m^2)
Malkasian *et al.* (1977)	208	9	5-Fluorouracil
Wasserman and Carter (1977)	188	15	Cyclophosphamide
Wasserman and Carter (1977)	172	10	Bleomycin
Piver *et al.* (1978)	88	10	Doxorubicin
Wasserman and Carter (1977)	77	16	Methotrexate
Wasserman and Carter (1977)	44	23	Vincristine
Wasserman and Carter (1977)	18	22	Mitomycin

B. Bleomycin

1. Intravenous Administration

Bleomycin has received extensive evaluation in the treatment of advanced cervical cancer, and its most effective dosing schedule continues to be a controversial issue. Wasserman and Carter (1977) reported only a 10% response rate in a collection of trials involving 172 patients (Table I). A variety of doses, administration routes, and schedules were used in those trials. The trial that has stimulated the most interest in the continuing development of bleomycin as an important agent in the treatment of cervical cancer involved its use by continuous intravenous infusion of 7 to 11 consecutive days in doses of up to 0.25 mg/kg/day. Krakoff *et al.* (1977) reported a 30% response rate to bleomycin in 32 patients using this infusion schedule. This relatively high response rate contrasts significantly to the activity of bleomycin reported by Wasserman and Carter (1977) in cervical cancer trials that used only bolus administration schedules. Despite the variability of response rates bleomycin's lack of myelosuppressive properties, unique mechanism of action, and proven synergism with cisplatin (the most consistently active agent in cervical cancer chemotherapy) recommend it for continued use in combination chemotherapy of cervical cancer.

2. Intramuscular Administration

Although there is considerable evidence that the efficacy of bleomycin is improved when it is administered by continuous intravenous infusion, this route presents some drawbacks in that repeated use generally requires continuous venous access (i.e., subclavian catheterization) and an external pump source. Thus, considerable expense and on-going nursing care are required to assure continuous drug delivery. To reduce the costs and labor associated with continuous intravenous administration of bleomycin, we have evaluated new, intermittent intramuscular, and subcutaneous dosing schedules for this agent.

Eighteen patients with gynecologic cancers were included in a pharmacokinetic study, which compared data for continuous intravenous, intermittent intramuscular, and subcutaneous dosing schedules (Alberts and Peng, 1979). A total bleomycin dose of 18 U/m² body surface area (BSA) was administered daily for 4 consecutive days by each administration route. For the intramuscular and subcutaneous dosing schedules, 6 U/m² was administered every 8 hr for 12 doses. Heparinized blood samples were obtained daily prior to the 8 a.m. dose and thereafter hourly for up to 8 hr. Following administration of the final dose on day 4 (or after termination of the continuous intravenous infusion), blood samples and 24-hr urine samples were obtained at varying intervals for as long as 240 hr. A previously published radioimmunoassay was used to measure bleomycin concentrations in both new plasma and urine samples (Broughton and Strong, 1977).

Figure 1 shows the plasma decay curves for bleomycin after continuous intravenous, intermittent intramuscular, and subcutaneous dosing. The continuous intravenous infusion route resulted in mean steady-state plasma concentrations of 0.28 ± 0.17 mU/ml, and the mean trough (i.e., concentration prior to each 8-hr dose) plasma concentrations associated with intramuscular and subcutaneous

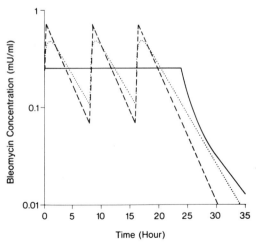

Fig. 1. Plasma disappearance of bleomycin during and following a 4-day continuous infusion of 30 U/day by three different routes in 18 patients: ——, continuous iv infusion; – – –, repeated subcutaneous injection; ·····, repeated intramuscular injection.

TABLE II   BLEOMYCIN DISPOSITION AFTER CONTINUOUS INTRAVENOUS
INFUSION VERSUS REPEATED SUBCUTANEOUS
OR INTRAMUSCULAR ADMINISTRATION[a]

Administration route	Mean trough plasma concentration (mU/ml)	Mean peak plasma concentration (mU/ml)	Plasma $t_{1/2}$ B (min)	Total plasma $C \times T^b$ (mU·hr/ml)	$C \times T^b$ ratios im or sc versus iv
Intravenous		0.28 ± 0.17	273 ± 141	27 ± 18	
Intramuscular	0.12 ± 0.04	0.55 ± 0.21	183 ± 33	26 ± 8	0.98
Subcutaneous	0.10 ± 0.10	0.71 ± 0.20	141 ± 31	25 ± 7	0.95

[a]Numbers represent mean $\pm$SD of data for up to 10 studies for each route.
[b]$C \times T$, Concentration–time products.

bleomycin dosing were 0.12 ± 0.04 and 0.10 ± 0.10 mU/ml, respectively (Table II). Of greatest importance, there were no significant differences in the cumulative plasma concentration–time products ($C \times T$) associated with the three different administration routes. Also, there were low but measurable concentrations of bleomycin in urine samples obtained daily 10 days after termination of either intravenous or intramuscular dosing, suggesting slow release of bleomycin from deep-tissue compartments.

We have concluded from these studies that it is possible to simulate the pharmacokinetics of continuous infusion bleomycin using intermittent intramuscular or subcutaneous dosing schedules. Because the subcutaneous route results in the development of subcutaneous fibrosis and skin discoloration at the drug administration sites in up to one-third of patients, we prefer to use intramuscular administration when considering an intermittent dosing schedule. The intramuscular dosing route lends itself to outpatient therapy and is, of course, considerably less expensive than continuous intravenous infusion schedules for bleomycin. Obviously, phase III clinical trials would be required to prove that the intramuscular dosing route is as efficacious as the various continuous intravenous infusion schedules.

C. Investigational Agents

A relatively large number of investigational cytotoxic agents have been evaluated in the last few years in patients with recurrent, advanced cervical cancer. Shown in Table III are data concerning three of the more active agents (Baker's antifol, dianhydrogalactitol, and ICRF-159), which have been evaluated in at least 25 patients. None of these drugs are receiving further clinical trials in cervical cancer; however, dibromodulcitol, a metabolite of dianhydrogalactitol, is under current investigation.

TABLE III   INVESTIGATIONAL AGENTS WITH ACTIVITY IN THE TREATMENT
OF CERVICAL CANCER

Reference	Number of patients evaluated	Response rate (%)	Agent
Arseneau *et al.* (1980)	32	16	Baker's antifol
Blum *et al.* (1980)	36	19	Dianhydrogalactitol
Conroy *et al.* (1980)	28	18	ICRF-159

III. COMBINATION CHEMOTHERAPY INCLUDING BLEOMYCIN

A. Chemotherapy after Recurrence or Progression of Disease Following Definitive Radiation Therapy or Surgery

1. Background

Bleomycin has been incorporated into numerous drug combinations for the treatment of recurrent or metastatic disease following the failure of definitive radiation therapy or surgery. Its frequent use in this setting has been justified by its lack of myelosuppressive properties and its known synergistic interaction with other drugs commonly used in the treatment of squamous-cell cancer of the cervix, such as cisplatin and vincristine. In these combinations, bleomycin usually has been administered by weekly bolus injection in doses of 10 to 15 U/m^2 or on a continuous intravenous infusion schedule in total daily doses of 5 to 30 U for 4 to 7 days.

2. Bleomycin–Mitomycin

A series of six trials of bleomycin–mitomycin combination chemotherapy have been reported following the remarkably high complete response rate of 80% obtained by Miyamoto *et al.* (1978) in a Japanese study (Table IV). The chemotherapy schedule called for 5 U of bleomycin to be administered as an intravenous infusion over 3 to 4 hr daily for 7 days. Mitomycin at 10 mg was administered on day 8. Courses were repeated every 2 weeks as tolerated. The five follow-up evaluations of the Japanese trial failed to show such optimistic response rates (Table IV). In fact, studies by Leichman *et al.* (1980) in the Southwest Oncology Group and by Greenberg *et al.* (1982) in the Northern California Oncology Group revealed objective response rates of only 16 and 18%, respectively. One possible explanation for the discrepancy in results between these studies using identical chemotherapy regimens relates to the various

TABLE IV   BLEOMYCIN–MITOMYCIN COMBINATION THERAPY OF
ADVANCED RECURRENT CERVICAL CANCER

Reference	Number of patients	Response rate (%)
Miyamoto et al. (1978)	15	93
Krebs et al. (1980)	20	40
Petrilli et al. (1980)	9	18
Leichman et at. (1980)	19	16
Greenberg et al. (1982)	18	18
Trope et al. (1983)	33	36

sites of recurrent disease in each patient population. For example, in the
Miyamoto trial (Miyamoto et al., 1978) only 3 of 15 patients had pelvic and
intraabdominal tumor masses.

3. Bleomycin–Mitomycin–Vincristine

At Wayne State University, Baker et al. (1976) evaluated a combination
treatment using mitomycin at 20 mg/m² every 6 weeks and vincristine at 0.5
mg/m² 6 hr before administering bleomycin at 6 U/m² by intravenous bolus
twice a week for 12 weeks. These investigators obtained a 48% overall response
rate in 27 patients. A follow-up phase III trial by the Southwest Oncology Group
compared this regimen with one containing bleomycin and vincristine in the
same doses given once a week for 24 weeks along with mitomycin at 20 mg/m²
every 6 weeks, and with a third regimen containing bleomycin as a continuous 4-
day intravenous infusion (30 U every day) every 6 weeks (Baker et al., 1978).
As shown in Table V, the highest overall response rate (60%) was observed in

TABLE V   BLEOMYCIN–VINCRISTINE–MITOMYCIN THERAPY FOR
ADVANCED, RECURRENT CERVICAL CANCER[a]

Bleomycin schedule	Number of patients	Response rate (%)	Response duration (months)
6 U/m² iv bolus twice weekly × 12 weeks	50	60	2
30 U day × 4 iv infusion q 6 weeks	41	39	4
6 U/m² iv bolus once weekly × 24 weeks	24	25	3

[a]From Baker et al. (1978).

the 50 patients who received bleomycin twice a week by bolus administration. However, this response rate was not significantly different from the 39% response rate observed in the 41 patients who received bleomycin on the continuous intravenous schedule. In addition, the regimen containing vincristine–bleomycin twice a week was associated with severe neurologic toxicity. Of interest was the finding that the mean duration of response tended to be almost twice as long in the patients administered bleomycin by intravenous infusion. The drug schedule that included only vincristine–bleomycin once a week proved statistically inferior to the other two regimens. Considering the response rates, response duration, and toxicity observed, the three-drug combination including bleomycin by continuous infusion appeared to be the most efficacious.

4. Bleomycin–Mitomycin–Vincristine–Cisplatin

A natural evolution of the bleomycin–mitomycin–vincristine (MOB) combination for advanced cervical cancer involved the addition of cisplatin. We previously reported results of treatment with the MOB plus cisplatin four-drug combination in patients who had relapsed following primary radiation therapy (Alberts *et al.*, 1981; Alberts and Surwit, 1983). The initial study involved 14 patients who received at least two full courses of MOB plus cisplatin, as outlined in Table VI. Bleomycin was administered by continuous intravenous infusion based on the relatively low degree of toxicity reported by Baker *et al.* (1978) in the Southwest Oncology Group trial, when the drug was administered by this schedule instead of by the twice weekly bolus schedule. Five of the 14 patients (36%) achieved a complete response, lasting 8, 20, 23+, 30+, and 34+ months. Three of these patients achieved complete disappearance of pulmonary metastases, one showed resolution of a large left-sided pelvic-wall mass, and one showed complete disappearance of all skeletal metastases documented at autopsy. The median survival was 8 months for all 14 patients and 20 months for the 7 responders. Three patients have remained long-term disease-free and appear to be cured of their disease.

The chemotherapy regimen was extremely well tolerated. There were no instances of severe or irreversible renal dysfunction or peripheral neuropathy. The mean lowest white blood cell and platelet counts were 4540 and 205,000 per

TABLE VI   THE MOB PLUS CISPLATIN REGIMEN
FOR ADVANCED CERVICAL CANCER

Drug	Amount
Mitomycin	10 mg/m^2 iv days 1, 43
Cisplatin	50 mg/m^2 iv days 1, q 3 weeks × 6
Bleomycin	30 U iv infusion days 1–4, 43–46
Vincristine	0.5 mg/m^2 iv days 1, 4, 43, 46

deciliter, respectively. Although severe or life-threatening thrombocytopenia occurred in only 36% of patients, it appeared to be the dose-limiting toxicity of this drug combination.

Vogl *et al.* (1981) have reported the results of a similar clinical trial of mitomycin, vincristine, bleomycin, and cisplatin for advanced cervical cancer in 16 patients. In contrast to the MOB plus cisplatin regimen, they administered bleomycin as a weekly 10-U intramuscular dose. Mitomycin, vincristine, and cisplatin dosing schedules were otherwise similar. Of the 13 evaluable patients, 7 had partial responses and 3 had complete responses. The median projected survival for the 10 responders was only 10 months, and no mention was made of long-term complete responders.

A possible explanation for the more prolonged survival in responders observed by Alberts *et al.* (1981, 1982) may be related to the use of bleomycin as a continuous 4-day infusion. Prestayko and Crooke (1978) observed that when bleomycin is given in a dose of 20 to 30 U as a continuous infusion over 4 days, a deep-tissue compartment is established. Thus, more durable complete responses may result from a favorable bleomycin dosing schedule.

A follow-up phase II randomized study by the Southwest Oncology Group has compared the MOB plus cisplatin regimen to mitomycin plus cisplatin in an attempt to evaluate the role of continuous infusion bleomycin in the four-drug combination. Although the trial has been closed to further patient entry for more than six months, it is still too early to draw final conclusions concerning the efficacy of bleomycin when combined with mitomycin and cisplatin. Furthermore, the phase II trial design is not likely to yield a definitive answer.

5. Bleomycin–Cisplatin with or without Other Agents

A relatively large number of phase II clinical trials have been reported in which bleomycin was combined with cisplatin and methotrexate, cisplatin and doxorubicin, or cisplatin and vinblastine. One such combination of bleomycin–cisplatin–doxorubicin, reported by Sorbe and Frankendal (1984), was used to treat 21 consecutive patients. They reported four complete responses (19%) and four partial responses (19%). Of considerable interest was the finding that the objective response rate was 14.3% for patients with tumors within previously irradiated pelvic tissues but 100% for patients with distant metastases (75% were complete responses). Several investigators have commented on the difficulty of treating pelvic-tumor recurrences with systemically administered chemotherapy. Following radiation therapy of definitive intent, the microvasculature in pelvic structures may be compromised severely, leading to poor or inconsistent drug delivery.

Another reported study by Friedlander *et al.* (1983) failed to reveal a difference in complete or partial response rates between patients with primarily pelvic and distant lymph nodal disease. However, 10 of their patients with locally advanced bulky cervical tumors were treated with three courses of chemotherapy prior to any radiation therapy. These investigators used a combination of cisplatin at 60 mg/m² on day 1, vinblastine at 4 mg/m² on days 1 and 2, and bleomycin at 15 U by intramuscular administration on days 1, 8, and 15, with courses of therapy being repeated every 3 weeks. Objective tumor responses occurred in two-thirds of 33 evaluable patients and included a complete response rate of 18%.

Of 23 patients with locally recurrent or distant metastatic cervical cancer following radiation therapy and/or surgery, 69% responded to chemotherapy, including 6 patients (26%) who achieved complete tumor regression. The median duration of tumor response from the start of chemotherapy was in excess of 24 weeks for the complete responders, with median survival duration for this group ranging from 24+ to 104+ weeks (median, >40 weeks).

By far the most interesting aspect of this study was the treatment with three courses of cisplatin–vinblastine–bleomycin for 10 patients with stage IIB to stage IV disease prior to the use of radiation therapy or surgery. Six of these patients (60%) achieved a partial tumor regression and 3 showed stabilized disease. Seven of the 9 patients who went on to receive radiation therapy achieved complete tumor regressions. Thus, this small pilot trial of chemotherapy prior to radiation therapy indicates that bulky pelvic disease may be eradicated in more than 75% of patients with the combination treatment. It is hoped that future clinical trials will focus more heavily on the use of combination chemotherapy prior to the use of definitive radiation therapy or surgery.

B. Chemotherapy prior to Definitive Radiation Therapy or Surgery

Based on the evidence that the MOB regimen (using continuous intravenous infusion bleomycin) was associated with apparent long-term disease-free survivals and possibly cures in approximately 20% of patients with recurrent and/or distant metastatic cervical cancer, we have conducted a pilot study at the University of Arizona Cancer Center of this combination chemotherapy given prior to radiation therapy of curative intent. The objectives of this pilot study were twofold: (1) to determine whether combination chemotherapy using mitomycin, vincristine, bleomycin, and cisplatin could be administered safely prior to radiation therapy of curative intent in patients with far advanced stages IIB (with positive paraaortic lymph nodes) through IVA disease, as well as to evaluate the safety of administering cisplatin during the course of radiation therapy, and (2) to evaluate the complete plus partial objective response rate to chemotherapy prior to the start of radiation therapy.

Two courses of the MOB plus cisplatin regimen (Table VI) were administered prior to definitive radiation therapy in 15 patients with squamous-cell carcinoma of the cervix. Cisplatin at 50 mg/m^2 every 3 weeks also was administered during the radiation therapy treatment. Patients showed either advanced bulky disease (stage IIB, 1 patient, stage IIIB, 9 patients, stage IVA, 1 patient) or pathologically proven positive paraaortic lymph nodes (stage IB, 3 patients; stage IIA, 1 patient). Radiation therapy consisted of 4500 rad whole pelvic radiation with cisplatin at 50 mg/m^2 being continued during radiation therapy at 3-week intervals. Paraaortic radiation therapy also was administered to four patients. External radiation therapy was followed by either a single interstitial implant or tandem and ovoids in all patients.

The MOB plus cisplatin chemotherapy was well tolerated, with no severe or life-threatening toxicities occurring. No significant bone marrow suppression or delays in radiation therapy were encountered. One patient developed a rectovaginal fistula following completion of radiation therapy.

After the completion of two courses of MOB plus cisplatin, 10 patients (67%) had responded, with 3 complete responses (20%) and 7 partial responses (47%). Nine patients remain alive without evidence of disease following the completion of radiation therapy. Six patients have died, 4 of whom had shown no response to chemotherapy. One of these 4 patients died with progression of the primary pelvic disease. Two patients showed recurrence of pelvic disease, and 1 showed recurrence of pelvic disease as well as distant metastases. Two additional deaths occurred in patients whose pelvic tumors had undergone a greater than 50% regression following chemotherapy. One of these patients suffered a recurrence of pelvic disease 11 months after the documentation of a partial response to chemotherapy. The second patient had evidence of distant metastases 5 months after the onset of partial response to chemotherapy.

Results of this pilot study and those of Friedlander *et al.* (1983) suggest that combination chemotherapy, including at least cisplatin and bleomycin, can be administered safely prior to definitive radiation therapy for advanced cervical cancer. Furthermore, these chemotherapy regimens can induce complete disappearance of bulky primary tumors in ~20% of patients.

Whether these chemotherapy–radiation therapy regimens are likely to increase the disease-free or overall survivals of patients with far-advanced disease can be determined only by future phase III randomized trials. Certainly this therapeutic approach provides a new direction in the treatment of patients who have only a 30–35% chance of surviving 5 years.

REFERENCES

Alberts, D. S., and Peng, Y.-M. (1979). *Proc. Am. Soc. Clin. Oncol.* **20,** 432.

Alberts, D. S., Martimbeau, P. W., Surwit, E. A., and Oishi, N. (1981). *Cancer Clin. Trials* **4,** 313–316.

Alberts, D. S., and Surwit, E. A. (1982). *In:* ''Mitomycin C: Current Impact on Cancer Chemotherapy'' (M. Ogawa, M. Rozencweig and M. J. Staquet, eds.), pp. 127–134. Excerpta Medica, Princeton.

Arseneau, J. C., Bundy, B., Dolan, T., Homesley, H., DiSaia, P. (1980). *Proc. Am. Soc. Clin. Oncol.* **21**, 424.

Baker, L. H., Opipari, M. I., and Izbicki, R. M. (1976). *Cancer* **38**, 2222–2224.

Baker, L. H., Opipari, M. I., Wilson, H., Bottomley, R., and Coltman, C. A., Jr. (1978). *Obstet. Gynecol.* **52**, 146–150.

Blum, J., Blessing, J., Mladineo, J., Mangan, C., Ehrlich, C., and Homesely, M. (1980). *Proc. Am. Soc. Clin. Oncol.* **21**, 416.

Bonomi, P., Bruckner, H., Cohen, C., Marshall, R., Blessing, J., and Slayton, R. (1982). *Proc. Am. Soc. Clin. Oncol.* **18**, 110.

Broughton, A., and Strong, J. E. (1977). *Cancer Res.* **36**, 1430.

Conroy, J., Blessing, J., Lewis, G., Mangan, C., Hutch, K., and Wilbanks, G. (1980). *Proc. Am. Soc. Clin. Oncol.* **21**, 423.

Friedlander, M., Kaye, S. B., Sullivan, A., Atkinson, K., Elliott, P., Coppleson, M., Houghton, R., Solomon, J., Green, D., Russell, P., Hudson, C. N., Langlands, A. O., and Tattersall, M. H. N. (1983). *Gynecol. Oncol.* **16**, 275–281.

Greenberg, B. R., Hannigan, J., Jr., Gerretson, L., Turbow, M. M., Friedman, M. A., Hendrickson, C. A., Glassberg, A., and Carter, S. K. (1982). *Cancer Treat. Rep.* **66**, 163–165.

Krakoff, I. H., Cvitkovic, E., Carrie, V., Yeh, S., and LaMonte, C. (1977). *Cancer* **40**, 2027–2037.

Krebs, H. B., Girtanna, R. E., Nordquist, S. R., Mineau, I., Helmkamp, B. F., and Livingston, R. (1980). *Cancer* **46**, 2159–2161.

Leichman, L. P., Baker, L. H., Stanhope, C. R., Samson, M. R., Fraile, R. J., Vaitkevicius, U. K., and Hilgers, R. (1980). *Cancer Treat. Rep.* **64**, 1139–1140.

Malkasian, G. D., Jr., Decker, D. G., and Jørgensen, E. O. (1977). *Gynecol. Oncol.* **5**, 109–120.

Miyamoto, T., Takabe, R., Watanabe, M., and Terasima, T. (1978). *Cancer* **41**, 403–414.

Petrilli, E. S., Castaldo, T. W., Ballon, S. C., Roberts, J. A., and Lagasse, L. D. (1980). *Gynecol. Oncol.* **9**, 292–297.

Piver, M. S., Barlow, J. J., and Xynos, F. P. (1978). *Am. J. Obstet. Gynecol.* **131**, 311–313.

Prestayko, A. W., and Crooke, S. T. (1978). *In:* "Bleomycin[:] Current Status and New Developments" (S. K. Carter, S. T. Crooke, and H. Umezawa, eds.), pp. 117–129. Academic Press, New York.

Sorbe, B., and Frankendal, B. (1984). *Obstet. Gynecol.* **63**, 167–170.

Trope, C., Johnson, J. E., Simonson, E., Sigurdsson, J., Stendahl, U., Mattson, W., and Gullberg, B. (1983) *Cancer* **51**, 591–593.

Vogl, S. E., Moukhtar, M., Calanog, A., Greenwald, E. H., and Kaplan, B. H. (1981). *Cancer Treat. Rep.* **64**, 1005.

Wasserman, T. H., and Carter, S. K. (1977). *Cancer Treat. Rev.* **4**, 25–26.

Chapter 19

BLEOMYCIN IN CERVICAL CARCINOMA: PROTOCOLS OF THE NORTHERN CALIFORNIA ONCOLOGY GROUP

Samuel C. Ballon

Department of Gynecology/Obstetrics
Section of Gynecologic Oncology
Stanford University School of Medicine
Stanford, California

Branimir Ivan Sikic

Department of Medicine
Divisions of Oncology and Clinical Pharmacology
Stanford University School of Medicine
Stanford, California

I. INTRODUCTION

Although a variety of cytotoxic drugs have demonstrated activity against squamous carcinoma of the uterine cervix, no single agent or combination of agents has produced a clinically meaningful increase in duration of response or survival (Wasserman and Carter, 1977). Patients with advanced or recurrent cervical carcinoma that is not amenable to curative surgery or irradiation are candidates for new and promising treatment programs.

Bleomycin is active as a single agent against a variety of squamous cancers, including those originating in the uterine cervix. In addition, bleomycin has proven attractive for use in combination with other agents because it infrequently causes myelosuppression. Miyamoto *et al.* (1978) reported greater than a 90% response to the sequential administration of bleomycin and mitomycin among 15 patients with metastatic cervical carcinoma. The Gynecology Committee of the

TABLE I   NCOG PROTOCOL 5C81
DOSE SCHEDULE

Bleomycin	5 U iv bolus days 1–7
Mitomycin	5 mg/m^2 iv bolus day 8
Repeat every 15 days	

Northern California Oncology Group (NCOG) initially sought to confirm these preliminary results.

II. NCOG PROTOCOL 5C81

Protocol 5C81 established a 22% response rate in 18 evaluable patients with advanced, recurrent squamous cancer of the cervix using 5 U of bleomycin by iv bolus on days 1–7 and 5 mg/m^2 of mitomycin by iv bolus on day 8, repeated every 2 weeks, as shown in Table I (Greenberg et al., 1982). A minimum of three and maximum of five courses were administered.

The median duration of response was 3.4 months, with a median survival time of 8.5 months for responders and 4.0 months for nonresponders. All four responses were partial and involved pelvic tumor in 2 patients, distant disease (lung, liver) in 1 patient, and pelvic plus distant tumor (supraclavicular lymph nodes) in 1 patient (Tables II and III).

Hematologic toxicity was both mild and infrequent. No patient evidenced leukopenia below 2000/mm^3, and only one patient showed a thrombocyte nadir below 90,000/mm^3.

Five episodes of severe, nonhematologic toxicity occurred: one case of severe gastrointestinal toxicity, (diarrhea, nausea, vomiting), one of cutaneous toxicity, and three cases of bleomycin pulmonary toxicity (two severe, one moderate). Pulmonary toxicity occurred after the administration of 210, 210, and 245 U of bleomycin.

TABLE II   SITES OF RECURRENT
TUMOR IN NCOG 5C81 STUDY

Site	Number of patients
Pelvis	8
Distant	4
Pelvis and distant	6
	18

TABLE III   RESPONSE AGAINST SITE OF
RECURRENT TUMOR IN NCOG 5C81 STUDY

Site	Number of patients	Response Number	%
Pelvis	8	2	25
Distant	4	1	25
Pelvis and distant	6	1	17
	18	4	22 (total)

III. NCOG PROTOCOL 5C91

In December 1980, protocol 5C91 was activated, using cisplatin, bleomycin, and mitomycin in patients with recurrent and metastatic squamous carcinoma of the uterine cervix (Picozzi *et al.*, 1985). Cisplatin was added because of its activity as a single agent in this disease, as well as its nonoverlapping toxicity with the other two drugs. The dose of bleomycin in this study was increased to 15 U/m^2/day and was given as a continuous 72-hr iv infusion on days 1 through 3, mitomycin was given as an iv bolus of 10 mg/m^2 on day 1 of alternate courses of therapy, and cisplatin at 50 mg/m^2 was given as an iv infusion on day 4 of each 21-day course (Table IV).

Twenty-eight patients were entered into this study, which closed in October 1982. Patient characteristics are presented in Table V, and sites of recurrent tumor are shown in Table VI. The overall rate of response was 21% (Table VII). Responses occurred in 1 of 11 patients (9%) with tumor confined to the pelvis. Four of 14 patients (29%) with both pelvic and extrapelvic tumor responded in all sites, and an additional 3 of these patients responded only in extrapelvic sites. One of 3 patients with only extrapelvic tumor responded. Thus, extrapelvic tumor responded in 8 of 17 patients (47%), but pelvic tumor responded in only 5 of 26 (19%).

TABLE IV   NCOG PROTOCOL 5C91
DOSE SCHEDULE

Bleomycin	15 U/m^2/day on days 1 through 3[a]
Mitomycin	10 mg/m^2 iv bolus on day 1[b]
Cisplatin	50 mg/m^2 iv infusion on day 4[c]

[a]Continous 72-hr iv infusion every 3 weeks.
[b]Every 6 weeks.
[c]Every 3 weeks.

TABLE V PATIENT CHARACTERISTICS[a] IN NCOG
5C91 STUDY

Prior therapy	Number of patients	%
Surgery	2	7
Radiation	15	53
Surgery and radiation	10	36
None	1	4
	28	100

[a]Mean age, 48.5 years; median Karnofsky status, 75.

This combination was relatively well tolerated; however, most patients required dose reduction of cisplatin and mitomycin because of myelosuppression. Only one patient experienced granulocytopenia below $1000/mm^3$. No significant thrombocytopenia was encountered. Moderate to severe nausea was frequent, and three patients developed alopecia. Other significant complications included one episode of acute, transient renal failure, one allergic reaction to cisplatin, one case of fatal aspergillus pneumonia, and one episode of exfoliative dermatitis secondary to bleomycin. No patient developed pulmonary toxicity from bleomycin.

IV. DISCUSSION

These studies were designed to test the ability to deliver combinations of cytotoxic agents to patients with advanced, squamous carcinoma of the cervix. In general, combination chemotherapy has been difficult to administer to this patient population because of prior high-dose pelvic irradiation, the prevalence of obstructive uropathy, and general debilitation.

The combination of bleomycin and mitomycin was relatively well tolerated,

TABLE VI SITES OF RECURRENT
TUMOR IN NCOG 5C91

Site	Number of patients
Pelvis	11
Distant	3
Pelvis and distant	14
	28

TABLE VII   RESPONSE AGAINST SITE OF RECURRENT
TUMOR IN NCOG 5C91 STUDY

Site	Number of patients	Response	
		Number	%
Pelvis	11	1	9
Distant	3	1	33
Pelvis and distant	14	4	29
	28	6	21 (total)

although 3 of 18 patients (17%) did develop pulmonary toxicity secondary to bleomycin administered as an iv bolus. The 22% response rate was associated with early relapse and had little impact upon overall survival.

The addition of cisplatin to these two drugs produced no significant improvement in patient outcome. Failure to achieve a higher rate of response could be secondary to a number of factors: (1) intrinsic tumor insensitivity to the agents employed, (2) the necessity of frequent dose reductions because of myelosuppression potentiated by previous pelvic irradiation, and (3) suboptimal drug delivery to previously irradiated pelvic disease sites as suggested by the differential responsiveness of extrapelvic versus pelvic tumor.

The absence of pulmonary toxicity secondary to bleomycin in 5C91 as compared with the 17% incidence seen in 5C81 (Table VIII) suggests that bleomycin administration by continuous infusion can reduce this risk from that seen with administration by bolus injection. However, these numbers are too small to achieve clinical significance.

In summary, bleomycin and mitomycin, without the addition of cisplatin, have minimal activity in patients with recurrent and metastatic squamous carcinoma of the uterine cervix. The development of more active agents remains a primary objective.

TABLE VIII   TOXICITY EXPERIENCED IN 5C81 AND 5C91

Toxicity	5C81	5C91
Hematologic	Mild, infrequent	Mild, infrequent
Gastrointestinal	Infrequent	Moderate, severe
Cutaneous	Infrequent	Infrequent
Pulmonary	Moderate, severe	None
Renal	None	Reversible, infrequent
Other	None	Alopecia, aspergillus pneumonia

REFERENCES

Greenberg, B. R., Hannigan J., Jr., Gerretson, L., Turbow, M. M., Friedman, M. A., Hendrickson, C. A., Glassberg, A., and Carter, S. K. (1982). *Cancer Treat. Rep.* **66,** 163–165.

Miyamoto, T., Yakabe, Y., Watanabe, M., and Terasima, T. (1978). *Cancer* **41,** 403–414.

Picozzi, V. J., Sikic, B. I., Carlson, R. W., Koretz, M., and Ballon, S. C. (1985). *Cancer Treat. Rep.* (in press).

Wasserman, T. H., and Carter, S. K. (1977). *Cancer Treat. Rev.* **4,** 25–46.

Section VII
PULMONARY TOXICITY

Bleomycin Chemotherapy
(B. I. Sikic, M. Rozencweig, and S. K. Carter, eds.)

Chapter 20

PULMONARY TOXICITY OF BLEOMYCIN*

Branimir Ivan Sikic
Department of Medicine
Divisions of Oncology and Clinical Pharmacology
Stanford University School of Medicine
Stanford, California

I. INCIDENCE AND RISK FACTORS

Pulmonary fibrosis is the major dose-limiting toxicity of bleomycin. The overall incidence of clinically apparent toxicities is 10%, with a 1% incidence of lethality (Muggia *et al.*, 1983). The risk for serious pulmonary toxicity increases markedly when the total cumulative dose of bleomycin exceeds 400 units. However, significant decreases in carbon monoxide diffusing capacity (DL_{CO}) have been observed in almost all patients treated with the PVB (cisplatin, vinblastine, and bleomycin) regimen for testicular carcinoma above a total bleomycin dose of more than 250 units (Comis, *et al.*, 1979). Moreover, fatal pulmonary toxicity has been reported to occur, although rarely, with total doses of less than 100 units.

Several risk factors have been identified that increase the potential for pulmonary toxicity. These include patient age over 70 years, thoracic radiation therapy (Catane *et al.*, 1979), preexisting pulmonary disease, impaired renal function

*Supported in part by National Institutes of Health grant CA-27478 from the U.S. Department of Health and Human Services.

(Bennett *et al.*, 1980), and an increased inspired oxygen concentration during anesthesia (Goldiner *et al.*, 1978). Patients who receive bleomycin either before, during, or after chest radiotherapy are reported to have an approximate 20% incidence of significant pulmonary toxicity, and a markedly increased lethality rate of 10% (Catane *et al.*, 1979). Fulminant and lethal pulmonary toxicity also has been reported when bleomycin was administered after renal failure had developed with cisplatin therapy (Bennett *et al.*, 1980). The risk for lung toxicity appears additive in patients with prior exposure to bleomycin who later receive additional bleomycin (Crooke *et al.*, 1978).

II. CLINICAL FEATURES

Most commonly, bleomycin pulmonary toxicity becomes manifest with the development of an insidious dry cough and dyspnea on exertion. A physical examination may disclose bibasilar rales, with radiographic evidence of increased interstitial markings, predominantly in the lung bases. However, a variety of clinical presentations of pulmonary problems are seen with patients receiving bleomycin therapy. Acute fever, dyspnea, and new pulmonary infiltrates occur quite commonly in immunocompromised hosts. Infection is the most likely diagnosis in this acute setting, and it is mandatory to perform a workup for pneumonia secondary to bacteria, viruses, *Pneumocystis carinii,* or other opportunistic organisms. Frequently, this includes performing an open or transbronchial lung biopsy.

Drug toxicity is most likely if the clinical presentation includes a nonproductive cough, basilar fibrosis on chest X-ray film, and absence of dyspnea and fever. The extent of the work-up depends upon the clinical suspicion for infection and may not require a lung biopsy. A reduced DL_{CO} is the most sensitive indicator of pulmonary toxicity in these patients (Comis *et al.*, 1979). It should be emphasized that even with biopsy, bleomycin pulmonary toxicity is a diagnosis of exclusion. Most patients who have received greater than 200 units of drug will have some of the typical histologic features of bleomycin effect on a biopsy. Therefore, it is important to rule out treatable infections as coexisting problems. Bleomycin should be discontinued if there is a suspicion that toxicity is present, or if significant pulmonary compromise has developed due to other causes.

Localized fibrosis simulating tumor nodules has been described after PVB therapy for testicular cancer (Nachman *et al.*, 1981). In the setting of an isolated nodule or nodules in patients who have shown preexisting pulmonary metastasis or tumors that metastasize to the lungs, tumor recurrence or persistence may be more likely than drug toxicity. A needle aspiration is inadequate to make the diagnosis of drug-related fibrosis; therefore, an open biopsy may be necessary.

Bleomycin also may produce a hypersensitivity pneumonitis, as observed by

Holoye *et al.* (1978). In their report of three patients, the presentation was more acute than normally is seen in bleomycin pulmonary toxicity, with fever, dyspnea, and asymmetric pulmonary infiltrates. Two of the three patients demonstrated peripheral eosinophilia, and the lung biopsies showed alveolar eosinophilia characteristic of hypersensitivity pneumonitis. The patients were treated with steroids and showed prompt resolution. This type of bleomycin toxicity is probably quite rare compared with the more common direct pulmonary injury. Other drugs that have been reported to produce a similar hypersensitivity pneumonitis include methotrexate and procarbazine (Muggia *et al.,* 1983).

III. PATHOGENESIS AND HISTOPATHOLOGY

The lung injury of bleomycin appears to be due to a direct toxic effect on endothelial and alveolar lining cells by free radicals generated by the bleomycin–oxygen complex (Muggia *et al.,* 1983). The lungs are particularly susceptible to bleomycin because of their very low levels of the inactivating enzyme bleomycin hydrolase. Fibrosis results as the end stage of pulmonary inflammation and

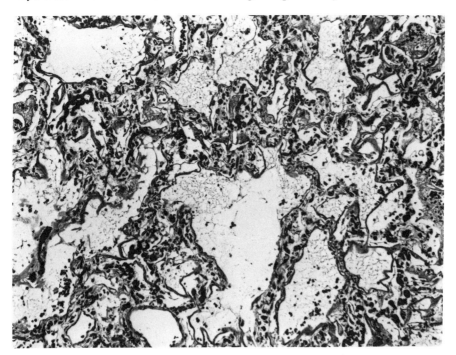

Fig. 1. The earliest histopathologic changes of bleomycin pulmonary toxicity on light microscopy include hyaline membrane formation and intraalveolar edema, due to damage to capillary endothelial cells and the type 1 alveolar lining cells (membranous pneumocytes). H + E, ×100.

repair. The histopathologic features of bleomycin lung toxicity include necrosis of type 1 alveolar epithelial cells, "atypical epithelial proliferation" of type 2 cells, increased numbers of alveolar macrophages, hyaline membranes, and interstitial fibrosis (see Figs. 1–4).

Bleomycin has been shown to produce pulmonary toxicity in many animal species (Sikic *et al.*, 1978a; Muggia *et al.*, 1983). The mouse model has been particularly useful in studying the pathogenesis of bleomycin lung toxicity as well as the effects of potential ameliorative agents, schedules of drug administration, and new analogs. The histologic changes in mice are identical to those in humans. The mouse model has been used to show that the risk of pulmonary toxicity is reduced by continuous infusion of bleomycin compared with bolus injection, as shown in Table I (Sikic *et al.*, 1978b). Vincristine has been shown to increase pulmonary toxicity when administered with bleomycin (Louie *et al.*, 1980). Several other agents had no effect on bleomycin pulmonary toxicity in this mouse model, including glucocorticoids, doxorubicin, methotrexate, vinblastine, and cyclophosphamide. Increased ambient oxygen concentrations

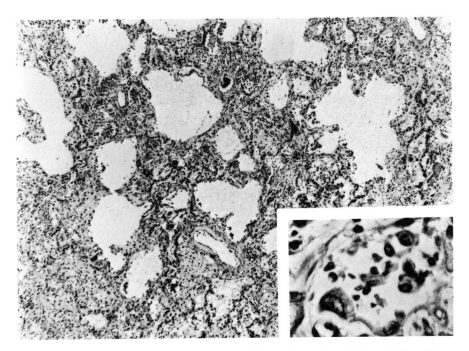

Fig. 2. The initial damage to alveolar lining cells is followed by an interstitial organization of the hyaline membranes by spindle-shaped fibroblasts and mononuclear cells. H + E, × 100. (Inset) Foamy macrophages fill air spaces, and atypical granular pneumocytes (type II) line alveolar septae. H + E, ×400.

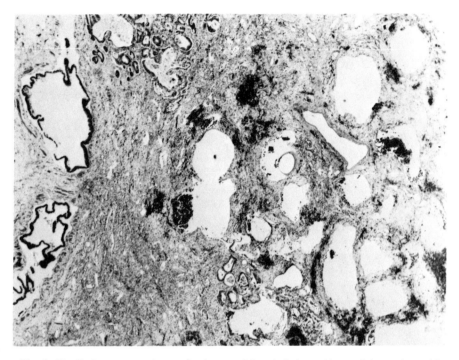

Fig. 3. The final common pathway of pulmonary injury includes architectural destruction, with interstitial fibrosis and the formation of end stage honeycomb lung. H + E, ×20.

greatly potentiated bleomycin lethality (Toledo *et al.*, 1982). It appears that cell-mediated immunity does not play a role in the pathogenesis of bleomycin pulmonary toxicity, since athymic nude mice appear to be as susceptible as strains with normal immune function (Szapiel *et al.*, 1979).

IV. CLINICAL MANAGEMENT

The most sensitive indicator of bleomycin pulmonary toxicity on pulmonary function testing appears to be the DL_{CO} (Comis *et al.*, 1979). A significant decrease in DL_{CO} of greater than 30% from predicted normal was observed in virtually all patients studied after receiving 250 units of bleomycin on the PVB regimen. When patients were used as their own controls, progressive decreases in DL_{CO} were seen with increasing doses of drug. Lethal toxicity was observed in one case when there was a greater than 60% decrease from predicted normal DL_{CO}. The DL_{CO} was a more sensitive indicator than the forced vital capacity, and a slight further decrease occurred over a 2- to 3-month period after the last

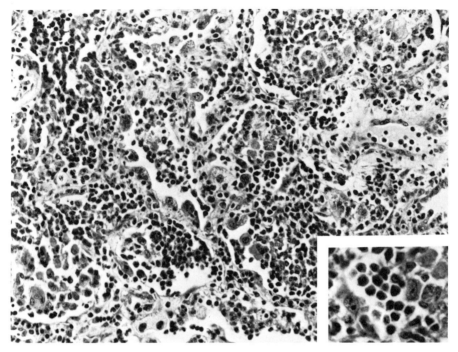

Fig. 4. A rare form of bleomycin pulmonary toxicity is a hypersensitivity reaction, manifested by fevers, asymmetric pulmonary infiltrates, and peripheral eosinophilia. There is airspace consolidation by variable numbers of eosinophils and macrophages (eosinophilic pneumonia). H + E, × 40. (Inset) Bilobed eosinophils and macrophages fill air spaces lined by reactive type II pneumocytes. H + E, ×400.

dose of bleomycin. Partial recovery was observed within 6 months of discontinuing the drug.

Minimization of bleomycin pulmonary toxicity in clinical practice requires an awareness of the risk factors. It is advisable to obtain both a chest X-ray film and a DL_{CO} measurement every 3 to 4 weeks when patients have received a total dose of more than 200 units of bleomycin. The drug should be discontinued if there are any symptoms or signs of pulmonary toxicity, including a decrease of the DL_{CO} to less than 50% of predicted normal. These recommendations are quite arbitrary and are based on a limited clinical data base. Further prospective studies are needed to determine whether they will have a major impact on reducing the incidence of severe pulmonary toxicity.

V. FUTURE DIRECTIONS

On the basis of data in the mouse model as well as uncontrolled clinical observations, continuous infusion appears to produce less pulmonary toxicity

TABLE I DECREASED PULMONARY
TOXICITY OF BLEOMYCIN IN MICE
WHEN THE DRUG IS ADMINISTERED
BY CONTINUOUS INFUSION[a]

Bleomycin schedule	Increase in lung collagen (%)
Bolus, 2× per week	20
Bolus, 10× per week	31
Continuous infusion	10[b]

[a]From Sikic et al. (1978b). The total dose of bleomycin was identical in the three schedules.
[b]Superior to bolus injection, $p < .05$.

than bolus injection of bleomycin (Sikic et al., 1978b; Cooper and Hong, 1981; Carlson and Sikic, 1983). It will be important to confirm these data with a randomized, controlled clinical trial, and such a comparison currently is being planned.

Also on-going are further trials of the predictive value of a DL_{CO} in preventing severe or lethal pulmonary toxicity. It has been shown in animal models that angiotensin-converting enzyme activity increases in serum after bleomycin treatment, presumably because of damage to pulmonary endothelial cells (Newman et al., 1980; Lazo, 1981; Lazo et al., 1981). The value of monitoring this serum enzyme to assess pulmonary toxicity also is being investigated.

Dehydroproline, an inhibitor of collagen synthesis, reduces bleomycin-related lung collagen accumulation in rats. However, clinical trials with inhibitors of pulmonary fibrosis have not been initiated.

Several analogs of bleomycin undergoing preclinical development may produce less pulmonary toxicity than bleomycin. Ideally, such a new bleomycin analog should retain the lack of bone-marrow toxicity of bleomycin and a similar or expanded spectrum of antitumor efficacy.

REFERENCES

Bennett, W. M., Pastore, L., and Houghton, D. C. (1980). Cancer Treat. Rep. 64, 921–924.
Carlson, R. W., and Sikic, B. I. (1983). Ann. Int. Med. 99, 823–833.
Catane, R., Schwade, J. G., Turrisi, A. T., Webber, B. L., and Muggia, F. M. (1979). Int. J. Rad. Oncol. Biol. Phys. 5, 1513–1518.
Comis, R. L., Kuppinger, M. S., Ginsberg, S. J., Crooke, S. T., Gilbert, R., Auchincloss, J. H., and Prestayko, A. W. (1979). Cancer Res. 39, 5076–5080.
Cooper, K. R., and Hong, W. K. (1981). Cancer Treat. Rep. 65, 419–425.

Crooke, S. T., Einhorn, L. H., Comis, R. L., D'Aoust, J. C., and Prestayko, A. W. (1978). *Med. Pediatr. Oncol.* **5,** 93–98.

Goldiner, P. L., Carlon, G. C., Cvitkovic, E., Schweizer, O., and Howland, W. L. (1978). *Br. Med. J.* **1,** 1664–1667.

Holoye, P. Y., Luna, M. A., MacKay, B., and Bedrossian, C. W. M. (1978). *Ann. Intern. Med.* **88,** 47–49.

Lazo, J. S. (1981). *Toxicol. Appl. Pharmacol.* **59,** 395–404.

Lazo, J. S., Catravas, J. D., and Gillis, C. N. (1981). *Biochem. Pharmacol.* **30,** 2577–2584.

Louie, A. C., Evans, T. L., and Sikic, B. I. (1980). *Proc. Am. Assoc. Cancer. Res.* **21,** 290.

Muggia, F. M., Louie, A. C., and Sikic, B. I. (1983). *Cancer Treat. Rep.* **10,** 221–243.

Nachman, J. B., Baum, E. S., White, H., and Cruissi, F. G. (1981). *Cancer* **47,** 236–239.

Newman, R. A., Kimberly, P. J., Stewart, J. A., and Kelley, J. (1980). *Cancer Res.* **40,** 3621–3626.

Sikic, B. I., Young, D. M., Mimnaugh, E. G., and Gram, T. E. (1978a). *Cancer Res.* **38,** 787–792.

Sikic, B. I., Collins, J. M., Mimnaugh, E. G., and Gram, T. E. (1978b). *Cancer Treat. Rep.* **62,** 2011–2017.

Szapiel, S. V., Elson, N. A., Fulmer, J. D., Hunninghake, G. W., and Crystal, R. G. (1979). *Am. Rev. Resp. Dis.* **120,** 893–899.

Toledo, C. H., Ross, W. E., Hood, C. I., and Block, E. R. (1982). *Cancer Treat. Rep.* **66,** 359–362.

Section VIII
OTHER USES

Bleomycin Chemotherapy
(B. I. Sikic, M. Rozencweig, and S. K. Carter, eds.)

Chapter 21

BLEOMYCIN: THE SEARCH FOR OTHER INDICATIONS

Arthur C. Louie

Bristol-Myers Company
Pharmaceutical Research and Development Division
Syracuse, New York

Bleomycin has been in clinical use for more than 15 years and has an established role in the treatment of testicular tumors, head and neck cancer, cervical cancer, and lymphomas. In addition, the absence of significant myelosuppression has led clinicians to use bleomycin for other tumor types, even with less evidence of activity. The question now arises of whether there are other indications for which bleomycin should be considered. If so, what data support these uses? Moreover, in which disease types should bleomycin usage be explored?

To answer these questions, reports from the medical literature have been collected regarding the use of bleomycin as a single agent and in combination to treat those tumor types not yet discussed in this volume. In this chapter, indications where bleomycin appears to have sufficient single-agent activity to warrant further trials will be discussed.

I. SINGLE-AGENT ACTIVITY OF BLEOMYCIN

Bleomycin monotherapy of cancer has been reported from a large number of trials primarily conducted during the 1970s. The studies were conducted in Japan, Europe, and the United States, and most are reports of small series of patients, usually less than 10 patients (Table I). The most extensive experience relates to the treatment of squamous-cell carcinomas, including tumors of the skin, penis, vagina, vulva, and anus. This is followed by studies of esophageal cancer and invasive bladder cancer, each with reports of more than 100 patients having received bleomycin monotherapy. Studies of single-agent bleomycin that include more than 20 patients were reported for the following tumor types: breast cancer, sarcoma, renal cell cancer, primary brain tumors, melanoma, superficial bladder tumors, gastrointestinal tumors, small-cell cancer, epithelial ovarian tumors, and Kaposi's sarcoma.

Among these tumor types, bleomycin has demonstrated major activity in treating squamous-cell carcinomas, and evidence of activity that should be followed up with subsequent trials exists for brain tumors, superficial bladder tumors, and Kaposi's sarcoma. Evidence of minimal activity, defined as an observed objective response rate of less than 20%, with a complete response rate of 0% or very low percentage, has been reported for esophageal cancer, invasive bladder cancer, sarcoma, renal cell cancer, melanoma, and epithelial ovarian tumors. For these tumor types, additional trials using different doses or schedules might be considered, but there is little evidence to suggest that major activity will be found. Bleomycin has been shown to be inactive (defined as an objective response rate of less than 5%, with no complete responses) in breast cancer, gastrointestinal cancers, and small-cell lung cancer. There are a variety of other tumor types that have not been tested sufficiently to make any assessment of probable activity. These include myeloma, choriocarcinoma, thyroid cancer, basal cell carcinomas, and a variety of childhood solid tumors, such as Ewing's sarcoma and neuroblastoma. One additional indication that will be discussed in this chapter is intracavitary instillation of bleomycin as palliative treatment for pleural or peritoneal effusions. A large number of patients have received such treatment, and successful palliation has been reported for many.

II. SQUAMOUS-CELL CARCINOMAS

Comparisons can be made between the Japanese experience and the European and American experiences with bleomycin for the treatment of squamous-cell carcinomas of the skin. Ikeda *et al.* (1976) reported a multiinstitutional study conducted in Japan. Among 78 evaluable patients, 19 had complete and 14 had

TABLE I BLEOMYCIN MONOTHERAPY

Tumor type	Number of patients (trials)	Number of CR	Number of PR	Response rate (%)	Activity	References
Squamous-cell carcinoma	311 (20)	42	88	42	+ + + +	Bajetta et al. (1982); Barlow et al. (1973); Bonadonna et al. (1976); Boonyanit and Vatananusarn (1973); Bristol Laboratories (1974); Cannon et al. (1970); Folke (1976); Haas et al. (1976); Halnan et al. (1976); Ikeda et al. (1976); Krakoff et al. (1977); Kyalwazi et al. (1974); Maiche (1983); Mishima and Matunaka (1972); Ohnuma et al. (1972); Rooyen et al. (1972); Shastri et al. (1971); Stephens (1973); Suzuki et al. (1970); Thuot et al. (1972)
Esophagus	134 (13)	2	14	12	+	Bonadonna et al. (1976); Bristol Laboratories (1974); Cannon et al. (1970); Haas et al. (1976); Halnan et al. (1972); Kolaric et al. (1976); Krakoff et al. (1977); Ohnuma et al. (1972); Ravry et al. (1973); Shastri et al. (1971); Stephens (1973); Van Dyk et al. (1972); Yagoda (1977)
Bladder (invasive)	111 (8)	3	5	7	+	Blum et al. (1973); Cannon et al. (1970); Edsmyr et al. (1984); Gad el-Mawla et al. (1978); Pavone-Macaluso et al. (1976); Thuot et al. (1972); Turner et al. (1979); Yagoda et al. (1972)

(continued)

TABLE I (*Continued*)

Tumor type	Number of patients (trials)	Number of CR	Number of PR	Response rate (%)	Activity	References
Breast	88 (6)	0	3	3	0	Band et al. (1977); Cannon et al. (1970); Cummings et al. (1981); Haas et al. (1976); Shastri et al. (1971); Van Dyk et al. (1972)
Sarcoma	77 (10)	1	5	8	+	Agre (1974); Bonadonna et al. (1972); Cannon et al. (1970); Haas et al. (1976); Hoogstraten et al. (1975); Krakoff et al. (1977); Oknuma et al. (1972); Shastri et al. (1971); Sonntag (1972); Thuot et al. (1972)
Renal cell	59 (6)	0	8	14	+	Bristol Laboratories (1974); Cannon et al. (1970); Haas et al. (1976); Hahn et al. (1977); Hoogstraten et al. (1975); Johnson et al. (1975)
Brain	38 (2)	5	17	58	+ +	Shastri et al. (1971); Takeuchi (1975)
Melanoma	34 (7)	0	3	9	+	Bracken et al. (1977); Cannon et al. (1970); Halnan et al. (1972); Hoogstraten et al. (1975); Krakoff et al. (1977); Shastri et al. (1971); Van Dyk et al. (1972)

Bladder (superficial)	32 (3)	9	37	++	Bracken et al. (1977); Sadoughi et al. (1973); Smith and McCollum (1976)
Gastrointestinal	29 (4)	0	0	0	Cannon et al. (1970); Haas et al. (1976); Hoogstraten et al. (1975); Moertel et al. (1972)
Small-cell lung cancer	26 (2)	0	0	0	Bodey et al. (1973); Pavone-Macaluso et al. (1976)
Ovary, epithelial tumors	24 (1)	1	17	+	Blackledge et al. (1976)
Kaposi's sarcoma	22 (4)	1	55	++	Agre (1974); Kim et al. (1979); Vogel et al. (1973); Yagoda et al. (1972)
Other tumors	34 (9)	3	24	NA[a]	Agre (1974); Cannon et al. (1970); Haas et al. (1976); Halnan et al. (1972); Kolaric et al. (1976); Mishima and Matunaka (1972); Takeuchi (1975); Vogel et al. (1973); Yim et al. (1979)
Other indications: intracavitary therapy	312 (7)	125	61	++++	Bitran et al. (1981); Cunningham et al. (1972); Gupta et al. (1980); Kyalwazi et al. (1974); Ostrowski and Halsall (1972); Paladine et al. (1976); Trotter et al. (1979)

[a]NA, Not available.

TABLE II   BLEOMYCIN MONOTHERAPY OF SQUAMOUS-CELL CARCINOMA:
SKIN (JAPANESE STUDIES)

Reference	Number of patients	Number of CR	Number of PR	Response rate (%)
Ikeda *et al.* (1976)	78	19[a]	14[a]	42
Mishima and Matunaka (1972)	2	1	1	100
	80	20	15	44 (total)

[a]Includes intravenous and intraarterial treatment.

partial responses. The overall objective response rate was 42% (Table II). In the American and European literature, the largest series were reported by Agre (1974), Haas *et al.*, (1976), and the EORTC (Pavone-Macaluso *et al.*, 1976). (Table III). Agre reported 9 partial responses among 38 patients. Haas, reporting for the Southwest Oncology Group, noted 1 complete and 8 partial responses in a group of 22 patients with ectodermal squamous-cell carcinomas (skin, vulva, and anus). When compared to other squamous-cell tumor types such as head and neck cancer, squamous-cell lung cancer, and esophageal cancer, which are all nonectodermal in origin, the response rates were considerably higher for squamous tumors of ectodermal origin (Table IV). The EORTC reported 13 patients with squamous-cell skin cancers treated with bleomycin as part of a much larger broad phase II study. In this series 7 patients achieved partial responses.

The cumulative experience from the American and European literature shows 3 complete and 34 partial responses among 91 patients for an overall objective response rate of 41%. This is in general agreement with the Japanese experience of 35 objective responses among 80 evaluable patients, for a 44% objective

TABLE III   BLEOMYCIN MONOTHERAPY OF SQUAMOUS-CELL CARCINOMA:
SKIN (EUROPEAN AND AMERICAN STUDIES)

Reference	Number of patients	Number of CR	Number of PR	Response rate (%)
Agre (1974)	38	0	9	24
Haas *et al.* (1976)	22	1	8	41
Cannon *et al.* (1970)	13	0	7	54
Stephens (1973)	8	1	5	75
Bonadonna *et al.* (1976)	5	0	2	40
Rooyen *et al.* (1972)	2	1	1	100
Shastri *et al.* (1971)	2	0	1	50
Oknuma *et al.* (1972)	1	0	1	100
Krakoff *et al.* (1977)	1	0	0	0
	91	3	34	41 (total)

TABLE IV   SWOG BLEOMYCIN PHASE II STUDY[a]

Squamous–cell cancer type	Number of evaluable patients	Number of CR[b]	Number of PR[b]	Response rate (%)
Head and neck	64	0	12	19
Lung	37	0	1	3
Cervix	26	0	2	8
Ectodermal[c]	22	1	8	41
Esophagus	8	0	1	12

[a]Adapated from Haas et al. (1976).
[b]Response duration for all squamous-cell cancers, 2 (1–7) months.
[c]Ectodermal: skin, vulva, anus.

response rate, although the Japanese report a much higher complete response rate.

Squamous-cell carcinoma of the penis, vagina, and vulva all follow the same pattern. The series are usually small and complete, and partial responses are often observed. Overall response rates appear to be 46% for squamous carcinomas of the penis and 49% for squamous carcinomas of the vulva and vagina (Tables V and VI). There is less experience with squamous carcinomas of the anus, and the response rate appears to be lower, with two complete and five partial responses among 31 patients (23%) (Table VII).

When squamous-cell carcinomas of the skin, penis, vulva, vagina, and anus are considered together, a total of 88 partial responses and 42 complete responses are recorded for 311 patients, for an overall response rate of 42%. The inevitable

TABLE V   BLEOMYCIN MONOTHERAPY OF SQUAMOUS-CELL CARCINOMA: PENIS

Reference	Number of patients	Number of CR	Number of PR	Response rate (%)
Kyalwazi et al. (1974)	15	3	4	47
Bristol Laboratories (1974)	15	1	4	33
Maiche (1983)	11	0	4	36
Halnan et al. (1972)	4	1	2	75
Ohnuma et al. (1972)	3	0	0	0
Folke (1976)	3	1	1	66
Bonadonna et al. (1972)	2	0	1	50
Rooyen et al. (1972)	1	0	1	100
Cannon et al. (1970)	1	1	0	100
Stephens et al. (1973)	1	0	1	100
Krakoff et al. (1977)	1	0	1	100
	57	7	19	46 (total)

TABLE VI   BLEOMYCIN MONOTHERAPY OF SQUAMOUS-CELL CARCINOMA:
VULVA AND VAGINA

Reference	Number of patients	Number of CR	Number of PR	Response rate (%)
Agre (1974)	19	2	8	53
Boonyanit and Vatananusarn (1973)	10	6	3	90
Krakoff et al. (1977)	6	0	0	0
Cannon et al. (1970)	5	0	1	20
Suzuki et al. (1970)	4	2	2	100
Halran et al. (1972)	3	0	1	33
Thust et al. (1972)	3	0	0	0
Barlow et al. (1973)	1	0	0	0
	51	10	15	49 (total)

conclusion is that bleomycin shows major activity as a single agent for this type of tumor, and this activity is consistently observed for all the subtypes of squamous-cell carcinoma, except perhaps for squamous carcinomas of the anus. In the United States, this is an approved indication for bleomycin.

III. PRIMARY BRAIN TUMORS

The largest study of bleomycin monotherapy for primary brain tumors was reported by Takeuchi (1975) and consisted of 36 patients. Patients were considered to have responded if there was improvement in clinical neurologic findings, reduction of elevated intracranial pressure, improvement of neuroradiologic findings, and the impression of improved survival duration. By these criteria, bleomycin was markedly effective in 5 patients and effective in 17 patients among 36 evaluable subjects. This study was reported in 1975, before the introduction of

TABLE VII   BLEOMYCIN MONOTHERAPY OF SQUAMOUS-CELL CARCINOMA:
ANUS AND RECTUM

Reference	Number of patients	Number of CR	Number of PR	Response rate (%)
Agre (1974)	25	2	4	24
Halnan et al. (1972)	3	0	0	0
Rooyen et al. (1972)	1	0	1	100
Shastri (1971)	1	0	0	0
Krakoff et al. (1977)	1	0	0	0
	31	2	5	23 (total)

TABLE VIII   BLEOMYCIN MONOTHERAPY OF BRAIN TUMORS

Reference	Number of patients	Number of CR	Number of PR	Response rate (%)
Takeuchi (1975)	36	5	17	61
Shastri (1971)	2	0	0	0
	38	5	17	58 (total)

computerized tomography scanning. As a consequence, complete documentation of tumor regression is not available for all patients. Nevertheless, it appears that neurologic improvement did occur in a significant proportion of patients, and these findings might be followed up with additional trials (Tables VIII and IX).

IV. SUPERFICIAL BLADDER TUMORS

Superficial bladder tumors that cannot be successfully excised surgically may be approached by instillation of chemotherapy into the bladder. Instillation therapy with bleomycin has been attempted with some success, although the cumulative experience is quite limited (Table X).

The largest series comes from the M. D. Anderson Hospital and was reported by Bracken et al. (1977). Patients were treated with weekly instillations of bleomycin for eight treatments. One month after the last treatment, patients were evaluated for response. No response was observed in 4 patients given 30 units of bleomycin dissolved in 60 ml of water, 4 patients given 120 units of bleomycin dissolved in 30 ml of water, or 1 patient given twice-weekly treatments of 45 units dissolved in 60 ml of water, while 4 complete responses and 1 partial response were achieved in 10 patients given 60 units of bleomycin dissolved in 30 ml of water (Table XI).

TABLE IX   BLEOMYCIN THERAPY OF BRAIN TUMORS:
JAPANESE STUDIES[a]

Number of patients	Markedly effective[b]	Effective[b]	Ineffective	Difficult to evaluate
36	5	17	11	3

[a]Adapted from Takeuchi (1975).
[b]Based on neurologic findings, intracranial pressure, neuroradiologic findings, and survival data.

TABLE X   BLEOMYCIN MONOTHERAPY OF SUPERFICIAL BLADDER TUMORS

Reference	Number of patients	Number of CR	Number of PR	Response rate (%)
Bracken et al. (1977)	26	7	3	38
Smith et al. (1976)	5	1	0	20
Sadoughi et al. (1973)	1	1	0	100
	32	9	3	37 (total)

V. KAPOSI'S SARCOMA

Only 22 patients with Kaposi's sarcoma have been treated with single-agent bleomycin; none of these series is larger than 10 patients. However, every report has noted objective responses, and one report (Kim et al., 1979) included a patient with a complete response (Table XII). The largest series was reported by Vogel et al. (1973) and consisted of 10 patients, of whom half had progressed after BCNU therapy. Partial responses were observed in six patients, and the duration of remission was 30–90+ days. The time to maximum regression of tumor lesions was usually 40 days. In this group, 1 patient died of pulmonary fibrosis.

There is now great interest in Kaposi's sarcoma, particularly in those cases associated with acquired immunodeficiency syndrome, and the number of effective agents used to treat this tumor is quite limited. Because bleomycin lacks significant myelosuppressive activity, it may be a very attractive agent to use in patients who are susceptible to opportunistic infections.

VI. INTRACAVITARY THERAPY

Palliative therapy of pleural and peritoneal effusions has little impact on survival in most cases, but it can be quite important for patient comfort and quality

TABLE XI   BLEOMYCIN INSTILLATION THERAPY OF SUPERIFICIAL BLADDER CANCER[a]

Results	30/60[b]	60/60[b]	60/30[b]	120/30[b]	45/30[c]
Complete response	0	3	4	0	0
Partial response	0	2	1	0	0
No change	4	2	5	4	1
	4	7	10	4	1

[a]Adapted from Bracken et al. (1977).
[b]Weekly instillation × 8 treatments.
[c]Twice weekly × 16 treatments.

TABLE XII   BLEOMYCIN MONOTHERAPY OF KAPOSI'S SARCOMA

Reference	Number of patients	Number of CR	Number of PR	Response rate (%)
Vogel et al. (1973)	10	0	6	60
Agre (1974)	6	0	2	33
Yagoda et al. (1972)	4	0	2	50
Kim et al. (1979)	2	1	1	100
	22	1	11	55 (total)

of life. Intracavitary bleomycin was first reported to be effective in preventing reaccumulation of effusions by Cunningham et al. (1972). They noted 16 complete responses among 28 patients. Responses cannot be evaluated by the usual tumor response criteria. The absence of fluid reaccumulation for a period of 30 days is required for complete response, and the standard for partial response is minimal fluid reaccumulation not requiring further thoracentesis or paracentesis for 30 days. A number of small series have resulted in consistent complete and partial response rates of 54 to 80% for bleomycin in this indication (Table XIII).

The largest series using intracavitary bleomycin comes from a multiinstitutional study performed in the United Kingdom (Ostrowski and Halsall, 1982). Patients were given 30–180 mg of bleomycin dissolved in 100 ml of normal saline following maximal drainage of their effusions. Thirty days after the treatment, patients were evaluated for reaccumulation of fluid. Of the 106 patients with pleural effusions who were treated with bleomycin and considered evaluable, 39 achieved complete responses and 27 achieved partial responses for a successful palliation rate of 62%. Among the 47 patients with peritoneal effusions, 8 achieved partial responses and 14 achieved complete responses, for a palliation rate of 47%. There were only 5 patients with both pleural and peritoneal effusions; among these patients 2 achieved complete responses and 1

TABLE XIII   INTRACAVITARY BLEOMYCIN

Reference	Number of patients	Number of CR	Number of PR	Response rate (%)
Ostrowski and Halsall (1982)	158	55	36	58
Paladine et al. (1976)	51	19	11	59
Cunningham et al. (1972)	28	16	0	57
Bitran et al. (1981)	25	20	0	80
Trotter et al. (1979)	22	—	16	73
Lippman et al. (1975)	15	11	0	73
Gupta et al. (1980)	13	4	2	54
	312	125	65	61 (total)

achieved a partial response. The overall rate of palliation in this trial was 58%, with 55 complete responses and 36 partial responses among 158 evaluable patients (Table XIV).

Intracavitary bleomycin was generally very well tolerated in this series; no side effects were reported for 79.5% of patients. Local pain and fever were the most common adverse effects of treatment and occurred in 10.5% of patients. Pain was more common with intraperitoneal bleomycin (21%) than intrapleural bleomycin (5%). Gastrointestinal side effects consisted mostly of nausea and vomiting and occurred in 5.5% of patients. Alopecia occurred in 1.5% of patients, but this is difficult to evaluate because 2 of the 3 patients received concurrent cyclophosphamide. Erythema was reported in 1 patient and dyspnea occurred in 1 patient. One patient died of an apparent myocardial infarction 4 days after receiving intrapleural bleomycin. The connection between this event and bleomycin therapy is tenuous (Table XV).

VII. RECOMMENDATIONS FOR FUTURE STUDIES

This review of bleomycin monotherapy indicates that bleomycin shows modest antitumor activity in a wide variety of tumor types. Bleomycin exhibits useful activity in the treatment of squamous carcinomas of the skin, vulva, vagina, penis, and anus. In addition, it is evident that palliation of pleural and peritoneal effusion can be achieved in the majority of patients with intracavitary bleomycin. Although the rate of palliation is high, further research might help to optimize the dose of bleomycin, volume of the instillation, duration of tube thoracostomy, and other technical details.

Activity has been reported for bleomycin treatment of superficial bladder tumors, Kaposi's sarcoma, and possibly brain tumors. In each case, clinical experience is very limited, but both complete responses and partial responses

TABLE XIV   INTRACAVITARY BLEOMYCIN AND EFFUSION REDUCTION[a]

Site of effusion	Number of patients	Number of CR	Number of PR	Response rate (%)
Pleural	106	39	27	62
Peritoneal	47	14	8	47
Pleural and peritoneal	5	2	1	60
	158	55	36	58 (total)

[a]Adapted from Ostrowski and Halsall (1982).

TABLE XV   INTRACAVITARY
BLEOMYCIN: SIDE EFFECTS[a]

Side effects	Incidence
None	159/200 (79.5%)
Pain and fever	21/200 (10.5%)
Gastrointestinal	11/200 (5.5%)
Alopecia	3/200 (1.5%)
Erythema	1/200 (0.5%)
Dyspnea	1/200 (0.5%)
Death	1/200 (0.5%)

[a]Adapted from Ostrowski et al. (1982).

have been reported, and the observed response rates are above 35%. Further trials are needed to confirm these observations. In the instance of instillation therapy of superficial bladder tumors, additional studies also should be conducted to optimize the technical details of treatment.

Not discussed but worthy of mention are several tumor types for which bleomycin experience is minimal (<10 patients reported). It is impossible to draw any conclusions about the activity of bleomycin from these reports, but for a few of these tumors, objective responses have been observed despite the limited clinical experience. Bleomycin monotherapy has been found to have some activity in choriocarcinoma (Yim et al., 1979), thyroid cancer (Haas et al., 1976), basal-cell carcinoma (Mishima and Matunaka, 1972), embryonal rhabdomyosarcoma (Yagoda et al., 1972), and endometrial cancer (Krakoff et al., 1977). Additional observations of bleomycin monotherapy for these tumor types will be helpful in assessing bleomycin activity.

VIII. BLEOMYCIN IN COMBINATION THERAPY

Bleomycin has been widely used as part of combination chemotherapy for the past decade. Most of these trials have used a disease-oriented approach, with no systematic attempt to demonstrate the contribution of the individual agents within each drug combination. In the treatment of small-cell lung cancer, a number of trials using bleomycin as part of four- and five-drug combinations have been reported since 1975 (Einhorn et al., 1976; Livingston et al., 1975; McMahon et al., 1975; Roberts et al., 1983; Samson et al., 1979; Schauer et al., 1977) Bleomycin was used in spite of single-agent data (Bodey et al., 1973) showing negligible activity for this tumor, and none of the trials have demonstrated bleomycin to be an important part of combination treatment.

Bleomycin has been used in a variety of combination chemotherapy programs for melanoma. Following the report of Nathanson and Wittenberg (1980), which indicated a 47% objective response rate in 34 patients treated with bleomycin, vinblastine, and cisplatin, a number of other investigators tried to duplicate these results (Bajetta *et al.*, 1982; Creagen *et al.*, 1982; NCICMG, 1984; York *et al.*, 1983). These trials produced response rates ranging from 0 to 28%, and again it is not clear that bleomycin contributed in any meaningful way to the treatment successes reported. The response rate in the treatment of melanoma with bleomycin as a single agent is only 9%.

Esophageal cancer has been the subject of a number of trials using bleomycin alone and in combination because of its squamous-cell histology and the need to control locally recurrent disease, distant metastases, and paraneoplastic syndromes. Despite the 12% cumulative objective response rate for bleomycin monotherapy, bleomycin is considered to be one of the most effective agents for treating this disease. Combination therapy trials have been attempted with cisplatin, doxorubicin, etoposide, and other agents (Forastiere *et al.*, 1983; Kelsen *et al.*, 1978; Kolaric *et al.*, 1980). The data available do not show the extent of bleomycin's contribution to the objective responses observed. This is important because many patients with esophageal tumors receive mediastinal radiation and consequently may be at higher risk of developing pulmonary complications following bleomycin therapy.

The absence of significant myelosuppression associated with bleomycin administration has led to its incorporation into chemotherapy combinations, even in instances whre the evidence for single-agent activity is minimal. Two assumptions have been made in these disease-oriented trials and should be examined. First, it has been assumed that bleomycin is relatively safe and that its incorporation will not produce significant harm to patients. Second, it has been assumed that bleomycin may contribute to the antitumor activity of the drug combination. On close examination, both assumptions are difficult to defend. It is clear that bleomycin has significant dose-related toxicity, particularly pulmonary toxicity. If the drug combination shows disappointing activity, it becomes very important to know which drugs contributed the most to antitumor activity, so that decisions can be made to design the next generation of studies. If the drug combination is active and is considered clinically useful, it becomes more likely that multiple courses of bleomycin will be given, resulting in a higher risk of bleomycin-induced complications. In either case, knowing the contribution of the individual drugs to antitumor effectiveness within the combination is useful and ethical.

Among those tumors for which bleomycin has demonstrated negligible or marginal activity, based upon single-agent studies, drug-oriented studies should be performed to establish a role for bleomycin prior to its acceptance as part of a new drug combination. This is the most direct way to produce the data base needed for the rational use of bleomycin in the future.

REFERENCES

Agre, K. A. (1974). *In* "New Drug Seminar on Bleomycin" (W. T. Soper, and A. B. Gott, eds.), pp. 66–81. National Cancer Institute, Bethesda, Maryland.

Bajetta, E., Rovej, R., Buzzioni, R., Vaglini, M., and Bonadonna, G. (1982). *Cancer Treat. Rep.* **61**, 1299–1302.

Band, P. R., Canellos, G. P., Sears, M., Israel, L., and Pocock, S. J. (1977). *Cancer Treat. Rep.* **61**, 1365–1367.

Barlow, J. J., Piver, M. S., Chuang, J. T., Cortes, E. P., Ohnuma, T., and Holland, J. F. (1973). *Cancer* **32**, 735–743.

Bitran, J. D., Brown, C., Desser, R. K., Kozloff, M. F., Shapiro, C., and Billings, A. A. (1981). *J. Surg. Oncology* **16**, 273–277.

Blackledge, G., Lawton, F., Mathe, G., and Umezawa, H. (1976). *Cancer Treat. Rep.* **68**, 549–550.

Blum, R. H., Carter, S. K., and Agre, K. (1973). *Cancer* **31**, 903.

Bodey, G. P., Gottlieb, J. A., Livingston, R., and Frei, E. (1973). *Cancer Chemother. Rep., Part 3* **4**, 227.

Bonadonna, G., DeLena, M., Monfardini, S., Bartoli, C., Bagetta, E., Beretta, G., and Fossati-Bellani, F. (1972). *Europ. J. Cancer* **8**, 265.

Bonadonna, G., Tancini, G., and Bajetta, E. (1976). *Prog. Biochem. Pharmacol.* **11**, 172–184.

Boonyanit, S., and Vatananusarn, C. (1973). *Proc. 8th Int. Cong. Chemother, Hellenic Society of Chemotherapy, Athens* **III**, 445–451.

Bracken, R. B., Johnson, D. E., Rodrique, L., Samuels, M. L., and Ayala, A. (1977). *Urology* **9**, 161–163.

Bristol Laboratories Updated Product Monograph (1974). "Blenoxane." Bristol Laboratories, Syracuse, New York.

Cannon, P. J., Wajsman, Z., Baumgartner, G., and Merrin, C. (1970). *Br. Med. J.* **2**, 643–645.

Creagen, E. T., Ahmann, D. L., Schutt, A. J., and Green, S. J. (1982). *Cancer Treat. Rep.* **66**, 567–569.

Cummings, F. J., Gelman, R., Skeel, R. T., Kuperminc, M., Israel, L., Colsky, J., and Tormey, D. (1981). *Cancer* **48**, 681–685.

Cunningham, T. J., Horton, J., and Olson, K. B. (1972). *Proc. Am. Assoc. Cancer Res.* **13**, 496.

Einhorn, L. H., Fee, W. H., Farber, M. O., Livingston, R. B., Gottlieb, J. A. (1976). *JAMA* **235**, 1225–1229.

Edsmyr, F., Anderson, L., and Esposti, P. (1984). *Urology* **23**, 51.

Folke, E. (1976). *In* "GANN Monograph on Cancer Research No. 19, Fundamental and Clinical Studies of Bleomycin" (S. K. Carter, T. Ichikawa, G. Mathe, and H. Umezawa, eds.), pp. 231–233. University Park Press, Baltimore, London and Tokyo.

Forastiere, A. A., Patel, H., Hankins, J. R., Van Echo, D. A., and McCrea, E. (1983). *Proc. Am. Soc. Clin. Oncol.* **2**, 480.

Gad el-Mawla, N., Hamsa, R., Chevlen, E., and Ziegler, J. L. (1978). *Cancer Treat. Rep.* **62**, 1109–1110.

Gupta, N., Opfell, R. W., Padova, J., Margeleth, D., and Sovadijian, J. (1980). *Proc. Am Soc. Clin. Oncol.* **21**, 189.

Haas, C. D., Coltman, C. A., Gottlieb, J. A., *et al.* (1976). *Cancer* **38**, 8–12.

Hahn, D. M., Schmipff, S. C., Ruckdeschel, J. C., and Wiernik, P. H. (1977). *Cancer Treat. Rep.* **61**, 1585–1587.

Halnan, K. E., Bleehen, N. M., Brewin, T. B., Deeley, T. J., Harrison, D. F. N., Howland, C., Konkler, P. B., Ritchie, G. L., Wiltshaw, E., and Todd, I. D. H. (1972). *Br. Med. J.* **4**, 635–638.

Hoogstraten, B., Haas, C. D., Hant, A., Talley, R. W., Rivkin, S., and Issacs, B. L. (1975). *Med. Pediatr. Oncol.* **1**, 95–106.

Ikeda, S., Hamamatsu, T., and Ishihara, K. (1976). *In* "GANN Monograph on Cancer Research No. 19, Fundamental and Clinical Studies of Bleomycin" (S. K. Carter, T. Ichikawa, G. Mathe, and H. Umezawa, eds).), pp. 235–254. University Park Press, Baltimore, London, and Tokyo.

Israel, L., Depierre, A., Choffel, C., Milleron, B., and Edelstein, R. (1977). *Cancer Chemother. Rep.* **61**, 343–347.

Johnson, D. E., Chalbaud, R. A. W., Holoye, P. Y., and Samuels, M. L. (1975). *Cancer Chemother. Rep.* **59**, 433–435.

Kelsen, D. P., Cvitkovic, E., Bains, M., *et al.* (1978). *Cancer Treat. Rep.* **62**, 1041–1046.

Kim, R., Guerrero, R. C., and Ho, R. (1979). *Cutis* **23**, 73–76.

Kolaric, K., Maricic, Z., Dujmovic, I., and Roth, A. (1976). *Tumori* **62**, 255–262.

Kolaric, K., Maricic, Z., Roth, A., and Dujmovic, I. (1980). *Oncology* **37**(Suppl. 1), 77–82.

Krakoff, I. H., Cvitkovic, E., Currie, V., Yeh, S., and LaMonte, C. (1977). *Cancer* **40**, 2027–2037.

Kyalwazi, S. K., Bhana, D., and Harrison, N. W. (1974). *Br. J. Urol.* **46**, 689–696.

Lippman, A. J., Cohen, F. B., and Custodio, M. C. (1975). *Proc. Am. Soc. Clin. Oncol.* **16**, 247.

Livingston, R. B., Einhorn, L. H., Bodey, G. P., Burgess, M. A., Freireich, E. J., Gottlieb, J. A. (1975). *Cancer* **36**, 327–332.

Maiche, A. G. (1983). *Br. J. Urol.* **55**, 542–544.

McMahon, L. J., Jones, S. E., Durie, B. G. M., and Salmon, S. E. (1975). *Cancer Lett.* **1**, 97–102.

Mishima, Y., and Matunaka, M. (1972). *Acta Dermatovener.* **52**, 211–215.

Moertel, C. G., Arena, P. J., Schutt, A. J., Rietemeier, R. J., and Hahn, R. G., (1972). *Cancer Chemother. Rep.* **56**, 207–210.

Nathanson, L., and Wittenberg, B. K. (1980). *Cancer Treat. Rep.* **64**, 133–137.

National Cancer Institute of Canada Melanoma Group (1984). *J. Clin. Oncol.* **2**, 131–134.

Ohnuma, T., Selawry, O. S., Holland, J. S., DeVita, V. T., Shedd, D. P., Hansen, H. H., and Muggia, F. F. (1972). *Cancer* **30**, 914–922.

Ostrowski, M. J., and Halsall, G. M. (1982). *Cancer Treat. Rep.* **66**, 1982.

Paladine, W., Cunningham, T. J., Sponzo, R., Donovan, M., Olsen, K., and Horton, J. (1976). *Cancer* **38**, 1903–1908.

Pavone-Macaluso, M., and EORTC Genito-urinary Tract Co-operative Group A (1976). *European Urology* **2**, 138–141.

Ravry, M., Moertel, C. G., Shutt, A. J., Hahn, R. G., and Reitemeier, R. J. (1973). *Cancer Chemother. Rep.* **57**, 493–495.

Roberts, J. D., Myers, C. F., Roland, T. A., and Krakoff, I. H. (1983). *Proc. Am. Soc. Clin. Oncol.* **2**, 197.

Rooyen, C. E., Yuce, K., and Haldane, E. V. (1972). *The Nova Scotia Medical Bulletin,* pp. 144–150.

Sadoughi, N., Johnson, R. A., Ezdinli, E. Z., and Bush, I. (1973). *JAMA* **226**, 465.

Samson, M. K., Baker, L. H., Fraile, R. J., Izbicki, R. M., Vaitkevicius, V. K. (1977). *Cancer Treat Rep.* **61**, 59–64.

Schauer, R., Sotto, J. J., Wiget, V., Perdrix, A., Bensa, J. C., Ribaud, P. (1977) *Europ. J. Cancer* **13**, 425–428.

Shastri, S., Slayton, R. E., Wolter, J., Perlia, C. P., and Taylor, S. G. (1971). *Cancer* **28**, 1142–1146.

Smith, P. H., and McCollum, C. N. (1976). *JAMA* **235**, 906–907.

Sonntag, R. W. (1972). *Cancer Chemother. Rep.* **56**, 197–205.

Stephens, F. D. (1973). *Med. J. Aust.* **1**, 1277–1283.

Suzuki, M., Murai, A., Watanabe, T., Nunakawa O, (1970). *Acta. Med. Biol.* **17**, 259–275.

Takeuchi, K. (1975). *Int. J. Clin. Pharmacol.* **12,** 419–426.

Thuot, C., Poisson, R., and Perron, L. (1972). *Union Medicale du Canada* **101,** 879–883.

Trotter, J. M., Stuart, J. F. B., McBeth, F., McVie, J. G., and Calman, K. C. (1979). *Br. J. Cancer* **40,** 310.

Turner, A. G., Durrant, K. R., and Malpas, J. S. (1979). *Br. J. Urology* **51,** 121–124.

VanDyk, J. J., Falkson, G., and Falkson, H. C. (1972). *S. Afr. Med. J.* **46,** 1921–1926.

Vogel, C. L., Clements, D., Wanume, A. K., Toya, T., Primack, A., and Kyalwazi, S. (1973). *Cancer Chemother. Rep.* **57,** 325–333.

Yagoda, A. (1977). *Cancer Res.* **37,** 2775–2780.

Yagoda, A., Mukherzi, B., Young, C., Etcubanas, E., LaMonte, C., Smith, J. R., Tan, C. T. C., and Krakoff, I. H. (1972). *Ann. Intern. Med.* **77,** 861–870.

Yim. C. M., Lumg, L. C., and Ma, H. K. (1979). *Gynecol. Oncol.* **8,** 296–300.

York, R. M., Lawson, D. H., and McKay, J. (1983). *Cancer* **52,** 2220–2222.

Section IX
NEW BLEOMYCINS

Chapter 22

PEPLOMYCIN AND TALLYSOMYCIN S_{10}b: TWO BLEOMYCIN ANALOGS

Arthur C. Louie
Robert C. Gaver
Marcel Rozencweig
Bristol-Myers Company
Pharmaceutical Research and
Development Division
Syracuse, New York

Raymond H. Farmen
Robert L. Comis
State University of New York
Upstate Medical Center
Syracuse, New York

C. R. Franks
Bristol-Myers International Corporation
Pharmaceutical Research and Development
Brussels, Belgium

I. INTRODUCTION

Bleomycin has demonstrated activity in a number of tumor types, including testicular cancer, lymphomas, and squamous-cell carcinomas of the head and neck, the skin, and the uterine cervix. This anticancer effect is not clearly dose-dependent, and an optimal mode of administration has not yet been established. The drug does not produce myelosuppression, which makes it attractive for combination chemotherapy regimens; however, bleomycin does produce cumulative and dose-limiting pulmonary toxicity.

Much effort has been devoted to developing bleomycin analogs, with hopes of demonstrating greater efficacy, an expanded or different spectrum of activity, and reduced adverse reactions with more manageable toxic manifestations or different dose-limiting factors. The terminal amine portion of the bleomycin molecule was found to contribute to both antitumor activity and pulmonary toxicity (Matsuda *et al.*, 1978a; Raisfeld, 1981; Tanaka, 1977). Further, it was suggested that antitumor activity and pulmonary toxicity might be separable, and that altering the groups on the terminal amine portion of the bleomycin molecule might lead to analogs with reduced potential for pulmonary toxicity. This line of thinking has provided both a rationale and strong incentive to fermentation chemists to develop additional analogs. Their efforts eventually led to the development of both peplomycin and tallysomycin $S_{10}b$.

II. CHEMISTRY

Analogs of bleomycin and tallysomycin can be produced through a number of procedures, including precursor-fed fermentation and semisynthetic methods (Tanaka, 1977). Precursor-fed fermentation is performed by adding certain diamines to the fermentation media. The fermentation process then adds the diamine to the terminal amine portion of the bleomycin or tallysomycin molecule, resulting in a new analog. Bleomycin analogs also can be produced semisynthetically. The bleomycin molecule is produced by fermentation and is then hydrolyzed enzymatically to bleomycinic acid. Analogs can be obtained through a conventional condensation reaction between bleomycinic acid and a primary amine. This procedure is convenient and was used to produce peplomycin in early reports.

Tallysomycins differ from bleomycins in that they have an additional amino sugar (4-amino-4,6-dideoxy-L-talose), a longer peptide chain, and a shorter terminal amino group. Analogs of tallysomycin have been produced by precursor-fed fermentation (Miyaki *et al.*, 1981a,b). For tallysomycin $S_{10}b$, 1,4-diaminobutane is added to cultures of *Streptoalloteichus hindustanis*. This results in the production of a tallysomycin with diaminobutane as the terminal amino group. The structures of bleomycin, peplomycin, and tallysomycin $S_{10}B$ are shown in Fig. 1.

Peplomycin (3-[(S)-1-phenylethylamino]propylaminobleomycin sulfate) has a molecular weight of 1571.67 and an empirical formula of $C_{61}H_{88}N_{18}O_{21}S_2$. It is a white to pale yellowish white amorphous powder that is freely soluble in water.

Tallysomycin $S_{10}b$ is available as a white to off-white solid lyophilized

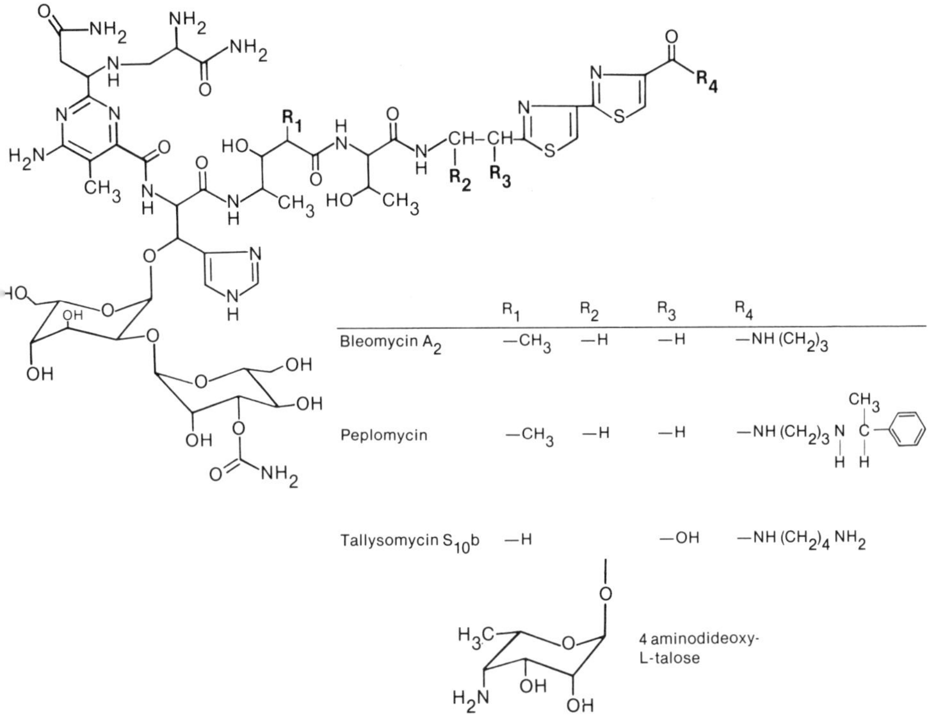

Fig. 1. Chemical structures of bleomycin A2, peplomycin, and tallysomycin $S_{10}b$.

powder with a molecular weight of 1546.62 and an empirical formula of $C_{59}H_{91}N_{19}O_{26}S_2$.

III. ANTITUMOR SCREENING ACTIVITY

Peplomycin activity has been compared with bleomycin in a number of animal tumor models and has been found to be more potent than bleomycin against HeLa S3 cells in culture (Matsuda et al., 1978b). Bleomycin and peplomycin show comparable activity against Ehrlich carcinoma in both the solid and ascitic forms (Matsuda et al., 1978b), the B16 melanoma (Sikic et al., 1980), the 20-methylcholanthrene-induced squamous-cell carcinoma in mice, and the AH66 rat ascitic hepatoma (Matsuda et al., 1978b).

There is evidence that the experimental antitumor activity of peplomycin is both schedule-dependent and route-dependent. Continuous ip infusions of peplomycin were reported to produce greater antitumor activity than multiple daily injections or single daily injections of equivalent total drug doses (Kato *et al.*, 1983; Ekimoto *et al.*, 1984). It also was noted that pulmonary toxicity occurred least in the continuous infusion group. Moreover, antitumor activity and pulmonary toxicity were greatest in animals treated by the iv route, and decreasing biologic activity was seen in animals treated intramuscularly, subcutaneously, and intraperitoneally, in that order (Ekimoto, *et al.*, 1984).

Initial studies revealed that tallysomycin A and tallysomycin $S_{10}b$ yielded comparable activity against B16 melanoma and Lewis lung carcinoma (Miyaki *et al.*, 1981a,b). The latter was more active against sarcoma 180 but less active against the P388 leukemia. The activity against sarcoma 180 was notable, with the median survival time (MST) of treated animals equal to 226% that of untreated controls (% T/C), and 6 of 16 animals surviving on day 45.

Subsequent experiments confirmed and extended these observations (Schurig *et al.*, 1984). Tallysomycin $S_{10}b$ was found to be equally active or somewhat more active than bleomycin against intraperitoneal P388/J leukemia, subcutaneous B16 melanoma, intravenous Lewis lung carcinoma, and subcutaneous Madison 109 lung carcinoma (Table I). Both drugs were minimally active or inactive against intraperitoneal P388 leukemia and inactive against intraperitoneal L1210 leukemia.

Tallysomycin $S_{10}b$ produced 90% inhibition in the human colon tumor xenograft model and 60% inhibition against human lung and colon tumors in the subrenal capsule assay (Table II). There also was slight activity against a subcutaneous human breast tumor in the same model. Overall, as compared to the parent compound, tallysomycin $S_{10}b$ exhibits approximately twice higher potency in murine systems where both drugs are active.

TABLE I   EXPERIMENTAL ANTITUMOR ACTIVITY OF
TALLYSOMYCIN (TLM) $S_{10}b$ AND BLEOMYCIN (BLM)[a]

		MST (% T/C)	
Tumor	Implant site	TLM $S_{10}b$	BLM
P388	ip	124	Inactive
P338/J	ip	150	131
L1210	ip	Inactive	Inactive
B16 Melanoma	sc	172	167
Lewis lung	iv	176	143
M109 Lung	sc	174	146

[a]From Schurig *et al.* (1984). MST, Median survival time; T/C, treated/control; ip, intraperitoneal; sc, subcutaneous; iv, intravenous.

TABLE II   EXPERIMENTAL ANTITUMOR ACTIVITY OF
TALLYSOMYCIN (TLM) $S_{10}b$ AND BLEOMYCIN (BLM)[a]

| Tumor | Implant site | MTW (% T/C) | |
		$TLM_{10}b$	BLM
CD8Fl mammary	sc	16	42
Colon 38	sc	9	14
CX-1	sc	7	28
	Subrenal capsule	28	≥113
LX-1	sc	≥77	≥56
	Subrenal capsule	39	≥62
MX-1	sc	21	27
	Subrenal capsule	47	46

[a]From Schurig et al. (1984). MTW, Median tumor weight; T/C, treated/control; sc, subcutaneous.

IV. MECHANISMS OF ACTION

The mechanisms of action of peplomycin and the tallysomycins are believed to be similar to those of bleomycin. Both classes of drugs bind to DNA and produce breakage of the sugar phosphate backbone, giving rise to single-strand DNA breaks and the release of free nucleotides, nucleosides, or bases (Haidle, 1971). DNA breakage occurs at specific sites on the DNA, and when single-strand breaks on opposite strands are close together, double-stranded DNA breaks may rise (D'Andrea and Haseltine, 1978). These are thought to be important in the cytotoxic action of bleomycin-type drugs.

A series of experiments based upon ethidium bromide staining patterns and nucleotide sequence analysis of the DNA fragments produced by bleomycin and its analogs showed that tallysomycin A fragments DNA at different sites than bleomycin A2 (Mirabelli et al., 1982, 1983). The differences in site specificity are probably due to the two new amino acids and the 4-amino-4,6-dideoxy-L-talose sugar moiety found in tallysomycin, rather than differences in the terminal amine moiety. Site specificity of DNA cleavage was found to depend to some extent on the tertiary structure of the DNA itself. It was proposed that these differences in action at the molecular level between bleomycin and its analogs may help explain differences in the biologic activity of the drugs.

In vitro experiments performed by Lown and Sim (1977) suggest that bleomycin-induced DNA damage involves the formation of a bleomycin–Fe(II)–oxygen complex, with the production of oxygen free radicals that produce the DNA breaks. Repair of this DNA damage may give rise to mutations (Podger and Grigg, 1983).

The way in which bleomycin and its analogs produce pulmonary fibrosis remains unknown. The structure–activity fibrogenic potential of terminal amine substituents recently was reassessed in a rat model of bleomycin-mediated fibrosis (Newman *et al.*, 1983). There is no evidence that the terminal amine moieties associated with bleomycin A2 and B2 by themselves are pulmonary toxic. Spermine, the polyamine associated with bleomycin A6, and spermidine, the polyamine associated with tallysomycins A and B and bleomycin A5, can produce lung consolidation, but the mechanism may be different from that of bleomycin. Therefore, it seems that the terminal amine portion of the bleomycin molecule can influence the potential for pulmonary toxicity through a change in the action of the entire intact bleomycin or tallysomycin molecule, even if it is not pulmonary toxic by itself.

V. PRECLINICAL TOXICOLOGY

Comparative preclincal toxicology studies of peplomycin and bleomycin indicated that the former produced less pulmonary toxicity, as evidenced by measurements of lung collagen contents estimated by hydroxyproline levels in the mouse and the hamster (Sikic *et al.*, 1980; Yoshida *et al.*, 1983) as well as through the relative histopathologic findings of fibrotic changes in the mouse and the dog (Matsuda *et al.*, 1978b). Peplomycin also was reported to produce higher BUN and transaminase elevations than those observed for peplomycin. Skin changes in the mouse were qualitatively similar for peplomycin and the parent compound (Sikic *et al.*, 1980). Peculiar central nervous system manifestations were described with the analog in this species.

Tallysomycin toxicity studies in mice showed dose-related nephrotoxicity at all dose levels (Buroker *et al.*, 1984). Measurements of serum chemistry values did not predict the histopathologic changes very well. Degenerative changes were seen in the epithelium of the proximal convoluted tubule, and there was cortical interstitial fibrosis. There was little evidence of repair four weeks after completion of drug exposure.

Pulmonary toxicity also occurred in these studies. Schurig *et al.* (1984) reported that relatively low doses of tallysomycin $S_{10}b$ appeared comparable to bleomycin in terms of pulmonary toxicity, as measured by whole-lung hydroxyproline content and pulmonary histopathology scores. However, as doses increased, bleomycin produced greater changes in both parameters. In rats, comparable effects were seen in lung compliance and vital capacity for tallysomycin $S_{10}b$ and bleomycin. In dogs, nephrotoxicity was dose-limiting in both the single- and multiple-dose schedules (Buroker *et al.*, 1984). Serum BUN and creatinine were extremely insensitive predictors of histopathologic changes in this species as well. Renal changes developed slowly and were progressive, and there was little evidence of significant repair at all toxic doses. Nephrotoxicity was schedule-dependent, with diminished toxicity in groups treated with five divided doses as compared with those treated with single doses. Pulmonary toxicity was observed in the dog studies, and at comparable doses in the single-dose experiments, tallysomycin S$_{10}$b and bleomycin were equally pulmonary toxic. Myelosuppression and cardiomyopathy were not observed.

VI. PHARMACOLOGY

Matsuda *et al.* (1978b) reported the organ distribution of peplomycin using a microbiologic assay. Highest levels were found in kidney, skin, lung, and stomach and were similar to levels observed after bleomycin administration. Unlike bleomycin, peplomycin could be detected in the brain and the liver. Neither drug was detected in the spleen.

Pharmacokinetic studies with radioimmunoassay were carried out in 3 patients treated with short iv infusions of peplomycin (Aherne *et al.*, 1982). The data were consistent with a biphasic plasma clearance, the terminal half-life being approximately 3 hr. The apparent volume of distribution calculated from the area under the curve averaged 12 liters, and the mean plasma clearance was 45 ml/min. Dialysis experiments revealed that 25–40% of the drug was protein-bound.

Pharmacologic studies of tallysomycin S$_{10}$b have used a sensitive and specific radioimmunoassay, which is based upon rabbit antisera, ^{125}I labeling, and dextran-coated charcoal to separate free and bound antigen. Preliminary clinical data appear to show a terminal plasma half-life of 12 hr, which is three to six times longer than that of bleomycin (Table III). The renal clearance is only one-fourth that of bleomycin (5 versus 21 ml/min/m^2), but the volume of distribution and total body clearance were similar to bleomycin. Tallysomycin S$_{10}$b seems to be cleared mainly by metabolism or nonrenal excretion, since, unlike bleomycin, relatively little unchanged drug can be recovered in the urine (10 versus 45–69%).

VII. CLINICAL STUDIES

Peplomycin has been the subject of extensive studies performed in Japan and Europe. A summary of the single-agent activity data is listed in Table IV.

TABLE III   COMPARATIVE DISPOSITION OF BLEOMYCIN (BLM)
AND TALLYSOMYCIN (TLM) $S_{10}b$ AFTER INTRAVENOUS BOLUS
ADMINISTRATION TO CANCER PATIENTS

Parameter	Mean values	
	TLM $S_{10}b$	BLM
Terminal elimination	12 ± 4	4.0 ± 0.6[a]
half-life (hr)		2.2 ± 0.1[b]
		2.0 ± 0.1[c]
Clearance (ml/min/m²)		
Total body	57 ± 23	80 ± 15[c]
		51 ± 10[a]
Renal	5 ± 3	21 ± 6[a]
Volume of distribution (liter/m²)	10 ± 6	18 ± 4[a]
		14 ± 1[c]
		11 ± 3[b]
Percentage of dose excreted	8 ± 5	69 ± 6[b]
as parent compound in		68 ± 3[b]
24 hr urine		45 ± 12[a]
Doses administered	1.25, 2.5, 5.0	15 U[b]
(mg/m²)		22–30 U[a]
		30 U[c]

[a]Alberts *et al.* (1978).
[b]Crooke *et al.* (1977).
[c]Hall *et al.* (1982).

Objective responses have been reported in head and neck cancer, lymphomas, squamous-cell carcinoma of the skin, and prostate cancer. This spectrum of activity is essentially similar to what has been reported for bleomycin. Toxicity was qualitatively similar to bleomycin, as well, with mild to moderate nausea/vomiting, fever, chills, a somewhat smaller percentage of skin changes, and definite pulmonary toxicity. Table V illustrates the clinical toxicity of peplomycin as reported in an EORTC study with 47 patients treated intramuscularly with 20 mg weekly or 10 mg twice weekly to a median cumulative dose of 160 mg (70–320 mg) (Depierre, *et al.,* 1981).

Clinical experience with tallysomycin $S_{10}b$ is much more limited; two phase I trials have been completed. H. Hansen and co-workers at the Finsen Institute (personal communication) treated patients using a twice-weekly schedule, with dose escalations starting at 1.25 mg/m² twice weekly. This trial recorded dose-limiting pulmonary toxicity, decreases in pulmonary diffusion capacity, and changes in chest radiographs in 3 of 4 patients receiving cumulative doses greater than 60 mg/m².

TABLE IV   CLINICAL ACTIVITY OF PEPLOMYCIN

Reference	Tumor type	Number of patients			Response rate (%)
		Total	CR	PR	
Oka (1980)	Head and neck	235	44	70	49
Mathé et al. (1982)		63		6	10
Depierre et al. (1981)	Lung (squamous cell)	47		1	2
Homma and Niitani (1980)		25		3	12
Sorensen et al. (1983)		21		1	[5]
Mathe et al. (1982)	Breast	53	1	5	11
M. Kimura et al. (1983)		8	1	1	[25]
K. Kimura et al. (1981)	Non-Hodgkin's lymphoma	36	7	5	33
Mathé et al. (1982)		21	2	5	[33]
Koiso and Niijima (1981)	Prostate	35		8	23
Yoshimoto et al. (1981)		9		3	[33]
Inuyama (1980)	Skin (squamous cell)	35	9	7	46
Mathé et al. (1982)		6	1	2	[50]
Mathé et al. (1982)	Hodgkin's disease	10		3	[30]
K. Kimura et al. (1981)		7	2	1	[43]
Mathé (1982)	Vulva	4	0	2	[50]

[a]Brackets indicate response rate for series with fewer than 25 patients.

R. L. Comis and the group at Upstate Medical Center (unpublished) used the weekly schedule and started dose escalations from 1.25 mg/m^2. Rales were detected in 2 patients who had received cumulative doses of 22.5 mg/m^2 and 37.5 mg/m^2. In the first patient no X-ray or diffusion capacity changes were observed.

TABLE V   PEPLOMYCIN-INDUCED TOXIC EFFECTS IN 47 PATIENTS[a]

Toxic effects	Number of toxic patients
Nausea and vomiting	15
Fever–chills	15
Skin changes	11
Lung	7(3)[b]
Pain at the injection site	6
Stomatitis	5
Leukopenia	4
Diarrhea	1
Alopecia	1

[a]From Depierre et al. (1981).
[b]Number of patients with World Health Organization (WHO) grade III–IV toxicity.

Other toxicities observed in both trials included nausea, vomiting, fever, fatigue, alopecia, and bleomycin-like skin changes. In both studies, tallysomycin $S_{10}b$ was generally well tolerated. It has been recommended that phase II studies initiate treatment at doses of 1.25 mg/m^2 twice weekly or 2.5 mg/m^2 weekly.

VIII. CONCLUSION

Peplomycin and tallysomycin $S_{10}b$ are analogs of bleomycin that have marked similarities to the parent compound in structure, experimental animal tumor activity, mechanism of action, and preclinical toxicology. Peplomycin pharmacology is very similar to that of bleomycin, but tallysomycin $S_{10}b$ is cleared primarily by metabolism or nonrenal excretion. Peplomycin has been studied extensively in Japan and Europe and appears to be active in a number of bleomycin-sensitive tumors. Its role in the treatment of prostatic cancer remains to be clarified. Clinical toxicities appear to be similar to those of bleomycin. There are insufficient data regarding improved antitumor activity or reduced toxicity to conclude that peplomycin is a successful analog. Tallysomycin $S_{10}b$ recently has completed phase I trials and appears capable of producing pulmonary toxicity. Phase II studies for this compound are about to begin.

REFERENCES

Aherne, G. W., Saesow, N., James, S., and Marks, V. (1982). *Cancer Treat. Rep.* **66**, 1365–1370.

Alberts, D. S., Chen, H. S. G., Liu, R., Himmelstein, K. J., Mayorsohn, M., Perrier, D., Gross, J., Moon, T., Broughton, A., and Salmon, S. E. (1978). *Cancer Chemother. Pharmacol.* **1**, 177–181.

Buroker, R. A., Comereski, C. R., Barnett, D., Hirth, R. S., Madissoo, H., and Hottendorf, G. H. (1984). *Drug Chem. Tox.* **7**, 259–272.

Crooke, S. T., Comis, R. L., Einhorn, L. H., Strong, J. E., Broughton, A., and Prestayko, A. W. (1977). *Cancer Treat. Rep.* **61**, 1631–1646.

D'Andrea, A. D., and Haseltine, W. A. (1978). *Proc. Natl. Acad. Sci. USA* **75**, 3608–3612.

Depierre, A., Lelli, G., Weber, B., Clavel, M., Rimoldi, R., Planting, A., Carriere, J., Kirkpatrick, A., Rozencweig, M., and Kenis, Y. (1981). *In* "Third NCI–EORTC Symposium on New Drugs in Cancer Therapy," abstr. 98.

Ekimoto, H., Takahashi, K., Matsuda, A., and Umezawa, H. (1984). *Gan to Kagakuryoho (Japan)* **11**, 853–857.

Haidle, C. W. (1971). *Molecular Pharmacol.* **7**, 645–652.

Hall. S. W., Strong, J. E., Broughton, A., Frazier, M. L., and Benjamin, R. S. (1982). *Cancer Chemother. Pharmacol.* **9**, 22–25.

Homma, H., and Niitani, H. (1980). *Cancer Treat. Rev.* **7**, 183–189.

Inuyama, Y. (1980). *Gan to Kagakuryoho (Japan)* **7**, 1498–1504.

Kato, T., Mizutani, M., and Ota, K. (1983). *Gan to Kagakuryoho (Japan)* **10**, 763–767.

Kimura, K., Ogawa, M., Wakui, A., Konda, C., Saito, T., Amaki, I., Sakai, Y., Masaoka, T., Kimura, I., Okada, Y., Ichimaru, M., and Yunoki, K. (1981). *Gan to Kagakuryoho (Japan)* **8**, 1701–1705.

Kimura, M., Koida, T., and Fukuda, T. (1983). *Gan to Kagakuryoho (Japan)* **10**, 665–669.

Koiso, K., and Niijima, T. (1981). *Prostate Supplement* **1**, 103–110.

Lown, J. W., and Sim, S. K. (1977). *Biochem. Biophys. Res. Comm.* **77**, 1150–1157.

Mathé, G., Armand, J. P., deVassal, F., Cappelaere, P., Keiling, R., and Chauvergne, J. (1982). *Cancer Chemother. Pharmacol.* **9** (suppl), 37.

Matsuda, A., Yoshioka, O., Yamashita, T., Ebihara, K., Umezawa, H., Miura, T., Katayama, K., Yokoyama, M., and Nagai, S. (1978a). *Recent Results Cancer Res.* **63**, 191–210.

Matsuda, A., Yoshioka, O., Takahashi, K., Yamashita, T., Ebihara, K., Ekimoto, H., Abe, F., Hashimoto, Y., and Umezawa, H. (1978b). In "Bleomycin[:] Current Status and New Developments" (S. Carter, S. Crooke, and H. Umezawa, eds.), pp. 311–331. Academic Press, New York.

Mirabelli, C. K., Huang, C. H., Prestayko, A. W., and Crooke, S. T. (1982). *Cancer Chemother. Pharmacol.* **8**, 57–65.

Mirabelli, C. K., Huang, C. H., and Crooke, S. T. (1983). *Biochemistry* **22**, 300–306.

Miyaki, T., Tenmyo, O., Kei-ichi, N., Matsumoto, K., Yamamoto, H., Nishiyama, Y., Ohbayashi, M., Imanishi, H., Konishi, M., and Kawaguchi, H. (1981a). *J. Antibiotics* **34**, 658–664.

Miyaki, T., Numata, K., Nishiyama, Y., Tenmyo, O., Hatori, M., Imanishi, H., Konishi, M., and Kawaguchi, H. (1981b). *J. Antibiotics* **34**, 665–674.

Newman, R. A., Hacker, M. P., and Sakai, T. T. (1983). *Tox. Appl. Pharmacol.* **70**, 373–381.

Oka, S. (1980). *Recent Results Cancer Res.* **74**, 163–171.

Podger, D. M., and Grigg, G. W. (1983). *Mutation Res.* **117**, 9–19.

Raisfeld, I. H. (1981). *Tox. Appl. Pharmacol.* **57**, 355–366.

Schurig, J. E., Rose, W. C., Hirth, R. S., Schlein, A., Huftalen, J. B., Florczyk, A. P., and Bradner, W. T. (1984). *Cancer Chemother. Pharmacol.* **13**, 164–170.

Sikic, B. I., Siddik, Z. H., and Gram, T. E. (1980). *Cancer Treat. Rep.* **64**, 659–667.

Sorenson, P. G., Rorth, M., Hansen, H. H., Dombernowsky, P., and Host, H. (1983). *Eur. J. Cancer Clin. Oncol.* **19**, 25–27.

Tanaka, W. (1977). *J. Antibiotics* **30**, 541–547.

Yoshida, A., Yamada, T., Hiramatsu, M., Kiuchi, H., Sekiya, S., Kawaguchi, T., Yamamoto, K., and Yu, S. Y. (1983). *J. Antibiotics* **36**, 1067–1075.

Yoshimoto, J., Masumura, Y., Asahi, T., Ozaki, Y., Suyama, B., Kaneshige, T., Tsushima, T., Mizuno, A., Ohmori, H., Ike, N., Josen, T., Kamei, Y., Takamoto, H., and Takahashi, T. (1981). *Gan to Kagakuryoho (Japan)* **8**, 1109–1117.

Bleomycin Chemotherapy
(B. I. Sikic, M. Rozencweig, and S. K. Carter, eds.)

Chapter 23

NEW ANALOGS AND DERIVATIVES OF BLEOMYCIN

Hamao Umezawa
Tomohisa Takita
Sei-ichi Saito
Yasuhiko Muraoka
Institute of Microbial Chemistry
Tokyo, Japan

Katsutoshi Takahashi
Hisao Ekimoto
Seiki Minamide
Kiyohiro Nishikawa
Takeyo Fukuoka
Tokuji Nakatani
Akio Fujii
Akira Matsuda
Research Laboratories
Nippon Kayaku Company, Ltd.
Tokyo, Japan

Since we discovered bleomycin (BLM) in 1963 (Umezawa *et al.*, 1963), we have pursued intensively its biologic, biochemical, and chemical studies involving this agent. In 1978, we determined the total structures of bleomycin (Fig. 1) (Takita *et al.*, 1978a) and its copper complex (Takita *et al.*, 1978b). Based on an understanding of these structures, it became possible to elucidate the mechanism of action on a molecular level. Bleomycin is a bifunctional compound that binds to and reacts at sites with DNA (Fig. 2) (Takita *et al.*, 1978b). The electrostatic charge of the terminal amine moiety directly affects the strength of the binding to DNA (Kasai *et al.*, 1978). The primary action of bleomycin appears to be DNA cleavage, which is caused by an active oxygen species on the axial ligand site of

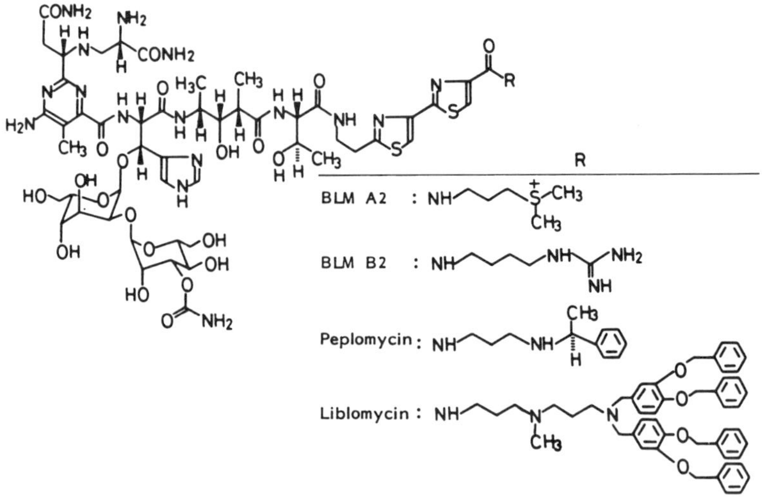

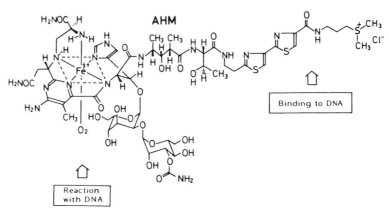

Fig. 1. Structures of bleomycin, peplomycin, and liblomycin.

BLM–Fe(II) complex (Sausville *et al.*, 1976; Kuramochi *et al.*, 1981). Moreover, the degree of toxicity, the distribution among organs, and the excretion differ among the bleomycins, which contain different terminal amines. This chapter describes recent synthetic studies of bleomycin, which have given new information on the mechanism of BLM action, and the selection of a new derivative, liblomycin (LIB), which promises to become a clinically useful and important agent.

Fig. 2. The mechanism of bleomycin action.

I. TOTAL SYNTHESIS OF BLEOMYCIN AND PREPARATION OF BLEOMYCIN ANALOGS

In 1981, we were successful in the total synthesis of bleomycin for the first time (Takita *et al.*, 1981), and in 1982, we reported an improved method of total synthesis (Saito *et al.*, 1982). Using these methodologies, we successfully reconstructed a BLM molecule from the fragments obtained by chemical degradation of BLM (Saito *et al.*, 1984). Thus, we have prepared a series of new bleomycin analogs that cannot be derived directly from natural bleomycins and that provide important information on structure–activity relationships.

During structural studies, we obtained the following modification and degradation products: bleomycinic acid (Umezawa *et al.*, 1973), iso-BLM (Nakayama *et al.*, 1973), decarbamoyl-BLM (Naganawa *et al.*, 1977), deglyco-BLM (Muraoka *et al.*, 1981), epi-BLM (Muraoka *et al.*, 1976), deamido-BLM (Umezawa *et al.*, 1974), depyruvamide-BLM (Muraoka *et al.*, 1977), and others. In observing the bioactivities of these products, we were able to determine which part of the structure is important for antitumor activity. Deamido-BLM is most interesting because it is formed by BLM-inactivating enzyme, which is widely distributed in various organs.

All of these products are modified at the peripheral parts, such as the terminal amine moieties, the sugar moieties, and the pyrimidine-2 substituents in a BLM molecule. Modification at the inner part, such as the (2S,3S,4R)-4-amino-3-hydroxy-2-methylpentanoic acid (AHM) moiety and the bithiazole moiety, is possible only be reconstructing the BLM molecule. To determine the role of the AHM moiety in BLM action, we prepared five analogs, in which the AHM moiety of BLM was replaced by 4-aminobutanoic acid, (3S)-4-amino-3-hydroxybutanoic acid, (4S)-4-aminopentanoic acid, (4R)-4-aminopentanoic acid, and (3S,4R)-4-amino-3-hydroxypentanoic acid. The bond lengths between the DNA-reaction and DNA-binding sites in these analogs are the same as that of BLM. The bioactivities of these analogs were tested by antimicrobial activity against *Bacillus subtilis*, cytotoxicity against HeLa cells, and DNA cleavage activity *in vitro*.

As shown in Table I, the analogs containing 4-aminobutanoic acid and (4S)-4-aminopentanoic acid did not show detectable antibacterial and anti-HeLa activities, although they showed DNA cleavage activity of approximately 10% of BLM. The analog containing (3S)-4-amino-3-hydroxybutanoic acid showed antibacterial activity to be 11% of BLM. However, the anti-HeLa and DNA cleavage activities were similar to those of the former two analogs. The analog containing (4R)-4-aminopentanoic acid showed antibacterial activity to be 16% of BLM, and anti-HeLa activity was 7.6 times weaker than that of BLM. However, DNA cleavage activity was approximately two times stronger than that of BLM. The analog containing (3S,4R)-4-amino-3-hydroxypentanoic acid showed almost the

TABLE I   BIOACTIVITY OF SYNTHETIC ANALOGS OF BLEOMYCIN

Analog	Antibacterial activity (*Bacillus subtilis*) (%)	IC_{50} (µg/ml) against HeLa cells	DNA cleavage activity (pBR322) *in vitro* (%)
(structure: CH₃ CH₃ / H N–C–C–C–C with OH, O)	100	1.18	100
(structure: H N–C–C–C–C, O)	0	>>10	~10
(structure: H N–C–C–C with OH, O)	11	>>10	~10
(structure: CH₃ / H N–C–C–C–C, O)	16	9.0	~200
(structure: CH₃ / H N–C–C–C–C, O)	0	>>10	~10
(structure: CH₃ H / H N–C–C–C–C with OH, O)	100	4.07	~100

same activities as BLM, with the exception of a slightly weaker anti-HeLa activity. This amino acid is contained in talisomycin, although the absolute configuration has not yet been reported (Konishi *et al.*, 1977).

From these results, it can be seen that the AHM moiety not only is the connective chain between the DNA-reaction and DNA-binding sites in a BLM-molecule, but also has an important role in antitumor activity. In particular, it was found that the methyl substituent including its absolute configuration should play an important role in bioactivity.

II. PREPARATION OF NEW BLEOMYCINS AND THEIR DERIVATIVES

A. Biosynthetic New Bleomycins

There are more than 10 natural congeners of BLM in the fermentation broth of BLM-producing microorganism. They differ in their terminal amine moiety (Fujii *et al.*, 1973). Biogenetically, these terminal amines originate from amino acids. Clinically used bleomycin contains BLM A2 (~70%), B2 (~30%), and other components in a small amount. We found that when the BLM-producing microorganism is cultured in a fermentation medium containing an unnatural amine, an artificial BLM that has the unnatural amine at the terminal amine moiety is produced. Unnatural amines that are well incorporated into the terminal amine moiety are shown in Table II (Fujii *et al.*, 1974). Structural requirements for incorporation of the amine are (1) it must have one primary alkyl amino group, and (2) it must have one or more other basic functions. Peplomycin (PEP), which has been used clinically, is produced by the addition of (*S*)-3-phenethylaminopropylamine (Fig. 1).

B. Semisynthetic Bleomycins from Bleomycinic Acid

Bleomycin that lacks the terminal amine moiety is called bleomycinic acid (BLM acid). A trace amount of BLM acid is found in the fermentation broth. We succeeded in finding a microbial enzyme that hydrolyzes BLM B2 into BLM acid and agmatine (Umezawa *et al.*, 1973). This new enzyme was isolated from the mycelium of *Fusarium anguioides* and characterized as acylagmatine amidase. We also established a chemical method for selectively cleaving BLM

TABLE II   UNNATURAL AMINES WELL INCORPORATED INTO THE TERMINAL
AMINE MOIETY OF BLEOMYCIN

*Starting material of liblomycin.

**Peplomycin (*S* configuration).

A2 to yield BLM acid (Takita *et al.*, 1973). Using BLM acid as the starting material, we prepared new semisynthetic bleomycins that could not be obtained by biosynthesis.

C. Bleomycin Derivatives Resistant to BLM Hydrolase

During our biochemical studies, we found BLM inactivating enzyme present in various organs. This enzyme hydrolyzes the carboxamide vicinal to the free amino group of BLM, and thus deamido-BLM is formed. We named this enzyme BLM hydrolase (Umezawa *et al.*, 1974). The enzyme recognizes BLM at its free amino group. Therefore, we imagined that modifications at this free amino group or the scissile carboxamide would lead to derivatives resistant to this enzyme. In fact, the *N*-methyl derivative was confirmed to be resistant to the enzyme without losing bioactivity, and the transformation of the scissile primary carboxamide to the secondary amide decreased susceptibility to this enzyme. Therefore, among these resistant BLM derivatives, a clinically useful BLM derivative might be found.

D. Chemical Synthesis and Modification

Besides reconstructing the BLM molecule through total synthesis, important new BLM analogs are being prepared by chemical modification of existing BLM. The *N*-methyl derivative obtained by reaction with formaldehyde–sodium cyanoborohydride is one of the examples, as already described. The N-alkylation of the terminal amine moiety of biosynthetic bleomycins produced lipophilic derivatives. Liblomycin (LIB), thus obtained, has been studied as a candidate for clinical investigation.

III. SCREENING OF DERIVATIVES FOR CLINICAL STUDY

Bleomycin has been used in the treatment of lymphomas, tumors of the testis, skin, head and neck, cervix, and other sites since 1968. Peplomycin (PEP), used clinically since 1981, has been selected as a second-generation BLM that has less pulmonary toxicity and a broader antitumor spectrum. The efficacy of PEP has been broadened through its use in treating prostatic and breast cancers. However, the pulmonary toxicity of PEP still remains dose-limiting. Therefore, after application of PEP in 1979, we initiated a new screening program to study derivatives that have stronger and broader antitumor spectrums and less pulmonary toxicity than PEP.

In the first step of the screening, *in vitro* tests of antitumor activity were carried out using HeLa and P388 cells. Among the 227 derivatives tested, 141 were selected by testing the growth inhibitory activity to meet the criterion of being stronger than one-third of the activity of PEP. In the second step, pulmonary toxicity was tested by ip administration in mice (the criterion: weaker than one-half of PEP). Also performed at the same time were *in vivo* tests of antitumor activity against mouse P388 leukemia, which is not very sensitive to PEP (the criterion: T/C > 150%), and *in vivo* tests of antitumor activity against Ehrlich ascites carcinoma, which is sensitive to PEP (the criterion: therapeutic index of more than one-half of PEP). Of the 141 derivatives tested, 39 met the stated criteria, and 10 of these derivatives were selected according to biologic and structural features and entered the third step. In this next step, the pulmonary toxicity was tested again by iv administration in mice. Animal tumor tests also were expanded to Ehrlich solid carcinoma, Lewis lung carcinoma (LL), B16 melanoma (B16), colon adenocarcinoma 26 (colon 26), and rat ascites hepatoma AH66F. Organ toxicities other than the pulmonary toxicity also were tested by q 1 day × 10 ip administration in mice. Three compounds were selected from the overall experimental results. In the final step, acute and subacute toxicity tests were performed in dogs. Also tested were antitumor activity against dimethyl-benzanthracene-induced mammary carcinoma in rats and antitumor activity against human gastric cancer and squamous-cell carcinoma heterotransplanted in nude mice. As a result of these tests, liblomycin (LIB) was selected as a candidate for clinical studies.

IV. LIBLOMYCIN

LIB has a bulky lipophilic group at the end of the terminal amine (Fig. 1). The lipophilic group is introduced by reductive N-alkylation of a biosynthetic BLM (see Table II). In radioimmunoassay, LIB hardly reacted with BLM A5–BSA-conjugate-induced antibody, which reacts not only with BLM A5 but also with PEP, BLM A2, and BLM B2. Furthermore, LIB was resistant to BLM hydrolase, which inactivates PEP, BLM A2, and BLM B2.

In Table III, *in vitro* antitumor activities of LIB are shown in comparison with those of PEP. LIB's activity against HeLa, P388, and AH66F cells is approximately two to six times stronger than that of PEP, but against AH66 cells (which are sensitive to PEP) LIB's activity is only 0.06 times the activity of PEP.

In animal tests against eight types of tumors, LIB was shown to be effective against seven tumors, but not effective against B16, against which PEP also was ineffective according to the criteria of the National Cancer Institute (Fig. 3). Among the seven tumors, LIB showed distinctly stronger activity than PEP against P388, L1210, and AH66F. LIB exhibited a remarkably strong activity

TABLE III *IN VITRO* ANTITUMOR
ACTIVITIES[a] OF LIBLOMYCIN
AND PEPLOMYCIN

Cells	Liblomycin	Peplomycin
HeLa	0.38	0.65
P388	1.6	9.0
AH66F	0.97	3.6
AH66	1.5	0.085

[a]IC_{50}, μg/ml.

against AH66F. The *in vivo* activity of LIB against AH66 was comparable to PEP, while the *in vitro* activity was much less than PEP, as shown in Table III.

In Fig. 4, pulmonary toxicities and *in vivo* anti-P388 activities of LIB, PEP, BLM, and other derivatives are shown. Pulmonary toxicity of PEP was almost one-third that of BLM, and pulmonary toxicity was not observed with LIB, even

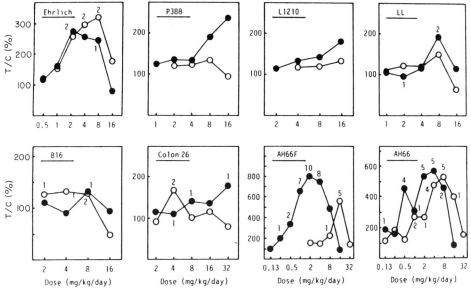

Fig. 3. Antitumor activities of liblomycin (●) and peplomycin (○) against murine transplantable tumors. Inoculum size and site, administration schedule, and observation period in each tumor system are as follows: Ehrlich ($n = 10$), 1×10^6 ip, qld $\times$ 10 (2 hr) ip, 75 days; P388 ($n = 10$) and L1210 ($n = 5$), 1×10^5 ip, q l d $\times$ 9 (day 1) ip, 30 days; LL ($n = 10$), 1×10^5 iv, q l d $\times$ 9 (day 1) ip, 60 days; B16 ($n = 8$), 5×10^5 sc, q l d $\times$ 9 (day 1) ip, 60 days; colon 26 ($n = 8$), 2.5×10^5, ip, q 4 d $\times$ 2 (day 1) ip, 60 days; AH66F ($n = 10$) and AH66 ($n = 6$), 1×10^6 ip, q 1 d $\times$ 10 (day 1) ip, 60 days. (Number n of animals used in a group are as given, and number of survivors are shown in the figure.)

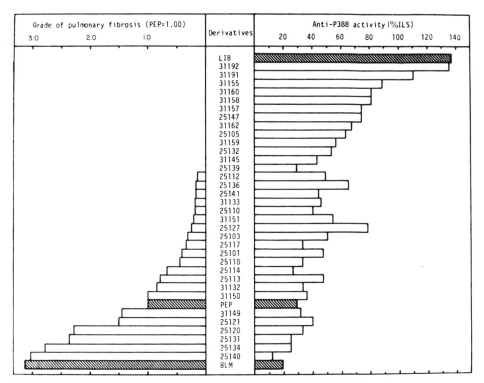

Fig. 4. Pulmonary toxicities and anti-P388 activities of liblomycin (LIB), peplomycin (PEP), bleo-mycin (BLM), and other derivatives. In the pulmonary toxicity test, each compound was adminis-tered ip to 15-week-old male ICR–SLC mice at a daily dose of 5 mg/kg for 10 days. Five weeks after administration, mice were sacrificed, lungs were fixed with neutral formalin solution, and histologic specimens were prepared. Grade of pulmonary fibrosis was expressed by scores given according to severity of toxicity, as previously reported (Takahashi *et al.*, 1979). Anti-P388 activity was tested, as shown in Table IV, and expressed by maximal value (%) of increased life span (ILS).

at 50 mg/kg total dose. A tendency has been observed that the stronger the antitumor activity against P388, the weaker the pulmonary toxicity. Figure 5 shows dose-response of LIB and PEP pulmonary toxicities. Histopathologic grade of the toxicity index of PEP was 1.67 at 30 mg/kg total dose and 2.65 at 50 mg/kg total dose; that of LIB was 0 at 50 mg/kg and 75 mg/kg total doses, and the first toxic sign (grade 0.07) appeared at the sublethal dose of 100 mg/kg total dose.

The LD_{50} values of LIB were 113 (iv, male mice) and 50 mg/kg (iv, male rats), and those of PEP were 51 and 246 mg/kg, respectively (Ito *et al.*, 1978). In an acute toxicity test in dogs, iv administration of 15 mg/kg of LIB was lethal, while that of 7.5 mg/kg did not cause death, and the minimal lethal iv dose of PEP was 30 mg/kg (Ito *et al.*, 1978).

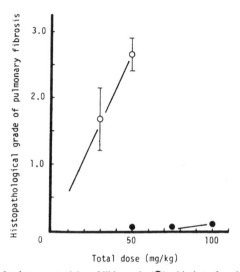

Fig. 5. Comparison of pulmonary toxicity of liblomycin (●) with that of peplomycin (○). Pulmonary toxicity was tested, as shown in Fig. 4, except that both compounds were administered iv. One point in peplomycin is a mean value ± standard deviation of five separate experiments. One point in liblomycin is the score of a single experiment. Eight to nine mice were used in a group in all experiments.

The pulmonary toxicity of LIB was compared with PEP in a subacute toxicity test in dogs. On the basis of the minimal lethal doses of LIB and PEP, the consecutive dose toxicity test was started at daily doses of 0.2 mg/kg and 0.4 mg/kg of LIB and at 0.8 mg/kg of PEP. However, as shown in Table IV, two dose escalations of LIB were required to cause death. A cumulative lethal dose of LIB was about 1.7 times higher than that of PEP.

Seventeen specimens of the lung from each dog were prepared for histopathologic observations. Table V shows the histopathologic findings of the lungs in dogs treated with LIB and PEP. In the dogs receiving PEP, pulmonary fibrosis was observed in all 34 specimens, but in the dogs receiving LIB, the fibrosis was not observed in any specimen. Alveolar wall thickening in the subpleura, which could not be diagnosed as fibrosis, was observed in 1 to 3 of 17 specimens in all dogs treated with LIB.

In the subacute toxicity test, toxicologic features other than pulmonary toxicity included tubulonephritis of the kidney by PEP, and follicle atrophy of the spleen, hemorrhage of the gastrointestinal tracts, and bone-marrow suppression by LIB. The LIB changes were observed only at the lethal dose. In addition to less pulmonary toxicity, a favorable feature of LIB was less stomatitis as compared with PEP.

TABLE IV SUBACUTE TOXICOLOGIC STUDY OF LIBLOMYCIN AND PEPLOMYCIN IN DOGS

Drug	Dog number	Sex	Total dose (mg/kg)	Total period (days)	Administration schedule[a] [dose (mg/kg) × days]	Terminus
Liblomycin	38	M	49.8	109	$0.2 \times 29 \to 0.4 \times 18 \to 0.8 \times 46$	Sacrifice
	39	F	49.8	109	$0.2 \times 29 \to 0.4 \times 18 \to 0.8 \times 46$	Sacrifice
	40	F	49.8	109	$0.2 \times 29 \to 0.4 \times 18 \to 0.8 \times 46$	Sacrifice
	44	M	82.8	86	$0.4 \times 19 \to 0.8 \times 18 \to 1.6 \times 38$	Moribund sacrifice
	45	F	92.4	94	$0.4 \times 19 \to 0.8 \times 18 \to 1.6 \times 44$	Death
	46	F	92.4	94	$0.4 \times 19 \to 0.8 \times 18 \to 1.6 \times 44$	Death
Peplomycin	55	F	54.4	79	0.8×68	Death
	61	F	49.6	72	0.8×62	Moribund sacrifice

[a]Liblomycin and peplomycin were administered im daily except Sunday.

TABLE V   HISTOPATHOLOGIC FINDINGS[a] OF LUNGS IN DOGS TREATED WITH
LIBLOMYCIN AND PEPLOMYCIN

Finding	Liblomycin total dose (mg/kg)						Peplomycin total dose (mg/kg)	
	49.8			82.8	92.4	92.4	54.4	49.6
	38[b] M[c]	39[b] F[c]	40[b] F[c]	44[b] M[c]	45[b] F[c]	46[b] F[c]	55[b] F[c]	61[b] F[c]
Fibrosis	−	−	−	−	−	−	+	+
Alveolar wall thickening	±	±	±	±	±	±	+	+
Foamy cells appearance	±	±	±	±	±	±	+	+

[a]−, Negative; ±, negligible; +, positive.
[b]Animal number.
[c]Sex.

From the animal experimental results described here, it is expected that LIB
will become a clinically useful agent with a broader anticancer spectrum than
bleomycin and without pulmonary toxicity.

REFERENCES

Fujii, A., Takita, T., Maeda, K., and Umezawa, H. (1973). *J. Antibiotics* **26**, 398.
Fujii, A., Takita, T., Shimada, N., and Umezawa, H. (1974). *J. Antibiotics* **27**, 73.
Ito, K., Irie, Y., Mitamoto, K., Yamashita, T., Tsubosaki, M., Matsuda, A., and Konoha, N.
    (1978). *Jap. J. Antibiotics* **31**, 719.
Kasai, H., Naganawa, H., Takita, T., and Umezawa, H. (1978). *J. Antibiotics* **31**, 1316.
Konishi, M., Saito, K., Numata, K., Tsuno, T., Asama, K., Tsukiura, H., Naito, T., and Ka-
    waguchi, H. (1977). *J. Antibiotics*.
Kuramochi, H., Takahashi, K., Takita, T., and Umezawa, H. (1981). *J. Antibiotics* **34**, 576.
Muraoka, Y., Kobayashi, H., Fujii, A., Kunishima, M., Fujii, T., Nakayama, Y., Takita, T., and
    Umezawa, H. (1976). *J. Antibiotics* **29**, 853.
Muraoka, Y., Fujii, A., Yoshioka, T., Takita, T., and Umezawa, H. (1977). *J. Antibiotics* **30**, 178.
Muraoka, Y., Suzuki, M., Fujii, A., Umezawa, Y., Naganawa, H., Takita, T., and Umezawa, H.
    (1981). *J. Antibiotics* **34**, 353.
Naganawa, H., Muraoka, Y., Takita, T., and Umezawa, H. (1977). *J. Antibiotics* **30**, 388.
Nakayama, Y., Kunishima, M., Omoto, S., Takita, T., and Umezawa, H. (1973). *J. Antibiotics* **26**,
    400.
Saito, S., Umezawa, Y., Yoshioka, T., Muraoka, Y., Takita, T., and Umezawa, H. (1982). *In*
    "Peptide Chemistry 1982" (S. Sakakibara, ed.), pp. 133–138. Protein Research Foundation,
    Tokyo.
Saito, S., Muraoka, Y., Takita, T., and Umezawa, H. (1984). *In* "Proceedings of the Annual
    Meeting Japanese Agricultural Chemical Society," p. 301.

Sausville, E. A., Peisach, J., and Horwitz, S. B. (1976). *Biochem. Biophys. Res. Comm.* **73,** 814.
Takahashi, K., Ekimoto, H., Aoyagi, S., Koyu, A., Kuramochi, H., Yoshioka, O., Matsuda, A., and Umezawa, H. (1979). *J. Antibiotics* **32,** 36.
Takita, T., Fujii, A., Fukuoka, T., and Umezawa, H. (1973). *J. Antibiotics* **26,** 252.
Takita, T., Muraoka, Y., Nakatani, T., Fujii, A., Umezawa, Y., Naganawa, H., and Umezawa, H. (1978a). *J. Antibiotics* **31,** 801.
Takita, T., Muraoka, Y., Nakatani, T., Fujii, A., Iitaka, Y., and Umezawa, H. (1978b). *J. Antibiotics* **31,** 1073.
Takita, T., Umezawa, Y., Saito, S., Morishima, H., Umezawa, H., Muraoka, Y., Suzuki, M., Otsuka, M., Kobayashi, S., Ohno, M. Tsuchiya, T., Miyake, T., and Umezawa, S. (1981). *In* "Peptides: Synthesis–Structure–Function," pp. 29–39. Proceedings of the 7th American Peptide Symposium.
Umezawa, H., Maeda, K., Okami, Y., and Takeuchi, T. (1963). *JP* 65-8117.
Umezawa H., Takahashi, Y., Fujii, A., Saino, T., Shirai, T., and Takita, T. (1973). *J. Antibiotics* **26,** 117.
Umezawa, H., Hori, S., Sawa, T., Yoshioka, T., and Takeuchi, T. (1974). *J. Antibiotics* **27,** 419.

Section X
SUMMARY AND PROSPECTS

Chapter 24

BLEOMYCIN: FUTURE PROSPECTS

Robert E. Wittes

Cancer Therapy Evaluation Program
Division of Cancer Treatment
National Cancer Institute
Bethesda, Maryland

I. INTRODUCTION

After many years of clinical trials with bleomycin, what can one say about this drug? Its spectrum is fairly broad; the drug shows appreciable activity in the lymphomas, testicular cancer, and squamous carcinomas of skin, penis, esophagus, head and neck, and vulva (Table I). Most oncologists consider the drug inactive in a variety of tumors of diverse histologies, including carcinomas of the kidney, breast, bladder, ovary, lung, as well as malignant melanoma, multiple myeloma, and the soft-tissue sarcomas (Table II). However, the activity of bleomycin is really indeterminate for many of these tumor types, because too few patients have been studied to fix the confidence intervals around the response rate with any precision. There is even less information for several other cancers, such as the carcinomas of stomach, prostate, pancreas, large bowel, liver, bile ducts, endometrium, and thyroid and CNS tumors.

Bleomycin has been given by many different routes. Trials have employed systemic (intravenous, intramuscular, subcutaneous) and regional (intraarterial, intrapleural) administration. Because of the absence of direct comparative trials,

TABLE I   SINGLE-AGENT ACTIVITY (BOLUS SCHEDULES)
IN RESPONSIVE DISEASES[a]

Tumor type	Number of patients	Responses (number)	Response rate (%)	95% Confidence interval
Testis	72	18	25	16–37
Lymphoma[b]				
NHL	238	111	47	37–50
HD	100	29	29	20–39
CTCL	22	18	82	60–95
Head and neck	431	94	22	19–27
Skin	65	26	40	28–53
Penis	29	17	59	39–76
Esophagus	137	31	23	16–30
Vulva	27	8	30	14–50

[a]Data compiled from several published studies in the literature.
[b]NHL, Non-Hodgkin's lymphoma; HD, Hodgkin's disease; CTCL, cutaneous T-cell lymphoma.

neither the optimal systemic route nor the optimal schedule has been clearly defined. Largely on the basis of a pharmacologic study performed at Memorial Sloan–Kettering Cancer Center several years ago (Krakoff *et al.*, 1977), oncologists have assumed that the therapeutic index of continuous infusion is superior to that of bolus administration. The drug has a fairly short serum half-life, and it exhibits phase specificity. Therefore, the potential superiority of continuous infusion is plausible but remains unsubstantiated by direct com-

TABLE II   SINGLE AGENT ACTIVITY (BOLUS SCHEDULES)
IN REFRACTORY DISEASES[a]

Tumor type	Number of patients	Responses (number)	Response rate (%)	95% Confidence interval
Renal	23	3	13	3–34
Cervix	172	17	10	6–16
Breast	38	2	5	1–18
Bladder	58	3	5	1–14
Ovary	15	1	7	0–32
Lung	76	2	3	0–9
Melanoma	12	1	8	0–38
Myeloma	10	0	0	0–31
Sarcoma	10	0	0	0–31

[a]Data compiled from several published studies in the literature.

parisons, or even by adequate single-agent data for continuous-infusion schedules in uncontrolled settings.

II. COMBINATION CHEMOTHERAPY

The fact that the drug does not exhibit clinically significant bone-marrow suppression as a dose-limiting toxicity probably accounts for its popularity in combination chemotherapy. A vast number of bleomycin-containing combinations have been explored clinically. The inclusion of this drug in combination therapy is easily understandable for those tumor types in which it has significant single-agent activity. It is somewhat less understandable for tumors, such as non–small-cell lung cancer, in which it has been incorporated into a large number of regimens, often in sequence with vincristine. The rationale for the use of bleomycin in this way was based on cell kinetic results in cultured cell lines (Barranco and Humphrey, 1971; Barranco, 1978); these results were translated into a large number of clinical protocols. Although initial results of sequenced vincristine and bleomycin appeared promising, numerous subsequent trials did not suggest a therapeutic advantage of combinations containing the sequence.

In any event, despite this very large experience, the uncontrolled nature of almost all of these trials simply does not permit a rigorous assessment of bleomycin's contribution to the efficacy of these regimens. Bleomycin is a component of potentially curative combinations in testicular cancer, the diffuse non-Hodgkin's lymphomas, and Hodgkin's disease. On the other hand, the lack of information about its role in these combinations is almost complete. With the important exception of the Hodgkin's disease studies in the Southwest Oncology Group (see Chapter by Coltman, this volume), the controlled trial that isolates the effect of bleomycin in cancer treatment evidently has not seemed worth the effort to most oncologists.

Some might argue that such trials are not important except to satisfy regulatory requirements of the Food and Drug Administration (FDA). Such trials are indeed pivotally important for FDA approval. In this regard, it is worth noting that current FDA-approved indications for bleomycin, single or in combination, include the lymphomas, testicular cancer, and carcinomas of the head and neck, penis, uterine cervix, and vulva.

Oncologists should clearly understand, however, that the information that is gained from pivotal controlled trials may have an impact on clinical decision-making. If an agent is incorporated into a combination but makes no measurable contribution to its efficacy, then patients treated with that combination are being exposed to potential toxicities that are not justifiable in terms of possible therapeutic gain. In addition, the uncritical incorporation of drugs into combinations by practitioners escalates medical care costs unreasonably. In an era when costs are being examined very carefully by third-party carriers, physicians may be called upon to justify their choices of treatment in ways that have no precedent.

III. BLEOMYCIN AND RADIOTHERAPY

Bleomycin has been studied as a radiosensitizer. As reported elsewhere in this volume by Fu, results in head and neck cancer have been mixed. The trial of the Northern California Oncology Group (NCOG) so far has shown no statistically significant differences between the group treated with radiotherapy alone and that treated with radiotherapy plus bleomycin during induction. In some ways, this trial is emblematic of the difficulties that the clinical cooperative groups have had over the years in accruing adequate numbers of head and neck cancer patients. Therefore, the NCOG trial should really be regarded as inconclusive rather than negative. In fact, the group treated with bleomycin does show a somewhat superior complete-response rate. That the difference lacks statistical significance may well be a function of the relatively small sample size of the trial. In any case, the positive studies of bleomycin as a radiosensitizer seem to have had little or no impact on patterns of standard primary treatment. I am not aware that anyone regards bleomycin given simultaneously with radiotherapy as standard treatment for any head and neck cancer. Except possibly for the results of a trial in India, the therapeutic advantage of this approach seems slim, if it exists at all.

IV. FUTURE DIRECTIONS

Where do we go from here? As noted, many very important questions about the clinical use of bleomycin remain unanswered. The sad fact, however, is that the opportunity to answer them probably has been irretrievably lost. Probably no physician would have any interest in studying the effect of subtracting bleomycin from potentially curative combinations at this point. Similarly, rigorous studies of schedule dependency probably would be very difficult to execute, given the alternate priorities of sponsors and investigators. The experience with bleomycin again makes it clear that opportunities for doing certain kinds of trials exist only during a particular interval in a drug's development; if those opportunities are not seized, the questions may never be answered.

A. Efficacy and Toxicity

In principle, future clinical research with bleomycin could be directed toward either enhancing the efficacy of the drug or decreasing its toxicity. As more becomes known about its detailed mechanism of action, rationally designed combinations with other agents may evolve. In certain *in vitro* systems, the combination of bleomycin and heat seems to be more effective than either modality alone (Hahn, 1979; Mizuno and Amagai, 1980). This lead has not been studied clinically in a systematic fashion, although some pilot data exist (Arcangeli *et al.*, 1979).

B. Analog Development

For other drug classes, the development of analogs has been extremely productive. Methotrezate has completely replaced aminopterin in the clinic. Cyclophosphamide, chlorambucil, and melphalan have almost completely replaced mechlorethamine and have largely fulfilled the goals of analog development in providing an increased spectrum, greater versatility, and better patient tolerance.

Except for acute leukemia, doxorubicin has replaced daunorubicin, and continued intensive efforts by medicinal chemists have yielded compounds that may retain the activity of doxorubicin with decreased toxicity. Carboplatin and iproplatin appear to have a pattern of dose-limiting toxicity different from cisplatin, with striking efficacy in at least some tumor types.

Of the many bleomycin analogs that have been synthesized, two have reached the clinic. A substantial and still-growing phase II data base is available for peplomycin. Evidence to date (see chapter by Louie *et al.*, this volume) suggests that this drug behaves clinically very much like the parent compound in terms of both efficacy and toxicity. Final judgments will obviously have to wait for completion of phases II and III. Tallysomycin has not yet received phase II evaluation in the United States. However, initial hope that this agent would lack the pulmonary toxicity of the parent compound appears to be waning rapidly.

C. Targeting Bleomycin

Previous efforts at targeting bleomycin, in order to maximize the drug concentration at the tumor cell and minimize exposure of normal cells, have focused on regional drug delivery. Bleomycin has been used rather extensively by the intracavitary route in order to inhibit the accumulation of third-space fluid. Existing clinical data support its utility, although controlled trials are few and endpoints notoriously difficult to define precisely. It is difficult to see how one might further improve the therapeutic index of ic administration. If the dose were to be increased, one might expect increased leakage of drug into the systemic circulation; in the absence of a means to protect target organs such as the lung, systemic toxicity would probably increase with dose. Since bleomycin has definite activity against squamous cancers and lymphomas, the possibility of conjugation with monoclonal antibodies specific against one or another of these tumor types is attractive theoretically. It seems likely to this nonchemist, however, that the synthetic problems involved in linking antibodies to this very complex molecule will be formidable.

D. Drug Resistance

The circumvention of natural or acquired drug resistance is an area of major contemporary emphasis. As reviewed by Sikic elsewhere in this volume, efforts to correlate effects of bleomycin on target tissue with the tissue levels of bleomycin hydrolase have met with only partial success. Attempts to relate tumor levels of hydrolase to therapeutic response have not been explored systematically in the clinic. Certainly, in many clinical circumstances, drug resistance is relative, and an increase in dose will produce clinical responses after failure to lower doses. Since the major limiting toxicities of bleomycin are potentially devastating and since no reliable technique of protection exists, this drug has not been a focus of high-dose studies clinically, nor should it be.

V. SUMMARY

In many ways, the clinical development of bleomycin has been a model for how *not* to study a new agent. There are gaping holes in our knowledge concerning the best way(s) of administering the drug and concerning its contribution to curative cancer therapy. These gaps are not likely to be filled for the variety of reasons just cited. The nature of the dose-limiting toxicities of this agent makes certain kinds of clinical experiments difficult or impossible at the present time. Analog development has not yet eliminated pulmonary toxicity as a potentially important clinical problem and, at least in the case of peplomycin, does not seem to have changed the spectrum of activity significantly. In the absence of fundamental advances of the kinds alluded to previously, the continued development of bleomycin probably will be limited in scope.

ACKNOWLEDGMENT

The author thanks William Soper and Candia Hench for expert technical and secretarial assistance.

REFERENCES

Arcangeli, G., Concolino, F., Maruo, F., Nervi, C., and Pavin, G. (1979). *Proc. Ann. Meet. Med. Oncol. Soc., 5th.*

Barranco, S. C., and Humphrey, R. M. (1971). *Cancer Res.* **31,** 1218–1223.

Barranco, S. C. (1978). *In* "Bleomycin[:] Current Status and New Developments" (S. K. Carter, S. T. Crooke, and H. Umezawa, eds.), pp. 81–90. Academic Press, New York.

Hahn, G. M. (1979). *Cancer Res.* **39,** 2264–2268.

Krakoff, I. W., Cvitkovic, E., Currie, V., Yeh, S., and LaMonte, C. (1977). *Cancer* **40,** 2020–2037.

Mizuno, S., Amagai, M., (1980). *Proc. Int. Symp. Cancer Ther. Hyperthermia, Drugs, and Radiation, 3rd.*

Bleomycin Chemotherapy
(B. I. Sikic, M. Rozencweig, and S. K. Carter, eds.)

Chapter 25

BLEOMYCIN IN CHEMOTHERAPY: SUMMARY AND CLOSING REMARKS

Edwin C. Cadman

Cancer Research Institute
University of California School of Medicine
San Francisco, California

I. CHEMISTRY

Bleomycin is an antibiotic isolated from *Streptomyces verticillus* in 1963 by a group of Japanese scientists (see Blum *et al.*, 1973). The primary mechanism of antitumor activity is considered to be the result of single-strand scission of DNA. Although certain parts of the bleomycin molecule can bind to DNA, the strand scission is most likely the result of local free radical formation (Bennet and Reich, 1979). The cells that seem to be most sensitive to bleomycin are those in the post-DNA synthesis (G_2) and mitotic (M) phases (Barranco, 1978).

II. PHARMACOKINETICS

Following an injection, the initial serum half-life $t_{1/2\alpha}$ of bleomycin is approximately 20 min. The terminal half-life $t_{1/2\beta}$ is between 2 and 4 hr. Nearly

80% of the drug is excreted within the first 24 hr, with 90% of that amount excreted within the first 6 hr. Therefore, it was not surprising to observe that in the presence of renal impairment, the elimination of bleomycin was reduced. Since pulmonary toxicity may be related to peak levels of the drug, there is concern that toxicity is enhanced in patients with renal failure (Ohnuma et al., 1974; Alberts et al., 1978; Crooke et al., 1977; Kramer et al., 1978). Because of rapid drug elimination, continuous infusion may be a more logical method of administration.

III. TOXICITY

Bleomycin has the unique capacity to induce pulmonary fibrosis. This toxicity can be detected clinically in 10% of patients and is estimated to contribute to the cause of death in ~1% of patients. Because it is devoid of bone-marrow-suppressive properties, oncologists tend to add bleomycin to many drug combinations. However, we do not yet totally appreciate the potential enhanced lung toxicity that may result when such combinations contain drugs that also may have subclinical pulmonary effects. Although the precise mechanism of this unusual toxicity is not completely understood, the result is an enhanced rate of collagen synthesis. Because this toxicity is associated with increased prolyl hydroxylase activity, inhibitors of this enzyme were tested and were found to be somewhat effective in reducing the pulmonary fibrosis (Vazques-Nin et al., 1979; Lin et al., 1980; Kelley et al., 1980; Counts et al., 1981; Phan et al., 1980; Clark et al., 1980; Riley et al., 1981).

IV. ANTITUMOR ACTIVITY

Bleomycin has been part of the curative combination therapy used for treating germ-cell tumors and lymphomas. It also appears to be uniformly effective in the treatment of all varieties of squamous-cell carcinomas. There is no doubt that as a single agent in early phase I and phase II clinical trials, bleomycin resulted in many documented responses. However, very few studies have been designed to test the impact of this drug when used in combination with other agents. The Southwest Oncology Group (SWOG) used regimens of low-dose bleomycin, high-dose bleomycin, and no bleomycin as the variables in one of their combination drug programs for Hodgkin's disease. There was no significant difference in response among the three groups. The SWOG also compared continuous infusion with bleomycin administered once or twice a week for the treatment of cervical carcinoma. The results achieved through twice-weekly and infusion programs were similar, while the weekly schedule showed the lowest response rate. There are hundreds of drug combinations that include bleomycin, but none of these studies were designed to evaluate the true contribution of bleomycin.

TABLE I   STUDIES USING BLEOMYCIN INFUSION

Investigator	Location[a]	Tumor	Response (%)
D. Alberts	Arizona/SWOG	Cervix	67
S. C. Ballon	NCOG	Cervix	21
R. B. Golbey	Memorial	Germ cell	90
D. Osoba	Toronto	Lung	43
M. B. Spaulding	Buffalo	Head and neck	87

[a]NCOG, Northern California Oncology Group; SWOG, Southwestern Oncology Group.

Several investigators now are using bleomycin as an infusion treatment based on the pharmacokinetic information mentioned (Table I). Although the drug doses and durations of infusion of these programs were variable, in each instance there were several complete remissions observed. While this is expected to occur in germ-cell tumors, it is quite unusual among the other tumors. In each of these trials, cisplatin also was used in the drug combinations. Certainly cisplatin has been used as a single agent often enough in lung and cervical cancer for us to realize that the response rates reported here are considerably better than what would be expected with the single agent. This suggests that perhaps cisplatin and bleomycin are synergistic. Thus, some basic research, inspired by these clinical results, may be indicated. Certainly a better understanding of these drugs and their interaction within cells would be beneficial for the design of future trials.

V. FUTURE CONSIDERATIONS

When considering new clinical investigations using bleomycin in the next few years, the following considerations are suggested as guidelines:

1. Are infusions better?
   a. What is the best dose?
   b. What is the best infusion duration?
   c. What is the toxicity observed?
2. Is bleomycin necessary for all drug combinations?
   a. What is the best schedule?
   b. How do combinations with and without bleomycin compare?
   c. What are the biochemical interactions with other agents?
3. Can pulmonary toxicity be prevented?
   a. At what dose and schedule?
   b. Which patients are biochemically susceptible?
   c. What are the protective agents?

4. Bleomycin analogs:
   a. What are the different reactive groups?
   b. Which shows less toxicity?
   c. Which achieves better antitumor activity?

VI. SUMMARY

Bleomycin is, indeed, a useful drug whose full potential is unknown. As with most clinical trials in oncology, we have been limited in our vision by the lack of basic scientific information necessary to maximize therapeutic decisions. As we learn more about the sites of action, the toxicity, the intracellular metabolism, effects of other drugs on bleomycin, and bleomycin's effects on other drugs, we will begin to use bleomycin in ways that could improve the treatment of cancer patients.

REFERENCES

Alberts, D. S., Chen, H.-S. G., Liu, R., Himmelstein, K. J., Mayersohn, M., Perrier, D., Gross, J., Moon, T., Broughton, A., and Salmon, S. E., (1978). *Cancer Chemother. Pharmacol.* **1,** 177–181.

Barranco, S. C. (1978). *In* "Bleomycin[:] Current Status and New Developments" (S. K. Carter, S. T. Crooke, and H. Umezawa, eds.), pp. 81–90. Academic Press, New York.

Bennet, J. M., and Reich, S. D. (1979). *Ann. Intern. Med.* **90,** 945–948.

Blum, R. H., Carter, S. K., and Agre, K. (1973). *Cancer* **31,** 903–914.

Clark, J. G., Overton, J. E., Marino, B. A., Uitto, J., Starcher, B. C., *et al.* (1980). *J. Lab. Clin. Med.* **96,** 943–953.

Counts, D. F., Evans, J. N., DiPetrillo, T. A., Sterling, K. M., Kelley, J., *et al.* (1981). *J. Pharmacol. Exp. Ther.* **219,** 675–678.

Crooke, S. T., Comis, R. L., Einhorn, L. H., Strong, J. E., Broughton, A., Prestayko, A. W., *et al.* (1977). *Cancer Treat. Rep.* **61,** 1631–1636.

Kelley, J., Newman, R. A., and Evans, J. N. (1980). *J. Lab. Clin. Med.* **96,** 954–964.

Kramer, W. G., Feldman, S., Broughton, A., Strong, J. E., Hall, S. W., Holoye, P. Y., *et al.* (1978). *J. Clin. Pharmacol.* **18,** 346–352.

Lin, P. S., Kwock, L., and Goodchild, N. T. (1980). *Cancer* **46**(11), 2360–2364.

Ohnuma, T., Holland, J. F., Masuda, H., Waligunda, J. A., Goldberg, G. A., *et al.* (1974). *Cancer* **33,** 1230–1238.

Phan, S. H., Thrall, R. S., and Ward, P. A. (1980). *Am. Rev. Respir. Dis.* **121,** 501–506.

Riley, D. J., Kerr, J. S., Berg, R. A., Ianni, B. D., Pietra, G. G., Edelman, N. H., Prockop, D. J., *et al.* (1981). *Am. Rev. Respir. Dis.* **123,** 388–393.

Vazques-Nin, G. H., Echeveria, O. M., and Pedron, J. (1979). *Cancer Res.* **39,** 4218–4223.